Awakening Intuition

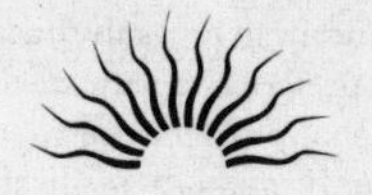

Awakening Intuition

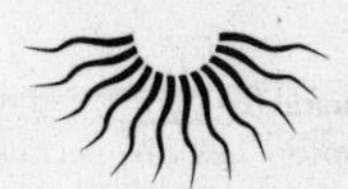

Using Your Mind-Body Network for Insight and Healing

Mona Lisa Schulz, M.D., Ph.D.

Foreword by Christiane Northrup, M.D.

THREE RIVERS PRESS
NEW YORK

The information in this book is not meant to be a substitute for medical care. Medical intuition does not diagnose illness nor does it prescribe specific medical treatment. It is not psychotherapy. If you have a medical or emotional problem, see your physician or other licensed practitioner in your area. You should only make a medical decision in this type of trusting partnership.

Human vulnerability to disease cannot be reduced to a single physical or emotional cause. Many genetic, nutritional, environmental, emotional, and other unknown reasons contribute to the development of illness and disease. Although many studies will be cited in this book that discuss specific emotional factors that contribute to illness, no study is perfect. There are limitations to any scientific inquiry. Patients should work with their health care practitioners to examine for themselves which problems, relationships, habits, and situations in their lives contribute to health or disease.

The medical intuitive readings presented in this book are composites of several similar readings. None represents a single identifiable individual. Sexes have been switched frequently, unusual names created, and locations changed. Any similarity to any real person's name or identity is coincidental.

Published by Three Rivers Press, 201 East 50th Street,
New York, New York 10022. Member of the Crown Publishing Group.

Originally published in hardcover by Harmony Books, 1998.
First paperback edition printed in 1999.

Random House, Inc. New York, Toronto, London, Sydney, Auckland
www.randomhouse.com

Printed in the United States of America

Design by Debbie Glasserman

Library of Congress Cataloging-in-Publication Data
Schulz, Mona Lisa.
Awakening intuition : using your mind-body network for insight and healing / Mona Lisa Schulz ; foreword by Christiane Northrup.
1. Intuition. 2. Healing. 3. Mind and body therapies. 4. Women—Health and hygiene. I. Northrup, Christiane. II. Title.
RZ999.S368 1998
613—dc21 97-46149

ISBN 0-609-80424-3

10 9 8 7 6 5 4 3 2 1

First Paperback Edition

To all of my mentors—
the physicians, scientists, and medical intuitives
who have helped me heal,
generously taught me everything they knew,
and then lovingly forced me out of the nest into the world
to do what I am supposed to do

ACKNOWLEDGMENTS

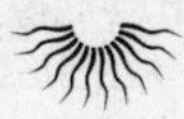

You wouldn't be holding this book in your hands right now if it weren't for a great number of people. No one creates alone. An egg needs sperm, Rocky needed Bullwinkle, and I needed an awful lot of help to do this. I thank the following.

My family for bringing me the challenges that inspired me to become a physician, scientist, and medical intuitive.

All the faculty at Brown University and Boston University who gave me the opportunity to shape and develop my intellect.

Margaret Naeser, Ph.D., Deepak Pandya, M.D., Edith Kaplan, Ph.D., Norman Geschwind, M.D., and M. Marcel Mesulam, M.D., whose collective work shaped how I see the brain and the mind as a neuroscientist. They taught me how emotion, memory, language, and behavior are created in the mind and in the brain.

Dr. George McNeil and all the other physicians, nurses, social workers, occupational therapists, and secretaries in the Psychiatry Department at Maine Medical Center, who helped sprout synapses in my brain and heart that helped me become a neuropsychiatrist. Thanks also to the Maine Medical librarians. To Judy Barrington, medical illustrator, who helped me take what was in the books and make it into pictures. Thanks to Mary Romano, for secretarial psychotherapy. To Marjorie Phyfe–Diane Boyce–Joyce Perry, M.S.W., who work so well together they are hyphenated. You women take your genius and help the most troubled patients put their lives back together.

To the physicians who have helped me heal—Dr. John Hall (who straightened me), Dr. Lee Thibideau (fused me), Dr. Flaherty (undeviated me), Dr. Christiane Northrup (tied me), and Dr. Jean Matheson (helped me wake up). To Fern Tsao (who needled me)—a master acupuncturist measuring 4 feet 9 inches and weighing in at 85 pounds soaking wet, her yin power would intimidate the faint of heart. To Bea Riordan, who listened to me cry, in person and on the phone, helped me to get support, and taught me how to support myself.

To Ruth Buczynski, Ph.D., for giving me a chance to speak at her wonderful conferences, even after I was described as "a person with a unique speaking style," and "an audiovisual nightmare with a speech impediment." Thanks to all the people at Hay House for giving me the opportunity to speak at the Empowering Women Workshops. The audiences are wonderful, and the speakers' dinners afterward are always a scream.

To Gina for wonderful food and Italian and Mediterranean companionship. To Paul, for hair psychotherapy. To Joanne Arnold, for teaching weight training to the vertebrally challenged. This woman works wonders with a dumbbell. I am also grateful to Mary Noyes, a business genius disguised in a high-end warm-up suit. Her "polite" banter and one-liners hide a heart made of gold. Thanks also to Jean Doane, for understanding my unusual financial profile as well as my unique capacity to have student loan deferment forms get lost in computerized black holes. And to Loretta Laroche, for giving me strange looks across crowded rooms. Her comic genius makes me almost incontinent.

To two red-headed moles (and one brunette with glasses) who secretively read my manuscript and gave me much encouragement when I really needed it.

To Zofia Smardz for donating the left hemisphere of her brain. I have only a tiny one of these. Without her wonderful capacity to capture my voice and put it to words on a printed page, this book would be only a single run-on sentence with lots of great pictures and diagrams.

To Diane Grover, for donating her frontal lobes. I don't have much of these either. She provides great organization and planning and tells me when to go where and how to act in socially appropriate ways once I get there.

To Charlie Grover, who runs the rest of my life from my home and does everything for me...except two things (he's Diane's husband).

To Winter Robinson, who introduced me to medical intuition. Appreciation for Louise Hay who is a self-made genius, who learned and teaches much about psychosomatic medicine and medical intuition, having learned it all without one student loan!

With deep gratitude to Caroline Myss, Ph.D., who, with great humor, brilliance, and tenacity, was my mentor, my "attending" during my "residency" in medical intuition training, and then unselfishly helped me get on the *Oprah Winfrey Show.* I am truly thankful for having been taught by one of the pioneers in energy medicine.

Thanks to Muriel Nellis, my agent, my literary godmother, who makes problems go *poof*. Her great love and candor guide me in the right direction with such comments as "Hey, toots, cut the jacket photos of the dead bodies."

Thanks to Joan Borysenko, Ph.D. We met at one of Ruth's speaker's dinners and realized that we had both shared the great pleasure and ecstasy of slicing rat brains in a lab. When I offered to do research for her wonderful book *A Woman's Book of Life* (Riverhead, 1997), she insisted that I write my own book and started the process immediately by handing me the phone to make the first call, right then and there.

With deep gratitude to Leslie Meredith, my editor at Harmony Books, of the Crown Publishing Group. She signed my book on the basis of what seemed to me to be a single story about a praying mantis and what she described as "something special." This is either intuition or impulsivity, or both. What this woman can do with a pencil and a manuscript over Italian food is truly awe-inspiring!

To Chris's kids, Annie and Kate. They have helped me get out my surrogate parenting needs. I have spent many a pleasant afternoon and evening working on a newsletter with Chris in a Mazda MPV, while driving them around from soccer game to theater rehearsal to tennis match. Balanced, grounded suburban living at twelve miles per gallon.

The amount of gratitude, love, and respect I have for Chris Northrup is incalculable. The first thing she said to me when I met her was, "What I need *from* you is the following..." Ironically, what this woman then proceeded to do *for* me cannot be described in words or pictures or calculated in numbers, dollars, or cents. She taught me everything she knows about women's health, gynecology, obstetrics, nutrition, feminism, politics (even when I feigned disinterest), and public speaking. Although I have a Ph.D. in Behavioral Neuroscience and have studied the brain and mind extensively, she has taught me that there is, in fact, a mind in the uterus. She is a true scientist in the most aesthetic form. I have laughed with this woman, I have cried, I have screamed, lost, won, I have learned, and then I have created. She introduced me to my editor, helped me meet my agent, wrote my Foreword, and forced me to put some things in this book that I was sure were unimportant or too scary to include. She has shared capuccino with me, eaten many a meal, and created several public displays of irreverence. Before I met her, I always did my research and created alone because this seemed simpler, less complicated, and safer. However, she has shown me that true partnership can in fact be accomplished between two bright, strong-minded, opinionated, emotional beings who also laugh a lot.

Finally to Emily and Dina, my cats who are always beside me. They scream when I am doing a difficult reading, hiss and spit when someone comes into my house who isn't good for me, and purr when someone comes in who is. They are truly part of my intuition.

CONTENTS

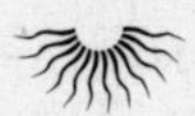

Foreword

by Christiane Northrup, M.D.

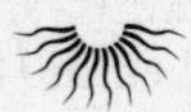

I've worked in a research partnership with Dr. Mona Lisa Schulz for more than five years now. Though I started out as her mentor when she was a medical student with a desire to learn the truth about obstetrics, gynecology, and women's health, we quickly moved from a student-teacher relationship to that of professional peers.

Together we have spent hours and hours laughing with and at each other, yelling at each other, and coming up with new ideas that both surprise and delight us. The fierceness of the discussions leading up to these inspirations and scientific discoveries—and the degree to which each of us holds her own in the process—can be frightening to the faint of heart—including, when they were younger, my own children. After all, before Mona Lisa's arrival into my life, they had never seen two grown-up women duking it out with quite the combination of intellect, intuition, and passion that each of us brings to the table.

During one such discussion in the summer before this book was scheduled for publication, when the title of the book had not shown itself yet, I was on the phone with Mona Lisa and our "director of operations," Diane Grover. We were refining and honing the particulars of our working relationship, and Mona Lisa was demanding a commitment from both Diane and me with her characteristic intensity. The conversation grew heated, and Diane and I became angry with her. We also realized that her intuitive insights, coupled with her intensity, were scary for us. As on many prior occasions, we had a feeling that we wouldn't be able to win this argument with her. As usual, we all hung in there and worked it through. And as usual, Mona Lisa had pinpointed the fears and weaknesses of all three of us with great accuracy and mental clarity. I acknowledged my own power, intensity, and scariness and realized that it expressed itself in a more inner (and cardiovascular) way than Mona Lisa's. Diane acknowledged that her fears tend to go into her gut when she feels trapped and caught in the middle—quite literally, the middle of her body. And as usual, by staying with it, we individually and collectively came to a new level of strength and commitment in our relationship. And I was given more insight into the magical world of medical intuition and how it works in our lives every day.

Here's what happened. On the summer morning of our conversation, Diane and I had walked out into my backyard, each with a portable phone. Mona Lisa was on call that day at the hospital, and there were some things we all needed to clean up with each other. So we held a three-way conversation. The morning was already hot, and I noticed that the grass under my feet was dry as I kicked at it with my bare toes. The intensity of our conversation and the dry grass under my feet got me to thinking about the primal energy of lightning and how it burns away the old. I had even suggested a week before that the word "lightning" be used somewhere in Mona Lisa's book title, since her energy and insight are lightning-fast and also because her presence is so apt to cause electrical problems when her emotions are running high.

While I was kicking the dry grass and noodling around with the concept of lightning, I noticed that Diane, phone in hand, had wandered into a wooded area of our property that was covered with deep grass...the sort of place she usually avoids completely because of her lifelong snake phobia. But there she was, addressing her own fears of being trapped while picking up old branches and throwing them over the bank—sort of a property cleanup happening simultaneously with a psychic cleanup. Or, if you will, a confrontation with inner demons while fearlessly venturing into the habitat of outer ones.

As the intensity of our conversation peaked and then gradually burned itself out, the idea of lightning kept coming back to me again and again. I couldn't get it out of my mind. Though one part of me was engaged in the final stages of the conversation and our new level of understanding, another area of my brain was inspired by the energy and purpose of lightning and how to capture this Mona Lisa–like energy—in a book title. Then I remembered the sequoia trees in the western United States and how their seeds require searing heat in order to crack their tough shells so that they can germinate new life. The heat required for this comes during forest fires that are ignited naturally by lightning, the force that provides the initial energy burst which gradually awakens the dormant seeds.

By daring to walk through the fire set by Mona Lisa's lightning, all three of us broke through some hard old shells and found seeds of new life ready to germinate in ourselves and in our relationship. Later that day I realized how apt the title *Awakening Intuition: Using Your Mind-Body Network for Insight and Healing* is. And once again I realized that I had fulfilled my role as an obstetrician-midwife for a new creation.

By reading this book and applying Dr. Schulz's lightning to your own tough seeds, you too can find healing, new growth, and a new life. Resist the urge to back away when things get hot. The universe itself began with a Big Bang—an explosion characterized by light and heat. The principles that run the universe every day haven't changed much. Things that are green and new and exciting sometimes require light and heat to crack them open.

If the doors of perception were cleansed, everything would appear to man as it is, infinite.

WILLIAM BLAKE

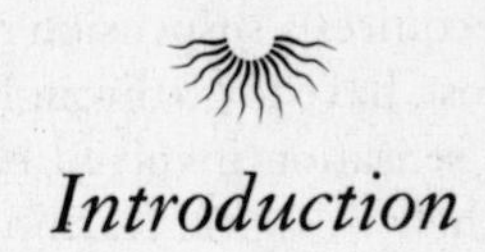

Introduction

I'm a physician who is also a medical intuitive. I do intuitive consultations over the telephone. A person calls and tells me his or her name and age—nothing more. Then, having never met or even seen the individual in question, I perform a long-distance "reading." I discern both the person's physical condition and the emotional state of his or her life, and explain how the two are linked together. Invariably, after I finish, the clients respond in one of two ways. Some gasp in surprise and say, "How do you do that? *I* could never do that. *I* don't have intuition." Others, unimpressed, state flatly, "I already knew that." While they did know it, *intuitively,* they didn't believe it—or admit or express it until I, a total stranger, expressed it to them in impersonal terms.

This is how it usually is. Many people either don't believe they have intuition, or they don't believe in intuition at all. They therefore don't trust or won't recognize the intuition that's through their bodies, throughout lives. I'm frequently asked, "Do you really believe there's such a thing as intuition?" Asking me that is like asking me if I believe in vitamin C, or whether I trust that there's a Hawaii. I've never been to Hawaii. Nor do I know specifically how vitamin C works. But I trust that they exist. As for intuition, I don't just believe it exists. I know it does. And contrary to the prevailing myth, it doesn't exist exclusively among a small band of individuals who possess some sort of extraordinary God-given power. Intuition is just another sense, like seeing or feeling or hearing. Moreover, it's a sense we all share. We are all intuitive.

I admit that accepting and acting on the presence and working of intuition in your life can require a leap of faith—the way we all have to take it on faith that Neil Armstrong and other astronauts truly walked on the moon. It requires a suspension of your natural disbelief. Many people, perhaps most, have to go through the act of intuiting and experience the amazing sensation involved before they can begin to implement intuition in their lives. Yet learning to decipher your own unique *language* of intuition can help you immeasurably in creating a happier, healthier life and a healthier body. For intuition is precisely that: another unique language created by the brain and the body to help us gain insight into and understanding of our past and to provide solutions for the future and help us create stronger, more pleasurable lives.

This is what this book will reveal to you: If you have a brain and a body, if you have memories, if you sleep at night (or any other time), then, by definition, you have to be—*you are*—intuitive.

And, most important, you can use your intuition to make your body healthier and your life more pleasurable.

When something significant happens to us in our lives, the emotionally charged experience gets encoded in the brain. We may not even know the true significance of this experience, yet it, and other emotionally charged memories, will affect everything we do in the future, from whom we choose for companionship to what we do for a living. By reclaiming the memories stored in our *brains,* we can understand rationally how the past continually influences our conscious minds and our everyday actions and realities.

We have other memories besides those in our brains. Memories and experiences and the emotions associated with them are also encoded systematically in all the tissues and organs of our bodies. These memories and emotions speak to us not via the rational processes of the brain, but by means of symptoms and disease in our bodily organs. A substantial number of scientific studies have indicated that certain emotional and psychological patterns are associated with diseases in specific organs; other studies support the link between specific memories and emotions and certain organ-specific diseases, such as breast cancer, coronary heart disease, and Parkinson's disease.

Our rational minds find it difficult to understand how painful memories and experiences can create distress and disease in our lives. Traditional or even alternative medical approaches and psychotherapy can't always help people who are ill or in pain. The key to healing lies in the unconscious. If we can become aware of the memories stored in our *bodies* and bring them to mind, we can gain a different, nonrational understanding of how the past influences the present and our conscious minds and actions. We can do it if we learn to tap into what I call the intuition network, to help us envision and create healthier lives, instead of allowing old memories and patterns of behavior to continue re-creating painful experiences.

I wish I could say that I learned the connection between memories, dreams, intuition, and healing in a college course or, better yet, through divine inspiration. As fate would have it, however, I had to reach an understanding of this connection the way I believe many, if not most, people do—through illness.

I've always been intuitive, but I haven't always wanted to be. My first recollection of possessing any intuitive skill is from my early childhood. Each evening after dinner, my father would go over the arithmetic tables with my older sister. He drilled her in addition, subtraction, and multiplication, and whenever she came up with the wrong answers, I would intuitively blurt out the correct answers, even though I was only five at the time. My father would look at me in shock and ask me how I knew what the right answers were. "I was just guessing," I would reply. The expression of disbelief on his face unsettled me; soon enough I began to equate guessing with disapproval. My parents were more inclined to chalk my remarkable ability up to brains, which, I quickly realized, they considered far preferable.

So from my earliest days, the message I received—and I believe it's the message most of us receive—was that intuition was bad, while intelligence was good. Intuition is suspected; intelligence is accepted.

This message was no doubt reinforced for me when my parents, concerned that I wasn't normal, took me in for a psychological evaluation at the age of seven. Although I received a clean bill of health, it was clear to me that what I had to do was to put aside my intuition and to work very, very hard at being "smart." That's just what I proceeded to do. The results, for the first four years of my schooling, weren't very encouraging. The very same math problems I had intuitively solved just a few years earlier now stumped me as thoroughly as they had my sister and kept me indoors at recess while all my friends played outside. Nevertheless, I didn't give up. I plugged away at applying my intelligence, and in fifth grade (perhaps thanks at least in part to some fervent prayers to God the summer before), everything seemed to click. My teachers informed my delighted parents that I was at the top of all my classes and that I was being moved into more accelerated courses.

I had learned that you didn't get points for intuition; you got them for having brains. From then on, I cultivated thinking and repressed intuition. Never having been one to do things in moderation, I worked so hard at earning points that I eventually earned enough for an M.D. and a Ph.D. It might not surprise you to learn that my Ph.D. is in neuroanatomy and behavioral neuroscience—the study of the brain and intelligence, that acceptable way of knowing and learning.

As I was racking up degrees and publications on my curriculum vitae, however, I also underwent an experience that gradually opened my eyes to the truth that my brains and intelligence could take me only so far. During my junior year at Brown University, I was diagnosed with a brain disorder similar to narcolepsy, a disease in which the brain receives a signal to sleep and dream immediately and transmits it to the body. In other words, you fall asleep unexpectedly no matter where you are or what you're doing, whether you're in the shower or shopping at the mall. Although I'd been falling asleep in strange places and at strange times all my life, I'd learned to live with the problem and to mask it to a degree. I had mastered the art of quickly piecing together, after I awoke, what had been occurring while I was "out." I'd learned, for instance, to play close attention to the conversation at dinner parties so I could pick up the thread if I unexpectedly nodded off for a minute or two over my plate. I would go to see the same movies three or four times so I could get their story lines down pat. (I saw *Amadeus* four times before it dawned on me that Mozart had led a less than happy life.) I actually fell asleep in the middle of my first date! I could fall asleep standing, sitting, even walking. My life was a constant reenactment of the famous scene in *The Wizard of Oz,* when Dorothy, the Lion, and Toto, running through a field of poppies, sink to the ground as they're overcome by the uncontrollable urge to sleep.

I was able to cover up the problem successfully for quite some time. I told myself that I was just tired and that people who knew me would learn to overlook my little idiosyncrasy.

Although I had believed I had everything under control, the stress of my studies intensified the sleep problem, which frightened those around me. I knew no other way of functioning and being in the world, but one roommate suggested I might need help when she saw me fall asleep while I worked out on an exercise bicycle. I was falling asleep more frequently and for longer periods. I could no longer mask what was happening. My intellect became less and less capable of controlling a process that was apparently taking place in some nonrational, nonintellectual center of my mind. Finally, I was persuaded to let myself be examined.

After the diagnosis of a sleep disorder like narcolepsy, I was placed on several trials of medicine, which had the side effect of jumbling my thinking. Concentrating, reading, and writing became very difficult. For the first time in my life, I could not survive on the strength of my intellect alone. The very thing I had relied on and worked so hard to develop was now inadequate for running my life.

I had to go back to guessing.

To intuition.

I took a medical leave of absence from school, moved to Boston, and took a job in a research lab. I knew I might have difficulty reading the directions to the experiments we'd be conducting, but I figured I'd wing it. I'd simply have to use my intuition.

In fact, I soon became known in the lab for being very intuitive. This was something my boss quickly learned to capitalize on. He soon figured out that even if he lost a file in the lab somewhere, I could invariably tell him where to find it. In other circumstances, he didn't find my ability quite so gratifying. We ran a lot of football pools in the office, and every Friday we'd go through the list of NFL teams playing that weekend, bet the winners, and pick the point spreads. My knowledge of football was absolutely zero, and everybody knew it. Yet I won so often that my colleagues finally eliminated me from the pool. I think the bet that put them over the edge was the time I picked Green Bay, which was 1–11, to win by 6 points over Dallas, the reigning Super Bowl champs. "How could you have known that?" my boss demanded sourly as he handed me fifty dollars.

I made it up to him soon enough, though. We were having trouble with a study in which we were attempting to create artificial gonorrhea cells, or liposomes. No matter what we did, the cells would repeatedly leak like sieves. My supervisor was annoyed and impatient. One day he loomed over my lab bench, the veins bulging at his temples. Punching his finger at me, he demanded, "What are you going to do about this?"

I looked up at him. "We'll try alpha-glucosidase!" I blurted—wondering even as I spoke what on earth alpha-glucosidase was, what it did, and, above all, where this wild idea had popped into my head from!

My boss clearly wondered, too. He glared at me skeptically. "What will that do?" he demanded. "Where did you get that idea?"

I asked him to leave me alone for a while, because I needed to take some time to write up a detailed experimental design that would fully address his questions and many others that would eventually come up. I went straight to the library and looked up alpha-glucosidase. After consulting several reference texts, I figured out how this enzyme might be used to design an artificial gonorrhea cell that wouldn't leak. I tried it in the lab, and it worked! Later that year, I presented a paper on the experiment at a scientific conference.

My boss was giddy with delight over my success. Although I was happy, too, I was full of questions. I still wondered from where the information to solve that problem had come to me. What, I wondered, was the source of intuitive information? But once again, instead of embracing intuition and resolving to answer those questions to my satisfaction, I pushed the whole issue aside.

Although I had continued to suffer from sleep attacks while working at the lab, I had learned to rely on my intuition to compensate for when my intellect was inaccessible. Now, however, my doctors came up with a drug that stopped the attacks altogether. I was elated. As I saw it, this meant that my life could go back to normal. I could read and write again. I could concentrate. I could stop relying on my intuition and go back to using my intellect, go back to "normal" ways of knowing. The operative word, of course, is "normal." I thought that intuition was a compensatory response to a disease. Diseases weren't normal, so intuition couldn't be normal, either. And I was determined, at all costs, to be a normal person.

I returned to Brown. My grade point average soared from 2.22 to 4.0, and I basked in the glow of my intellectual success. Meanwhile, I turned my back on the great gift that disease had given me—the knowledge that there was more to life than intellectual abilities.

I was soon to learn, however, that if you don't learn the lesson your intuition teaches you through an illness the first time, it will return and hit you with a bigger hammer.

In my case, the hammer was quite literal, and it came in the form of a truck. Two weeks after I graduated from college, I was running my customary miles across a suspension bridge when a panel truck came up behind me and struck me. According to the police report, I flew 80 feet down the length of the bridge. My pelvis was broken in four places, and I suffered several broken ribs, a collapsed lung, and a shattered shoulder blade.

The doctors immediately speculated that I had had another sleep attack, which would mean my medicine was no longer working. Once they took a look at my blood work, though, they realized I had a far greater problem. My body wasn't tolerating the medicine. The blood cells were dying, and my liver was becoming inflamed. I pleaded with the doctors to keep me on the one medication that gave me back my intellect. They refused. If my blood cells kept dying, they said, then I would die.

This time, I got the hint. I accepted the message my body was sending me. I knew I had to go back to using intuition.

My sleep attacks returned, because the new medication the doctors gave me didn't work as well as the first. Acupuncture, exercise, and diet helped control them, and I was able to keep them to a minimum by coming to understand that ignoring certain emotions would exacerbate the problem. Worrying about money, for instance, increased the attacks. So did a bad relationship; choosing to be alone, in contrast, decreased them. This was my first introduction to the truth that my body was speaking to me, intuitively, about emotions and issues in my life that needed to be addressed and resolved.

A lot of my energy was going into controlling my health. One day, a friend suggested that I have a reading by a medical intuitive. Skeptical and reluctant, I met with a woman I'll call Marisa. To see her, I took a bus trip to Boston with two hundred dollars cash in a paper bag—all the money I had at the time. I was desperate to find help. I expected to meet with an overweight, elderly Gypsy type who would read my palm and tell me I would marry a handsome man, have many children, and enjoy years of good fortune. Instead, Marisa seemed perfectly normal, wore no beads or feathers, and had no crystals or any other of the pseudospiritual trappings I had expected.

Marisa sat with me and gave me a simple message. She calmly told me that I could learn to stop my sleeping spells with my mind. In fact, she said, most of my mind's ability and my emotions were frozen. Unless I unfroze my emotions and got my mind and body in sync, I would never heal.

Her pronouncement shook me up, but it felt fairly accurate.

Because it was a pretty general kind of statement, however—all of us have vast unused potential in our brains—I pushed her to tell me something concrete and specific about my past. Marisa looked up and away from me and began to describe an episode from my childhood when something traumatic happened to me in a closet. Of course, lots of children can say they've been locked in closets or frightened by closets, but Marisa's description of my particular closet was so meticulously detailed that she simply bowled me over. She described the closet's unique color, design, hinge mechanism, and intricate woodwork and moldings. Convinced that she had really seen into my past, to where my body had been, and to the source of some of my deepest challenges, I had to stop her from going further.

Marisa couldn't give me specific advice about how to unfreeze my emotions, but she refused to accept any money from me. This impressed me profoundly. I left her office feeling stunned and chilled by the truth of the reading, which I could feel in my body. I boarded the bus back to Providence and took my paper bag of cash to a bookstore, looking for information about ways to bring my mind and body into sync. As I browsed among the shelves, one title seemed to leap out at me: *You Can Heal Your Life,* by Louise Hay. I bought the book and began practicing her visualizations, phrases of positive reinforcement that you repeat to yourself over and over. For the next two months, I'd look at myself in the mirror and say things like "I deserve good health now," and "I deserve the best and accept it now," and "I love and approve of myself just the way I am." Basically I taught myself (and, I guess, every cell in my body in the process) how to love and accept myself, how to forgive, and how to believe that I deserved health. To my complete astonishment, it worked. My sleep attacks almost completely went away. During the day I remained awake and was fully able to read, write, and concentrate. Very gradually, under the supervision of several friends who were health professionals, I weaned myself off all medicines.

Marisa had also told me that I had a "frozen lake" of intuitive ability and unused potential in my mind. While I knew that I needed to learn to appreciate all of my mind's perceptual abilities, not just my "normal" intellect, and learn to appreciate and respect intuition, it wasn't until two years later that I began to do so in a concerted way. I had begun my medical school clerkships in a very busy, poorly staffed, undersupplied inner-city hospital. On my first day, I was told to go down to the emergency room to meet my first patient, a fifty-six-year-old woman named Betty. I was to take her history, find out why she was in the hospital, and do a physical exam. As soon as I heard the patient's name, I found myself envisioning what was going on in her physical body. At the same time, I saw what was going on in her emotional life that would help set the scene for the illness in her body. In my mind's eye, I saw Betty as around 5 feet 4, obese, and experiencing pain in the upper right side of her abdomen. She believed it might be her gallbladder. I realized the pain was occurring around the setting of some family responsibility that Betty was ambivalent about discharging.

Wanting to plan ahead, I checked in the reference books in the on-call room about how to investigate right abdominal pain. I wrote down all the possible diseases that could cause this symptom and determined which tests I would need to order to make a diagnosis. These included liver function tests, especially an amylase, and an abdominal ultrasound.

I arrived in the emergency room to see that Betty, my patient, was a middle-aged overweight woman clutching the right side of her belly. She had been on her way to a family reunion and was very upset that she would disappoint her family if she was not able to attend. Some of her liver function tests were elevated, and an ultrasound of her belly revealed gallstones. I was elated. I had done my first medical intuitive reading!

Using my intuition helped me organize myself better in the hospital. I ended up being faster, more efficient, and able to leave the hospital sooner than others. Moreover, I was using my intellect *and* my intuition in a productive and fulfilling fashion. My intuition, working with my intellect, made me a better physician.

We all have certain fixed ideas by which we come to live, ideas that experience has made us believe are true. Some of them are self-limiting: "I'll always struggle." "There will never be enough money." "No one will ever understand me." "I'll always be alone." At some key moment, these limiting ideas are physicalized. They become physical symptoms that challenge us to examine ourselves and our lives. I believe, as many mind-body doctors do, that disease is a signal to look for imbalance in our lives, to reevaluate where we are and where we're going. One way to reevaluate is by learning the language of disease and the mind-body emotions that correspond to certain physical symptoms. We need to learn how to interpret the life challenge that our bodies present us by learning our bodies' unique language of intuition.

For a long time, I thought I wouldn't find acceptance in life unless I could be like everyone else. I let that fear rule my life for many years. I wouldn't acknowledge the emotions of shame and anxiety that had kept me in a holding pattern of repression and denial of who I really was. It wasn't until I became seriously ill, until my intuition spoke to me through body symptoms and body distress, that I acknowledged the unexpressed emotions behind that distress and moved to change my life.

Emotions are a major component of each person's intuitive network, his or her internal intuitive guidance system, which pinpoints and highlights what's wrong in our lives and urges us to address it. Albert Einstein formulated a famous equation: $E = mc^2$. Energy equals matter accelerated. He was talking about physics, but his formula applies equally well to intuition and health. Many medical intuitives, in reading clients, see their bodies in terms of so-called energy fields. They stand on the energy side of Einstein's theorem. But I would call myself an emotional intuitive, and I'm more concerned with the other side, with matter accelerated. That, in my view, is the consequence of unreleased and unacknowledged emotions. The very word "emotion" derives from the Latin for moving out, or moving forward. If we don't recognize and express our emotions, as I did not for many years, if we don't move them out and move ourselves forward, then the emotions will do the moving for us. They'll accelerate mass in our bodies, causing cells to move in ways that may take on the pattern of disease. The energy of disease is only released by the emotions we keep contained and unexamined inside us, like a radioactive nuclear core.

It's hard for many people to accept that this might be so, that emotional situations in our lives, or memories of emotions stored in our organs, can affect our very bodily health. And yet look at the strange ways in which disease strikes. Thirty people go to a picnic where some bad hamburger is served, but only ten get ill, even though everyone ate the same meat. Why did the *E. coli* bacteria cause a reaction in those ten, but not the other twenty? Is it just coincidence? In a famous experiment, a scientist and his laboratory staff drank vials of liquid containing cholera bacteria and waited to see what would happen. You'd naturally imagine that everyone would immediately come down with cholera. But in fact only some of the staff became ill. Others were completely unaffected. The conclusion drawn from this is that the cause of the illness is not simply the bacteria, but the way in which the bacteria interact with the immune system of those persons who fall sick.

In life, if you focus on possibilities, they become probabilities. How you perceive the world and everything in it affects how the world influences you. A belief that you're not safe and secure and the world is a dangerous place, feelings of helplessness and hopelessness, have been associated with increased susceptibility to illness and reduced immunity. Memories from past emotional experiences, trapped in your tissues, memories associated with certain emotions you've never fully resolved, thus affect your physical health. If you focus on the world as being unsafe, if you believe "I will always get sick," then you may in fact be more likely to get sick than someone who believes the world is full of germs, but who has no sense of being hopeless and helpless.

In this book, you'll see how such memories in the brain and the body, activated by your intuition, are your soul's attempt to move you to change your life, to nudge you in directions that will lead to greater happiness and health. Since I became a medical intuitive, I've seen the proof of this countless times. I've seen it as well in regular medical practice. Consider this case of stroke. The patient was male, a heavy drinker, full of anger and rage, who would regularly beat his wife, but felt guilty about it afterward. He had had a stroke to one side of his brain, to the very area of his brain that connects rage with movement. He was unable to move half his body in response to his emotion. Eventually, the stroke reversed, and he was able to move again.

His intuition had sent him a message, a warning signal about his behavior. He had been given a chance to change, to adjust and improve his life, stop hurting his wife. Unfortunately, he didn't listen to the intuitive message. He ignored the warning signals of his intuition network and kept abusing his own body and his wife. And what happened? He had a second stroke. This time, he blew out the same area on *both* sides of his brain. This was remarkable because, anger being such a primal and important protective emotion, there are many routes in the brain along which it can travel. It's like the highway system around New York City; if one highway's backed up, there are at least seven other routes you can try. Yet every one of this man's anger routes was blocked by the stroke. It was as though he had given himself a frontal lobotomy. Now all he could do was sit in a chair, unable to move, unable to feel any emotion. It seemed as though, because he had failed to act on his intuition, his soul took over and simply excised his problematic behavior, making him appear numb to any emotions or deficits in his situation.

In another instance, I was able to learn how a patient could help herself by applying her intuition to her problem. Early in my clerkships, I was assigned a forty-eight-year-old patient named Sheila, a divorcée with failing kidneys. I quickly established a rapport with her, since I was the only medical student able to draw blood from her veins successfully. One afternoon she told me about her life. She had been married for twenty-four years to a man named Joe. Together, she and Joe had raised three children. They took pride in having worked their way out of poverty. Sheila had been happy and fulfilled by her life as a wife and mother and her career as a legal secretary. She was looking forward to sharing a long, productive, and enjoyable life with her husband once her children were grown and gone from home.

Soon after her last child went off to college, Sheila discovered that her husband was having an affair with a woman half her age. He moved out to be with the other woman, leaving Sheila alone for the first time in her life. Six months later, her kidneys failed. She had to leave her job because of her health and wound up losing her house when her debts got out of hand.

Sheila's physicians placed her on steroids, which caused her to become diabetic. My job, as her student physician, was to regulate her diabetes. I privately believed that the stress and betrayal of her husband's affair had played a role in her loss of kidney function. But as a medical student, I felt it wasn't my place to focus on this aspect of her illness. My job was to provide quality medical care based on her symptoms, blood tests, and other laboratory data.

I felt my job was also to listen to her grief and witness her pain. One afternoon Sheila was watching a TV talk show while I was drawing her blood for what seemed like the millionth time. Ironically, the topic of the show that day was men who cheated on their wives. As I drew the last tube of blood, Sheila began to make comments about the men on the show.

"See that guy there? That guy's no good," she said. "His wife should kick him out."

I looked up from my work. The man on the TV did, in fact, look like a real loser, and I agreed with her.

Then Sheila said: "You know, I've just figured out why my kidneys failed. My whole life, I never thought I could live without a man. After my husband left me, I wondered whether or not I could survive. And then my kidneys started to die. I didn't deserve how my ex-husband treated me. I felt betrayed, but I still didn't think I could live without him.

"But you know," she said—and there was a firmer note in her voice than I had heard before—"that was two years ago. Somehow I've learned to live on my own. I've survived, and I'm stronger now than when I was married. I think I'm going to be okay now."

Sheila's kidneys soon began to function again. She was able to get off steroids, and her diabetes went away as well.

Sheila had spent her whole life in the belief that she could exist only with a man. That was all she had ever known. Then, due to fate or some other mechanism, her husband left her, placing her in a situation that would challenge her conviction that she could live only as a devoted wife and mother. Sheila was forced to face her fear of being alone by her disease, kidney failure. Then, by means of her own intuition, she was able to listen to the message behind her disease, the language through which her body was communicating that all was not okay with her life. She came to peace with this life crisis and moved on, stronger and wiser for the experience.

I have learned the intricate relationship between intuition, memories, dreams, and the body through disease and health, through my work as a scientist, through my work as a physician, and, finally, through my work as a medical intuitive. Most important, I've seen others begin to use intuition in their own lives to heal disease and accept personal challenges in emotional growth.

You, too, can learn the language of your body. By learning to read body sensations, body movements, and body memories, the signals of distress and disease, you can become a body intuitive.

In this book, you will learn how the memories stored in our brains and our bodies are communicated to us through feeling, sensation, pain, and disease. You'll learn how dreams help us chart possible futures out of disease and crisis. Finally, you'll learn to understand your own unique language of intuition and how it can empower you to create a healthier, happier life.

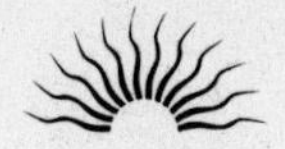

Part One

THE INTUITION NETWORK

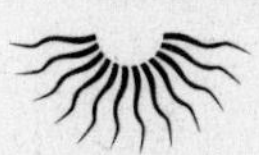

ONE

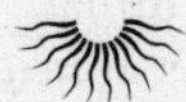

The Commonest Sense: The Truth about Intuition

I felt like some watcher of the skies,
When a new planet swims into his ken.
JOHN KEATS

One of the first nights I was on duty as an intern in the emergency room, the place was a zoo. Patients were coming in out of the dark with complaints as ordinary as the flu and as urgent as shock and trauma.

I was low man, or woman, on the totem pole. The attending physician issued my instructions. The paramedics had brought in an elderly lady who had collapsed at home in front of her clothes dryer. The attending had examined her, and she seemed all right. Her vital signs were stable. She appeared to have recovered from her fainting or dizziness, or whatever had caused her collapse, and she was resting quietly. He could discharge her, the attending said, but since there was no one at home to care for her or monitor her, he thought it best to keep her in the hospital overnight as a so-called social admit.

My job was to have her admitted and send her upstairs to the floor. I walked out into the corridor, where people were scurrying around on various errands, and headed for my patient. As I approached her gurney, I began to get a vague, fuzzy, yet insistent feeling that seemed to cut through all the noise and commotion around me. I just had a sudden conviction, seeming to come out of nowhere, that contrary to the physical evidence, all was not right with this patient.

I wanted her to get an EKG. Don't ask me why. Her chart indicated no history of heart trouble, and the examining physician hadn't noted any signs of cardiac problems. The orderlies were getting ready to move her upstairs. On an impulse, I hid her chart to knock them off the track—a patient can't go anywhere without the all-important chart. Then I hurried back to the attending.

"Um," I began, clearing my throat, "I know you said there's nothing wrong with this patient, but just in the interest of thoroughness, couldn't we order an EKG?" He looked at me. He gave me a slightly patronizing smile. I could just see him thinking: "Compulsive intern!" Everybody thought I was compulsive. Maybe that's why he indulged me. Okay, he said, he'd order up an EKG. And I took off.

For some reason, it seemed urgent to check medical records. I flew up two flights of stairs, my feet taking me there as if of their own accord, as if they knew something my brain didn't. As it turned out, my feet were full of wisdom. In the medical records department, I found some previous charts for the elderly lady and pulled them. And there it was in black-and-white. The physical evidence for my hunch. The records revealed that the patient had a history of heart problems even as, downstairs, a brand-new EKG was showing her to be in the middle of a full-blown heart attack.

The woman was rushed to the ICU. My gut feeling not only helped save the woman's life, it also saved the attending physician from making a serious error and the hospital from losing a patient.

What happened to me that night in the emergency room is not an uncommon experience. I had had an intuitive "hit." Most people have had something similar happen to them at some point in their lives, on the job or elsewhere. We've all heard the stories about people who got a gut feeling, changed their travel plans at the last minute, and miraculously avoid a plane crash. Or people who have a sudden, inexplicable sense at a certain moment in the day that something somewhere is not right, only to learn later that something happened to a loved one or a friend at that very moment. Even more common are the everyday hunches we get, about how to perform a certain task, when to ask for a raise, whether or not to ask someone out on a date, when to call home to check on a child, and when to avoid or delay any number of ordinary, daily activities. And then, of course, there are the dreams we have at night—sometimes prophetic, sometimes symbolic, but frequently providing remarkable insights into the events of our waking hours.

WHAT IS INTUITION?

Whether we call them hunches, gut feelings, senses, or dreams, they're all the same thing—intuition, speaking to us, giving us insight and knowledge to help us make sound decisions about any number of actions we take. Intuition occurs when we directly perceive facts outside the range of the usual five senses and independently of any reasoning process. As one scientist defined it, intuition is "the process of reaching accurate conclusions based on inadequate information."[1] This describes precisely my experience in the emergency room. I made a correct decision on the basis of insufficient—really, nonexistent—data. On a purely rational level, I shouldn't have gone running off to look at medical records. No concrete indications of any kind suggested that this was necessary. In fact, going off like that could have gotten me into trouble. My brain was telling me to admit the patient and attend to my other duties, but my body was running around looking for seemingly meaningless EKGs, pursuing nothing but a vague hunch. Yet somehow, in a manner totally unconnected to the facts, and without reasoning it through, I had perceived something that did in fact turn out to be true.

Where did that perception come from? Scientists are still struggling to pinpoint the answer to this question.[2] One theory holds that people with exceptional intuitive skills in given fields are simply experts tapping into vast mental libraries of information, memories that they keep stored in their minds.[3] According to this explanation, an aviation expert who can diagnose a malfunction in an aircraft that has stymied everyone else is able to do so because a single detail will trigger a recollection of having fixed a plane with a similar problem in the past. This causes him to pull out the appropriate technical manual from his memory stacks, thumb through it mentally, and—bingo!—apply the suggested solution. This is an elegant theory, but it has a lot of flaws. For one, it doesn't explain my experience with the heart attack patient in the emergency room. At that point, I didn't have a library in my mind. I had a couple of file cards, maybe. Nothing in my experience could have signaled to me on any rational or cognitive level what was happening with that patient.

Moreover, it's possible to know something intuitively without ever having subscribed to the appropriate journal, much less having amassed a library on the subject. My friend and colleague Caroline Myss was working at a publishing house when she discovered her abilities as a medical intuitive. She knew nothing about the body and had never shown any interest in it. Yet as soon as she tapped into her medical intuition, she was able to give people amazingly accurate readings of their health based on no more information than a client's name and age.

People who routinely rely on intuition in their work or profession don't consciously think about where the information is coming from or why it helps them do what they do. They just take it and apply it. One of the most intuitive groups of people I ever ran into were the nurses in the hospital intensive care unit. The one time I had duty in the ICU as an intern, I walked up to a nurses' station where it seemed that every conceivable patient alarm and buzzer was going off—and, believe me, there are lots of monitors and alarms in an ICU. Calmly sitting in front of the brightly lit monitor board were three or four nurses, completely ignoring the clamor. One was happily eating pork fried rice, another was busy with chicken wings, and a couple of others were dipping into a box of Dunkin' Donuts. I was astounded. Didn't they know those buzzers could mean patients in crisis? Why weren't they responding? In their place, having a slight case of post-traumatic stress disorder, I would have been dashing around the unit checking on every patient with a ringing buzzer. And of course I would have been exhausted within ten minutes.

Those nurses somehow knew when the buzzing and beeping around them was serious and when it wasn't. Even as I watched, another alarm went off, and a nurse looked up at the board, dropped her chicken wing, and ran down the hall. This time a patient *was* in crisis. And the nurse had apparently discerned that from not much more than the sound of a beeper and the sight of a flashing light. This phenomenon was repeated again and again. Almost invariably, although they ignored most of the alarms that went off, the nurses responded whenever a real crisis threatened. Again I was amazed. But when I asked them how they knew when they should react and when they could afford not to, they looked at me blankly. Every one of them shrugged and answered: "I don't know. I just *know.*"

What doctor hasn't heard a nurse repeat that phrase time and again? Like my lady in the emergency room, a patient will appear objectively stable or on the mend, but the nurse who has cared for him all night will insist that he's getting worse or is on the verge of crisis.

"How do you know?" the doctor will ask, looking for objective data. "Let's look at the vital signs, the lab results, the X-rays." And the nurse can only respond, "I just know." Intuition is a right-hand aid of nurses, but neither they nor anyone else can tell you where it comes from.

In an extensive study of nurses and intuition, nurse and researcher Patricia Benner ascribed the intuitive process of nurses in clinical situations to "skilled pattern recognition." This is another version of "libraries of the mind." Once again, this theory concludes that previously acquired knowledge, an expertise based on memory and prior experience, is the basis and the source of intuition. A nurse detects something in a patient that rings a tiny bell in her mind and reminds her of a previous similar case that leads to her hunch about the current patient's condition.

One of Benner's own nurse cases, however, contradicts this neat theory. It involves a case of pulmonary embolism.[4] As it happens, pulmonary embolism, a blood clot in the lungs that's nearly always fatal if undetected, is one of the hardest things in Western medicine to diagnose. There are virtually no common symptoms and very often no discernible signs that a patient is in danger of a PE. A patient can have absolutely clear lungs and yet suddenly suffer a PE and die. It manifests differently in every individual. In medical school you're essentially taught always to consider the possibility of PE if you have a patient who's just generally "not right" and you can't figure out why. But fundamentally it's one of the most fatal medical problems and, tragically, one of the easiest to miss.

The nurse whom Benner observed saw a patient with cerebral edema, or fluid on the brain. His fluid intake had been restricted, and he was resting quietly. But the nurse was concerned. "Somehow I knew he was going to have a rough time," she reported. There it was—the intuitive hunch. "Somehow I knew he was on the highway to a pulmonary embolism." But what a hunch! How did she make the unbelievable leap to that extraordinary conclusion? It was a case of pole-vaulter cognition. This patient didn't have a problem with a clot in his lungs; he had cerebral edema. It wasn't even a case of right church, wrong pew; this nurse didn't even seem to be in the right state! The only possible symptom that she could relate to pulmonary embolism was having overheard the patient's wife say earlier in the day that he was anxious. That night the nurse couldn't stay away from the patient's room, even though he was assigned to someone else's care. Like my feet carrying me to the medical records department, her feet moved her over to his room to investigate. She found him "sort of pale and anxious," and even though he was still conscious, she called the doctors, and sure enough, just as the doctors arrived, the patient began to die. The doctors coded, or resuscitated, him. The pulmonary embolism was caught, and the patient was saved.

In trying to explain her need to check on the patient, the nurse could only say, "I had a suspicion there was something wrong with him, and maybe that's sort of an inside thing."

An inside thing.

An inside suspicion. Meaning intuition.

The word "intuition" derives from the Latin *intueri,* meaning to look within. Intuition is something we see and hear and feel within, an internal language that facilitates insight and understanding. As such, it's much more immediate than pattern recognition, which is based on external information. In fact, pattern recognition may be an important part of intuition, the part that comes from the right side of the brain. But intuition actually comes from a whole network, a cast of characters present in the brain and the body. Similarly, memories and experiences—those stored in the brain and those encoded in the organs of the body—have a vital function in our intuitive understanding. But the initial sense, that first gut feeling you get when intuition goes to work, is something else. Scientists like Benner and others have tried to rank it as a cognition, a part of the rational mind, the thinking brain. But intuition is a perception, of seeing or hearing or feeling rather than thinking. When I do a reading on a client, I have only his or her name and age to start with. I know nothing more about the person, so I can't, at first, be proceeding on the basis of pattern recognition, recognizing parts of this person's life that are similar to those of other people I've met. Not until I've perceived certain things about the client through intuitive perception can I begin to recognize patterns in the information.

The ancient Greeks believed that intuition was attributable to the gods, that when something as incomprehensible as an intuitive insight came to them, it came directly from the heavens. After formulating his famous theorem, the Greek mathematician Pythagoras immediately went out and sacrificed a thousand oxen to the god Apollo as thanks for having taught him this rule.

Modern-day scientists, especially those of us who study the brain, would generally dismiss this idea. We tend to believe that the source of all human function, behavior, and knowledge is housed in that complex and multifunctional organ. But occasionally something happens to challenge this conviction. I have a Ph.D. in neuroanatomy and behavioral neuroscience, and I wrote my dissertation on the structures of the motor system in the brain. I can probably say without exaggeration that I've read nearly everything that's been written about neurological control of the body's movement since just about the beginning of time. Until recently, as far as I was concerned, the brain controlled movement and that was that. No exceptions. If a certain part of the brain was damaged, the movement controlled by that part would cease or be impaired. This was something I knew. I had studied it, learned it, observed it. I was sure of it. Once you do the Ph.D., you're called a scientist, an authority.

Then I saw something that humbled me.

A man who had suffered a seizure was brought into our hospital. He was hooked up to an electroencephalograph, but over four days the machine detected no seizures in his brain. Two previous MRIs (magnetic resonance images) had likewise indicated no significant anomalies in the brain. The doctors concluded that his first seizure had been due to a conversion, or psychiatric, disorder rather than a physical one, and they prepared to discharge him.

I had seen him only once and had been surprised to see a large, raw scrape down the right side of his face. He had apparently received this injury from the fall in his first seizure, but in psychiatry we rarely see a person hurt himself in a conversion seizure, since these episodes are not usually very violent, not really "real" seizures at all. I took note of this. A few days later I was headed out to lunch past the nurses' station. This patient was also walking past with his wife. Suddenly he fell to the floor in another seizure.

I went in to evaluate him after it was over. At this point the patient who is having true brain-induced seizures is usually sleepy, semicomatose, and confused. To orient him, I asked him what the date was. He looked at me. Then he replied: "It's three...four...two, four, six, eight, who do we appreciate?" He wasn't oriented, indicating he'd had a true seizure. But he had come out with a very complex phrase, of a sort you wouldn't expect from someone in a post-seizure state. Now I was a little confused myself. The only diagnosis I could come up with was that his was a true seizure disorder with some psychiatric phenomena overlaid. I also suggested further testing for any other possible physical problems, because I felt something was not right with this patient.

Fortunately, the doctors taking care of him did another MRI. What they discovered was a shock to us all. The man had a grapefruit-size tumor, a huge midline mass across the center of his brain, which had apparently grown in the six months since his last MRI. It was so large that it had taken over the motor areas of his right and left brain, the white matter beneath them, and the language area of his left brain—virtually everything. Tumor cells are not supposed to be functional. We had been taught that this patient should have been a near-vegetable—paralyzed, nearly mute, incontinent. Yet, apart from a little confusion, he appeared almost completely normal and functional. In fact, the neurologists claimed that he *was* normal. They had observed him walking and talking, had confirmed that his reflexes were good, his sensations normal, and he had no signs of dementia.

The question arose: What was operating this man? At this stage he clearly had abilities that couldn't be ascribed to biology. Something outside him was in control, providing locomotion for his body. Something else was driving the bus. I was reminded of those bumper stickers you see on the highway that say "God is my copilot." In this man's case, it seemed to be the truth. Certainly this experience made me reevaluate everything I knew about movement. I had thought it came from the brain. Now I had to believe something outside the man might have been driving him forward, something beyond normal sense and reason, sight, sound, mind, and body. Could it have been his soul?

Intuition works in this same way, as an autopilot. We've always believed the brain is the repository of knowledge that we take in consciously on a rational level, but is it possible that the brain is also a *transmitter* of knowledge that comes to us unconsciously on a nonrational level? Think of my experience with alpha-glucosidase in the lab. I had never heard of this enzyme, yet its name came to me, whole and unbidden, at the precise moment when I could receive it and make use of it.

In *A New Science of Life,* Rupert Sheldrake writes about the theory of morphogenic fields—invisible fields that surround and connect all matter and communicate growth and change. He describes laboratory studies in which it took twenty trials to teach one hundred rats in one location to perform certain tricks. A month later, one hundred rats in another location were able to learn the same tricks in only two trials. Sheldrake theorized that the first studies caused a change in the morphogenic field, allowing the second group of rats to tap into it. Well before Sheldrake, Jung believed that we might gain intuitive insights by "tapping into the collective unconscious."[5]

That might explain my stumbling onto alpha-glucosidase in a big-city lab in the twentieth century. But it still leaves Pythagoras, back in ancient Greece, living at a time when there was not so much knowledge in the morphogenic field, thanking the gods for his theorem. He realized that the knowledge had come from somewhere outside himself, but he had to listen to his inner voice, his intuition, perhaps the language of his gods, to hear the message. Intuition is a language from our soul, from our gods, just as it was to Pythagoras. It's like the Walkman in your pocket, which can forever provide you with news and information, as long as you turn it on and listen to the station. Like the radio station that feeds a Walkman, the station that broadcasts to our intuition is something external. It's a god outside of us—the soul or the divine consciousness, if you will. The divine consciousness speaks to our human consciousness, offering us quick, keen insights into the problems of everyday life and suggesting potential solutions through the language of intuition—the language of the soul.

BLACK MARKET KNOWLEDGE

Intuition inspires us to become creative in our lives and in the ways we view our lives. For most of us, the first step toward hearing the language of intuition requires that we become open to accepting another, seemingly illogical way of perceiving and receiving information. This is problematic for a lot of people. Because of the mysterious nature and origins of intuition, combined with the rationalism of our modern culture, most people either distrust intuition or disbelieve it entirely. Even if they believe in it, people tend to think of intuition as uncommon, a special ability that only a small number of unusual individuals possess. They think of it as some kind of mystical power. "Mystical" is a word with heavy connotations of spirituality and apartness. Using it in connection with intuition would set the intuitive up as a hierophant, a religious authority with access to knowledge not available to the rest of us mere mortals. None of this applies to the reality of intuition.

A mystic may very well be an intuitive, but that doesn't mean that being intuitive makes you a mystic. I have an aunt who is a short, stocky Portuguese immigrant lady with all the robust, earthy qualities of our ancestry. She doesn't look mystical, yet she's one of the most intuitive people I've ever known.

As a medical intuitive, I've bumped up against the popular misconception of intuition as a kind of magical or supernatural power that should be put in the service of people in crisis who are seeking understanding or control over their situation. People request readings in the hope that I'll be able to change the outcome of a situation or otherwise affect the course of a given condition. Dealing with these hopes is always sobering and very difficult. Recently I had a request for a reading from the family of a four-month-old boy with a genetic bowel disorder. Doctors had told the family the baby's only chance at a decent life was a colostomy. They planned to remove his colon and replace it with a bag to trap his wastes outside his body. The family turned to me in desperation, thinking I could tell them something or do something to make this course of treatment unnecessary. But I couldn't, and I can't. That's not what I do. Even though intuitive knowledge can be very healing, getting an intuitive hit is not what heals the person. Reading this child might even have been damaging. The fact is that there's a certain mystery to a case like this baby's. We don't know why genetic disorders occur, or what purpose they serve. Some people believe that genetic disorders in babies are due to past-life issues or bad karma. Yet for me to say that to a sick child's family in a time of high emotion could make matters worse and, at the least, wouldn't help. The intuitive practical information I could give them probably wouldn't be appropriate in this crisis, and they wouldn't be ready to hear it. They were hoping against hope that there was something they could do beyond the course already offered to them, which was following the medical and surgical advice of their doctors, praying, and appealing to the soul of their child. I couldn't tell them to do any more than that.

It's counterproductive to think of intuition and intuitiveness in terms of separateness or superiority, or in terms of the supernatural, or even of the offbeat and bizarre. Intuition is simply a sense that's common to each and every one of us. It's neither a magic power nor just the crazy hunches of eccentrics. It's a real down-to-earth capacity that is available to anyone willing to tune in his transmitter and listen in to what's being broadcast. The information it offers us is practical, and it can immeasurably improve and enrich our lives. In this light, intuition is common sense operating on the most fundamental, spontaneous level.

Numerous studies have shown that the use of intuition in any number of fields is often what separates the men from the boys—that is, the experts from the amateurs.[6] It's the quantum quality that gives an individual an edge over others in his field and boosts him into the "expert" stratosphere. It explains why certain stockbrokers seem to have an uncanny knack for picking investment winners, why certain publishers know which books will be best-sellers, and why certain detectives can zero in on crime suspects whom no one else even considers. A study of intuition in the business world separated a group of businessmen into "high" and "low" intuitives depending upon their ability to identify playing cards blindly. Those who scored high in intuition were later shown to make significantly better decisions concerning simulated managerial problems than the low scorers.

The Benner study of nurses also concluded that those who were best in their profession applied intuitive judgment to their clinical decisions.[4] And yet Benner and other researchers have consistently found that all the experts actually devalue their own intuitive judgment. Unless they can find concrete evidence to support it, they distrust their intuition. One nurse in the study reported being drawn into the room of a patient who was not her responsibility. She felt he was "going sour" and called a code, even though he was still breathing and had a pulse. When the doctor came in, the nurse couldn't give him a specific reason for feeling that the patient was in trouble. She thought his heavy breathing indicated respiratory distress, but other nurses and the doctor agreed the patient was merely oversedated. The nurse backed down, but as she went home that night, she told a colleague that she would bet her last paycheck that the patient was going to die. And in fact he did. The next day the nurse kicked herself, as so many of us do when we fail to heed the intuitive voice. "I wasn't as assertive as I should have been," she declared. How many times have you said something similar after the fact? "I *knew* I should have done such-and-such." "I had a feeling that was going to happen." "I should have trusted my instincts."

Because intuition involves making decisions on the basis of inadequate facts, we tend to think that the knowledge it brings us isn't legitimate. However certain we may be of the accuracy of our intuitive judgment, more often than not we wilt in the face of demands for proof that can't immediately be found. Intuition, as Benner puts it, is viewed as a "black market" version of knowledge.

But black market money is still money. In fact, sometimes it can go a lot farther than the legal currency. Once when I was traveling in Brazil, the value of the cruzado, the national currency, was plummeting, and I decided to make an exchange on the black market. I was in a small town, and the villagers sent me down the road to—believe it or not—the coffin store. I don't know whether it was a front, but in the back, the owner handed over literally a bucket of money for the dollars I gave him. It was wonderful. I got a lot more bang for my buck than I would have on the legitimate market.

It's the same with intuition. The extra information it gives us is unavailable "legitimately" but it can be invaluable. Its practical application in everyday life can have important and enlightening consequences. Intuition's relationship to creativity has been well documented. It's astounding to think how many things might never have been discovered if their discoverers hadn't listened to their intuition. Take the case of Henry Jacobs.[7] In 1930, Jacobs was a medical student at the University of Chicago. On a particularly beautiful autumn day he found himself slightly miffed to be on call while everyone else was out enjoying the university football game. He wandered into the hospital lab, sat down on a bench, and found himself staring at shelves of chemical reagents. For some reason, he reached up and took down three bottles at random, without reading their labels. He put them on the table in front of him and continued to gaze at them absently for a while. Then he looked at the labels. The substances he had pulled down were cobalt chloride, choline chloride, and sodium ferrocyanide. He didn't know what their chemical properties were, but he felt impelled to mix them together. Bravely, he proceeded to do so. He poured the cobalt into the choline and added the ferrocyanide. The result was an emerald green liquid that ultimately became the basis for the colorimetric method of measuring potassium in the blood, a basic medical test that's performed on thousands of people every single day of the year.

I had a similar experience in the research lab in Boston. The very first day I reported for work, my supervisor handed me an aggreganometer for aggregating blood platelets, along with a tube of baboon blood platelets, some aspirin, and instructions for an experiment. My assignment was to get the platelets to aggregate, or clump together, and then to demonstrate how the aspirin inhibited this aggregating process. Because I'm dyslexic, and impulsive, too, I had trouble calming down enough to read the protocol, which went extensively into buffers and pH's. I'd never done well in those in school, anyway, so I just ignored what the instructions said. (That, of course, is not always the wisest thing to do. I did it once in college, and they had to evacuate the building after I accidentally released some toxic chemicals into the air.) The instructions also called for using distilled water in the experiment, and I remember quite distinctly thinking, "Water's water. What's the difference if it's distilled or not?" So I mixed the aspirin with tap water. I got the platelets to aggregate, and then I threw in the tap water with the aspirin. The aggregating stopped.

At the end of the day I showed my supervisor my results. He looked at me unbelievingly. "It worked," he said, sounding amazed. "Yes...?" I said, not understanding why he was so surprised. "We've never gotten it to work before," he said. "How did you make the buffer?" When I told him about the tap water, he couldn't believe it. But we analyzed the pH of Boston's tap water that day, made another successful buffer, and I had my first publication—after one day in the lab!

Skeptics might say that what Jacobs and I did was just an accident. But Jacobs himself described his experience as the direct consequence of intuition guiding his actions and leading him toward a new knowledge. I had the same sense of having been given internal guidance. Like Keats, and Jacobs, I felt the sudden sensation of something new, unexpected, and brilliant flying into my inner field of vision, broadening my knowledge and my range. Working in that intuitive field feels like what the poet called "touching the face of God." It's truly a transcendent experience. It's as if your soul touches the heavens, and a new creation is conceived.

A host of other scientists and inventors—from Pythagoras to Thomas Edison to Jonas Salk—have credited intuition with helping to spur their accomplishments.[8] In later life, Salk, who discovered the polio vaccine, wrote an entire book on intuition. He maintained that creativity depended upon the interaction of intuition and reasoning.

In the same way, we should all be receptive to intuition's role in our lives. As one scientist wrote, "Intuition is a universal ability that is reflected not only in the creations of great scientists but also in the daily hunches of individuals."[9] It can reveal amazing things to the humblest among us.

RECOGNIZING INTUITION

You can be awake, asleep and dreaming, or in a state of consciousness in between when intuition comes to you. Henry Jacobs believed intuition to be preceded by detachment, slight melancholy, and a sort of trancelike state, like the one he felt he was in when he made his discovery in the lab. You may have had that feeling yourself, when you were wandering around, maybe a little upset about something, or daydreaming, and you suddenly stumbled upon something unexpected. But intuition can certainly hit you when you're in the full force of conscious activity, like my experience in the emergency room. Afterward, though, as Jacobs maintained, you are positively exhilarated.

Intuition has several general characteristics:

Confidence in the process of intuition
Certainty of the truth of intuitive insights
Suddenness and immediacy of knowledge
Emotion/affect associated with intuitive insight
Nonanalytic, nonrational, nonlogical
Gestalt nature of knowing
Associated with empathy
Difficulty putting images into words
Relationship to creativity[9]

Intuitive hits are sudden, immediate, and unexpected ideas. They seem illogical and have no clear line of thought. They frequently come out of the blue. Nevertheless, they bring with them a feeling of confidence and a certainty of their absolute indisputability. Often, even when we're not outwardly confident about our intuition, when we're devaluing it, like the nurses in the Benner study, our bodies are expressing confidence in its information. I didn't have the confidence to tell the attending physician about my hunch in the ER, but my legs moved and my feet took me to the medical records department anyway. My body was responding to the intuition coming to me. What we need to do is to note and listen to the signs and symptoms the body sends our way. This is the intuitive language of the soul as it speaks to us through our bodies.

Intuitive insights involve emotion. They're hard to describe in words, or more accurately, they reveal themselves first as a gestalt, as hunches that are difficult to put words to. The left brain, however, quickly begins to fill in words and details, making the intuition marketable and easy to communicate. Intuition is also associated with empathy.

The body also has a language of intuition that speaks through symptoms of health and disease, through dreams, and in the form of visions and voices, body sensations, and emotions. Intuition is processed multimodally in the body and the brain and through dreams, in the form of sights, sounds, tastes, and smells and in the form of body sensations, movements, and emotions. It's sometimes called the sixth sense, but I avoid using this term because it implies a sort of bonus sense that not everyone gets to claim—like earning extra points on an exam—when in fact we all have intuition. And this term also suggests that intuition exists outside of and separate from the other senses. In fact, the opposite is true.

We all have vision and hearing related to external things in the world of which everyone is conscious. Intuition is an internal form of perception of things that are not directly in front of us in the world. It's an inner sight, a form of hearing, body sense, and emotion. It is actually common to all the other senses and an enhancement of them. What differentiates intuition from the other senses is the unique form of expression it takes in each individual. The mechanisms of sight, hearing, taste, touch, and smell are exactly the same in everyone. But no two people experience intuition in exactly the same way. Five medical intuitives reading the same individual would describe the information they received in five entirely different ways.

Some intuitives are clairvoyant. This means that intuition comes to them visually, through images they see in their mind's eye. Edgar Cayce, probably the most famous medical intuitive of the twentieth century, was a clairvoyant.[10] One of the first times I did a reading, I imagined myself inside a person's body, looking around. I put myself right in the abdominal cavity, by the aorta, and looked up. The aorta looked like a tree to me. It looked massive. The arteries to the abdomen, the pelvis, and so on were its branches and roots, jutting out at right angles. I got so close to it in my mind's eye that I could actually see the texture of the aorta's "bark."

Now when I do a reading of a person, I first see myself standing in front of the person, checking the individual's head, eyes, ears, nose, and throat. Then I step inside, into the esophagus, and head south. I go for a ride, traveling through the various organ systems and visually examining their condition. This is a form of empathy, imagining yourself in another person's shoes. If you have empathy, if your heart is open to receiving information, you'll find you receive more of it. Jonas Salk described his own intuitive process similarly.[8] When doing his research, he said he would imagine himself as an immune system and try to reconstruct what it would be like to engage with a virus or cancer cell. This extreme form of empathy allowed him to acquire new insights and design his experiments accordingly.

Other people are clairaudient: they receive intuition through sounds. When I examine a client's heart during a reading, instead of looking at it, I listen to it, to the rhythm of its beating. Remember that I'm miles away, on a telephone line, so I'm doing this in my head. Some people hear random and dissociated words coming into their minds. I receive both images and sounds.

Still other intuitives are clairsentient. They receive intuition through actual sensations in their own bodies. Another medical intuitive and I were once put in a room and asked to do readings of a person in another state on the other side of the country. I immediately envisioned pain in the lower cervical vertebrae of the neck (C6, C7, T1) and numbness in the fourth and fifth fingers of both hands. Meanwhile, the other intuitive said she felt fuzziness. "Something's wrong with my hands," she said. I took her hands and touched each finger and had her tell me which ones felt fuzzy and numb. She reported no sensation in the fourth and fifth fingers of both hands. This corresponded exactly to what I had intuited visually as problems in the patient's vertebrae, causing numbness in the corresponding fingers. The other intuitive had transported herself into that person's body and therefore experienced the patient's sensory loss in her own hands.

I've had spinal problems for years myself, and to this day I get numbness in my hands whenever I speak on the phone with a certain person with whom I've had turbulent relations in the past. Do you think my body is trying to tell me something?

Some intuitives experience déjà vu in which space and time become confused; others have precognitive episodes, where they know ahead of time that something will happen in the future. Intuitive information is coming at us all the time, every day in every way. Most of us, though, go through life with the volume turned to low on that intuition transmitter in our hip pocket. We learn to ignore it most of the time. We're so out of touch with our intuition that we don't even recognize it when it comes. For instance, I spent a weekend at a friend's house a while ago. On Friday night I was in my room getting ready for bed when I suddenly heard shouts coming from my friend's room down the hall. Alarmed, I rushed in to see what was wrong. My friend Mildred was lying on the bed, shouting at the air, screaming at something invisible to go away. "What's going on?" I managed to cry, shaking her by the shoulder. Mildred stopped screaming and turned to look at me. She seemed to wake up out of a kind of daze, her eyes focused, and she shrugged. "Oh, don't worry," she said. "This happens all the time. We'll talk about it in the morning." And she turned over and went to sleep.

Mildred has spent much of her adult life going to psychics, astrologers, palm readers, tea leaf readers, channelers, and crystal readers in her attempts to become more intuitive. She has done everything but dial 1-900-MAKE-ME-INTUITIVE. The next morning, over breakfast, she told me that from the age of twelve she had suffered nightly terrors between 10:00 and 11:00 P.M. She would go into a dreamlike state somewhere between sleep and waking and find that a group of people or objects on her ceiling would appear out of nowhere with the intent to injure her in some way. Not uncommonly, she'd even get up during one of these dreams and take the paintings off her bedroom wall and put them under the bed so they wouldn't harm her. In the morning, her husband would ask her what in the world she was thinking. He even tried to get her to go to a sleep specialist to get rid of her problem. Mildred resisted because, being a physician herself, she knew that modern medicine would not offer her an interpretation of this experience, but merely try to medicate it away. I suggested to Mildred that her night terrors were actually part of her intuition network and pointed out to her that the area in the brain that deals with intuition is also associated with fear, paranoia, and dreamlike states. It seemed to me that Mildred was having exactly the types of visitations that others go to intuition workshops to try to make happen in their lives, but Mildred was terrified of them and had been spending a lifetime *trying to get rid of them!* Meanwhile she tried fervently to import intuition, to get in touch with her soul, through other people.

An even more remarkable aspect of Mildred's intuition became clear to me a short while later. She took part in a heart stress study in which she was required to wear a Holter monitor to measure the rhythm and rate of her heart for twenty-four hours. She did it dutifully and sent the monitor off for analysis. A week or so later, when she received the printout of her heart rate from the institute conducting the study, she asked me to look at it and explain it to her, since she's not good at interpreting graphs. I couldn't believe my eyes. There's a history of heart disease in Mildred's family, and sure enough, I noticed arrhythmic peaks on the graph. But the amazing thing was when they occurred: at around 11:00 P.M. and again at around 4:00 A.M. When did she have her visitations? At around 11:00 P.M. (Four in the morning is another significant hour for intuition.) The gaps in her heartbeat allowed the visitations to slip in.

I stared and stared at that graph. I was so excited I was shaking. All at once I had an incredible sense of how we get intuition: *We get it through the holes in the soul—through our physical problems.* In fact, the soul speaks to the human consciousness through sensations of health or disease in the body. Since learning that her night terrors didn't have to be terrifying, Mildred has changed how she deals with them. Now, instead of resisting them, she is paying attention to the information they give her. During one recent episode, for example, she told me that she felt that the presences in the room were filming certain aspects of her life for a bigger project. She was also aware that her house was an experiment. This made sense. Mildred had recently completed a film project and was looking for further work in this medium. In addition, she was reevaluating and healing her relationships, including those with her children and husband. These relationships were represented by her house.

Successful as we may be at blocking intuition most of the time, there are times when the message seeps through, sneaks through our defenses and our reluctance to hear it. Illness, disease, and other troubles create a hole through which we get information in spite of ourselves. The information comes through these apertures. I'm narcoleptic, and my information comes through leaky electrical wiring in my brain. Mildred's came through leaks, or holes, in her heart. If you have diverticulitis, it may come through your bowel. If you have acne, it may come through your skin. But you don't have to lose a leg or have an accident to gain intuition. Even if you're generally healthy, intuition may be entering through any change in the natural rhythm of your body—the menstrual cycle, for example, or changes in sleep—or through any subtle change in organ function. Or it may be speaking to you through your dreams. This is the wiring of intuition.

This realization was a turning point for me as a physician. If you are a doctor, patients come to you with disease or symptoms of disease and ask you to eliminate these in order to make them whole again. They want you to plug up their holes. Yet it's through these holes that information about other matters in their lives—about experiences, emotions, or patterns of being that may be causing them anguish or unhappiness—is making itself known. Only by listening to this information about what's good and bad, strong and weak, right and wrong in their lives can we help our patients achieve true health and real peace. And patients need to listen carefully to each emotional or physical symptom, allow themselves to receive its message, and then act on that information. I began to wonder about my role as a physician, about caring for people's symptoms without helping them listen to the intuitive messages behind their diseases, without teaching them to understand the language of their souls.

Let me give you an example. One day, a female masters swimmer in her late thirties came into the Boston hospital where I worked. She was experiencing debilitating panic attacks. These came over her especially when she had to board a plane, which was often, since she traveled all over the world to athletic meets. She was very concerned about these attacks because they were restricting her willingness to travel and she feared they would affect her ability to compete in her sport. I sat there listening to her and thinking that this was precisely why she was having the attacks. Her bodily consciousness was telling her mental consciousness to get out of what she was doing, to make some changes in her life, to connect with something beyond her immediate life experience.

The doctors at the clinic ran some tests on her. Her heart checked out fine, but her hormone tests were another story. They indicated severe estrogen and testosterone depletion and hormone changes due to the fact that her body reserves were shot. She was completely lacking in androgens, an important sex steroid, and her hormone balance was totally out of kilter. In fact, this commonly happens in female athletes. This physical evidence told us, plain as day, that this woman was doing much too much competing. It told me she should slow down, but she didn't want to hear this. The irony of her situation was intense. One type of medical treatment for her condition was to prescribe androgens. In addition, she could take clonazepam to ease her panic attacks, but taking steroids and drugs is prohibited by the rules of the athletic world and would knock her out of competition in a sport over which she had reigned for years. In other words, the things that could help her physical symptoms were the very things that would remove her from the area of life that was most important to her.

I was convinced that her soul was speaking to her in a metaphor for her life. It was telling her that running from whatever she was trying to avoid wasn't working for her anymore. I wish I could say she got the message. Instead, she opted to try a nutritional treatment in the hope that this would balance her hormones. As far as I was concerned, even the best treatment in the world for her physical symptoms would have been little better than spackling up holes. Her intuition, I was convinced, would find another hole to worm its way through to her.

If we merely treat what ails us symptomatically, we'll only get into more trouble down the road. When symptoms go away, we forget about them and stop worrying about what might have caused them. Lounging on a beach in the Bahamas, you don't get those migraine headaches anymore, so you think, Well, problem solved. But as soon as you get back to the office, the hammer descends, twice as painfully and twice as often as before. That's what happened to me when I was hit by the truck.

That this happens is understandable. Very often we don't want to listen to our intuition because, like the athlete, we don't really want to hear what it's telling us. Through intuition, your brain is allowing you to hear things you don't want to hear. Intuition is the ability to gain access to thoughts that are not usually present in your external environment, knowledge that you don't usually *want* to see or act on but which is essential to your well-being. Ignoring what your intuition is trying to tell you through your body is like ignoring a rattle that occurs in your car at low speed. You may just drive faster, roll up the windows, and think the rattle has disappeared, but it is still there. And one day the engine will fall out.

THE INTUITION NETWORK

So how do we learn to hear our intuition, to understand its language and put it to use? We tune in to the intuition network.

This is that personal internal transmitter I've talked about. It's actually bigger than the Walkman in your pocket; it's your entire body, including your brain and every other organ, any one or combination of which may be the foundation for the unique manner and language in which your intuition speaks to you.

The brain is the chief interpreter and processor of intuition. The right hemisphere, which controls the nonverbal, image-bound processes, provides the gestalt, the general overall sense that is the initial spark of intuition; the left hemisphere, where the verbal and communications skills reside, fills in the details and gives intuition its verbal form. The temporal lobe, meanwhile, is a major channel of the intuition network for visual and auditory information as well as for memories and dreams.

Dreams are another part of the intuitive guidance system. Information about the organs in the body, about how they are processing health or disease, comes up in our dreams. The language of intuition has its own dream symbols; while some are universal, many are unique to each individual, and we all have to learn to interpret the unique language of intuition speaking to us through our dreams.

Memories and their attendant emotions are stored and encoded both in our *brains* and in our *bodies.* The wisdom we've gained and the traumas we've experienced are processed verbally in the brain. They're also processed nonverbally, often through stress, in the body. The brain communicates constantly with other organs, and they in turn communicate with us. The uterus, for instance, talks to you through the menstrual cycle, your stomach may communicate with you when you experience butterflies onstage, and your skin may have talked to you when you were under the stress of puberty. When intuition comes, the brain releases endorphins and neuropeptides to all the nerves, the blood vessels, the heart, the lungs, the gastrointestinal tract, and all the other organs. And a systematic organization of specific emotions and memories in the brain is being transferred to specific organs in the body. This is all part of our intuition network, our intuitive guidance system.

We all have a brain: a right hemisphere, left hemisphere, and temporal lobe. We all have dreams. We all have a body. We all have memories. An intuition network is in place inside every one of us.

If we listen to it, we can build a happier, healthier life. As wonderful a prospect as this is, I know it's also frightening to many people. Changing our perspective, the way we view ourselves and express ourselves, is far more terrifying than just sticking with the status quo, even if it makes us feel unfulfilled, unhappy—or ill.

I see the truth of this all the time, in large ways and small. I tried to read a friend's tarot cards for fun one weekend. On a Friday night, I laid them out, and the ace of pentacles, reversed, came up. The ace means a new beginning, pentacles mean money, and the upside-down direction of the card indicated that something was definitely in the offing that Claudia needed to change in her financial life. The card's appearance was a little alarming, since it can often signify bad luck in the financial area. My friend Claudia, however, reached over, folded up the deck, and said, "I'm tired. This isn't right. I don't want a reading right now." I was a little worried that she didn't want to focus on this hint of trouble, but I didn't push it. The next day was beautiful and sunny, and we got together to walk to the harbor. I pulled out the cards again, and as I laid them out, sure enough, the ace of pentacles, reversed, showed up again. Claudia just shook her head and said, "Maybe I'm not supposed to know about this," as she again closed the deck.

"Don't you want to figure it out?" I pushed her. "Maybe you can avoid some problem if you just sit with it a minute." Claudia shrugged and changed the subject. She really didn't want to know, the way most of us don't want to face and deal with difficulties that could affect our lives adversely. Yet, listening to our symptoms and heeding the signs that are given us offers us the opportunity to change what is wrong in our lives, to prepare for problems or adapt to them, to reach for something better, to influence outcomes.

The next day, Claudia went to her ATM to make a withdrawal. To her dismay, her account was overdrawn by a couple thousand dollars. As the machine spit back her card and flashed "Transaction denied" on the screen, she realized that the ace of pentacles, reversed, had been telling her of the need to look more carefully at her finances. Specifically, she needed to address issues she had with her money manager.

Today Claudia consults the tarot before she makes any business transactions or deals. She knows the cards aren't the source of her intuition, but they act as a helpful imagery channel for where she needs to give attention to her life. The cards are the jumper cables for her own intuitive engine.

That is the real power of intuition—that it gives us, at every moment, the capacity to change our destiny.

TWO

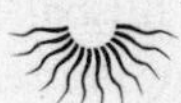

When the Gods Come Calling: The Intuition of Dreams

The Egyptians, the Greeks, and the people of other ancient cultures believed that the gods visited them in their dreams while they slept. They believed these divine visitors brought them solutions to the problems they faced during waking hours.[1] Centuries later, Sigmund Freud said he believed that dreams come from our own unconscious, expressing while we sleep wishes that we can't acknowledge or accept while awake.[2]

The ancients and Freud weren't actually that far apart in their thinking about dreams. They were both saying that dreams are a primary source of intuition, a channel through which crucial guidance is broadcast and vital images televised to us about matters that are critical to our lives.

Everyone sleeps and everyone dreams. Even if you think you don't dream, the truth is that you do. The key to getting intuitive information from dreams is to remember your dreams. You must also be willing to listen to and accept the information they broadcast to you.

One day a couple of years ago a nurse I worked with approached me a little hesitantly. I could see she wanted to talk to me about something that was troubling her, but she seemed uncertain about broaching the subject. Finally she said in a low voice, "You work in intuition, don't you?" Yes, I said, and she asked if she could run a dream she'd been having by me.

We sat down in the nurses' station, and she told me about a dream that had come to her several nights in a row but with a different ending each time. On the first night she found herself in a boat on a river, moving away from a burning house, heading for some new destination in her life. But she felt a strong pull to go back for her children, who were still in the house with her husband. On the second night she was running through the fire in the house searching desperately for her children so that she could take them with her to this new place she was heading.

"Then, on the third night," she said slowly, emphasizing each word as though she thought I wouldn't believe her, "honest to God, the fire was like a wall between me and my kids on one side, and my husband on the other." She looked at me expectantly. "What do you make of that dream?" she asked. "What does it mean?"

It was amazing how strongly this nurse's intuition was speaking to her through her dreams. To me, the dreams were vivid manifestations of problems in her marriage and her relationship with her husband. Of course, I couldn't tell her this outright. When I work with people intuitively, all I can do is to nudge or guide them in the direction of an understanding of what their own intuition is telling them. Not surprisingly, though, the nurse was unable—or rather, unwilling—to hear the message, just as most people are.

"Do you have any problems or issues with your—" I began, but before I could finish, she blurted, "Husband?" I nodded, and surprisingly, she seemed taken aback and even a little defiant, even though she had anticipated what I was going to say. She admitted she had begun to think that she might need to separate from her husband. But the dreams, she insisted, didn't have anything to do with that. In fact, she didn't want to discuss them in terms of her relationship with her husband at all. She knew that the dreams carried some sort of message for her, but *that* message made her uncomfortable. It wasn't the one she wanted to hear.

She thought perhaps the message of the dreams was that she should change careers. We talked about this on and off for several months, with me trying only to guide her toward the real issue, but she never changed her mind.

Eventually our ways parted. Over the next year, instead of pursuing her problems with her husband, the nurse went on a vocational search, trying on different jobs one at a time, pursuing various possible futures. At the end of a year she called me to report that she had realized, through her career search, that she wasn't growing with her husband, and that she needed to change her marital situation. She had filed for divorce.

The nurse's dreams had been very strongly suggesting this possible future outcome to her much earlier. While she slept, her intuition had created a series of scenarios for her to consider as solutions to her marital problems and her relationship with her husband. She could leave on her own, one dream said. But then she would miss her children, the second dream told her. She could take the kids and go, the third dream revealed, and end the marriage—which, of course, is what she eventually did. But not without resisting pretty hard at first, because her intuition was telling her something it wasn't easy for her to hear, something she preferred not to face squarely. So she busied herself in her waking life trying to create her own different solutions and ignoring the intuition of her dreams. Fortunately for her, she finally did make the changes her intuition had been signaling to her all along. Despite the divorce, her story had a happy ending, because by taking the action her intuitive guidance system had been urging and making the necessary changes in her life, she may well have avoided the risk that her unresolved problems could take root in her physical body, causing illness and disease. Her story is a clear illustration of the way intuition comes to many people. You don't have to lose a leg or develop a heart arrhythmia for intuition to reach you with its messages. Lots of us get intuition through our dreams, a primary link in the intuition network.

PATHS TO THE FUTURE

Researchers and scientists through the decades have posited that dreams are a problem-solving mechanism of the brain.[1,3] While we sleep, our minds, through dreams, try out various solutions to the problems of our lives. We try on each solution in the dream state the way we try on shoes in front of a mirror. "How does this fit?" our dreams ask. "Will this work for me? What will happen if I do this?" Dreams let us know all the potential choices we have in our lives. With their different endings, they tell us the result or outcome of each solution we might try. That was what was happening in the series of dreams my nurse colleague had. Her dreams were like practice runs her brain was conducting to find a way out of the problem that was being intuitively revealed to her.

It seems paradoxical, but more of your brain is awake when you're asleep than when you are in a conscious state.[1,3] When you're awake, only about 10 percent of your brain is firing at any given time. But when you're asleep, the whole thing lights up. Everything starts firing madly. If you think of the brain as a computer, it's as though the RAM, the memory capacity, were suddenly quadrupled. At the same time, your brain's activity is free from interference from people in the outer world telling you you're wrong and from your inner self telling you that something is impossible.

When we're awake, the brain's frontal lobe, which houses critical thinking and judgment, is always telling us that most things we want to do are ridiculous, so why bother. The frontal lobe is our grand censor. But when we're asleep, it's suppressed.[1] Remember that when Elvis Presley appeared on Ed Sullivan's program, the network censors made sure we could see him only from the neck up on the television screen. But of course most of Elvis's mass appeal was from the waist down. Those network censors were like frontal lobes, censoring Elvis's potential. But imagine now that those censors suddenly got bounced, lost their jobs, and we were able to see Elvis unleash his potential and do his act in all its uninhibited, full-bodied glory!

That's what happens when we're dreaming. When you're asleep, the frontal lobe can't stop you from dreaming about doing things you'd be completely inhibited from doing during the day. Say you have a crush on someone, a great-looking person you have a nodding acquaintance with at work. During the day you may toy with the idea of approaching this person and striking up a closer relationship, but your frontal lobe instantly clamps down on these thoughts and nips them in the bud. "No," it makes you say, "it would never work. He would never like me. He's a surgeon and I'm a psychiatrist; surgeons think psychiatrists are weird," and so on, through the whole litany of inhibitive behavior you learned growing up. When you're awake, the superego is in control, telling you to be careful, warning you not to make an idiot of yourself. But at night the brain finally turns off that noisy naysayer. In your dreams one night you see yourself going up to the good-looking object of your fantasies and saying, "How'd you like to go downstairs to the cafeteria and have one of those lovely hot dogs they serve?" (Freud would have had a field day with this symbolism.) The frontal lobe is disconnected, so you don't hear your mother saying, "No, no, he's not the right one for you." If you're a man, you're not reminded of that girl in high school who broke a date with you, saying she was sick, and then went out with the captain of the football team instead. Feeling encouraged by the progress you made in the first dream, you might go a little further the next night, inviting your crush out for a good dinner in a nice restaurant. Encouraged by the outcome of that dream, you make dinner at your place the next night. And the night after that…?

Even while your dreams are creating various scenarios for you to pursue, your sleeping body is also trying out various ways to achieve your heart's desires. Although most actual movement is suppressed during sleep, the body's neurons are still firing, often in ways that correspond to the content of your dreams.[1,4] So when you walk up to your dream person in your dream, the neurons in your legs are actually firing and laying down a real neuronal pathway in your brain that you might be able to follow in the waking future.

All of this has been confirmed by physical experiments performed by scientists trying to find out why we dream and how dreams function in our lives. One study measured and mapped the flow of blood to various areas of the brain during the REM, or rapid eye movement, phase of sleep, which is when most dreaming takes place.[5] Fascinatingly, it showed that dreams were associated with increased neuronal activity in very distinct areas of the brain. The areas that lit up during dream periods were those having to do with *emotionally charged memory,* both in the *brain* and in the *body;* intense *emotional states; body sensations;* and inwardly directed attention. Meanwhile, those areas having to do with being judgmental and exercising criticism were shut down. We call this the brain-stapling technique, when the frontal lobe is literally disconnected from the rest of the brain so that it can't prevent us from going after our hearts' desire. This study concluded that REM sleep is important for processing emotional components of *memory,* including *body memory.* Emotionally charged memories, both in the brain and in the body, are an integral part of the intuition network. When you dream, certain areas of your body can communicate information to you about the past or the present. They send you emotional information about what needs to be changed in your life. In fact, Freud agreed with these brain researchers when he said: "Dreams are a conversation with oneself, a dialogue of symbols and images that takes place between the unconscious and conscious levels of the mind."[2] This theory has always been controversial, but based on their results, the authors of the study wryly concluded that "Freud must be smiling."[5]

During sleep, in short, our minds have access to powers that we don't usually recognize when we're awake, powers of greater thought and creative ability. While we dream, we have potentially unlimited access to intuition. Dreams provide a way of obtaining information on what's going on in our lives, our emotions, and, significantly, our bodies. And if we listen to them, they give us the opportunity to change whatever is causing us conflicts, problems, or illness and work to heal it.

DREAMS AND THE BODY

In ancient Greece, the god of medicine was named Asclepius, or Aesculapius.[1,6] The ill and diseased traveled to his temples in search of treatment and cure. There some patients would be led by Asclepius's priests through a variety of ceremonies and undergo ritual purification. Afterward, in a state of psychic excitement, they would lie down to sleep, as the priests and acolytes covered them with the skin of a sacrificed ram. It was believed that as they fell asleep, the remedies for their illnesses would come to them in their dreams. The priests would then interpret these therapeutic dreams.

Other patients would consult the temple's dream oracles, who were something like early medical intuitives. The oracles would enter a dreamlike or trancelike state (which modern medicine would likely diagnose as a form of seizure or sleep disorder) to "incubate" the patients' dreams and receive information about the patients' emotional lives, their illnesses, and possible remedies for them.

It's no surprise that the Greeks sought information about illness and health in dreams. Aristotle, the great philosopher, was one of the first to maintain that the beginnings of illness could in fact be felt in dreams well before actual symptoms appeared in conscious time.[1] That rattle in your bodily engine would be clanking loudly in your dream ears while still undetectable to your waking ears.

This belief about the relationship between dreams and the body has been widely held by men of science and medicine for centuries. In the Middle Ages, a physician named Artemidorus[7] described the case of a man who dreamed on two separate occasions that his ear was being beaten with a stone and who soon developed a serious ear inflammation on the very side he had dreamed about. "Dreams," Artemidorus said, "are like magnifying glasses that can detect small beginnings of our physical illnesses." This is a wonderful description. It reminds me of the scenes in *Alice in Wonderland* where she grows gigantic after eating a mushroom labeled EAT ME and then shrinks down into a tiny little thing when she drinks out of the bottle marked DRINK ME. Her world is distorted, either very big or very small. Everything is exaggerated and surrounded by fear and foreboding. This is often the way things appear in our dreams. In order for the problems being telegraphed in dreams to make their way through to our consciousness, they have to be blown up and surrounded by a lot of emotion, like a Steven Spielberg movie. In dreams, our brains, like magnifying glasses, exaggerate the metaphors of our problems so that we will see them, hear them, and pay attention to them.

Body organs are better able to communicate with us at night than when we are awake. Dreams that predict illness, or prodromal dreams, were discussed by scientists as early as the mid-nineteenth century.[8] The German philosopher Arthur Schopenhauer described the organs' connection to specific nerves (the sympathetic nervous system), which in turn are connected to the brain.[9] At night, with the effects of the external world muted, the messages from the organs through the nervous system more readily reach the brain, he said. Think of this again in terms of our being like radio or television receivers. Like cable television, we have dozens of channels into what's going on in our world; we might have a channel to finances, one to our family, one to work, one to worries, and so on. During the day, as we rush around, we're constantly switching from channel to channel as various issues come up. The channel to our bodies, though, is like educational TV. We tend to skip right over it, not wanting to pause for a lecture or a documentary. At night, though, that becomes the only channel available. You tune in to it in spite of yourself. And the message gets through in the form of dreams, which come from your body. The only way you can filter out this message is by not remembering your dreams. But the dream and the message will still have an impact. Have you ever fallen asleep with a television show on, and then incorporated parts of it into your dreams? This is like the reverse of what happens when you forget dreams when you wake up. You've tuned out the program, but its message has been incorporated into your consciousness anyway. It filters in and affects your conscious moods and your mind, and influences your daily decisions.

In fact, if we don't fully experience, remember, and heed our dreams with all their intuitive information, telling us what needs to be changed in our emotional lives, then we risk the health of our physical bodies. This was dramatically demonstrated by a study of pregnant women and their dreams.[10] Researchers discovered that women who had dreams of anxiety and conflict during their pregnancies tended to have a short and uncomplicated labor of less than ten hours. In contrast, women who didn't have such dreams, whose dreams were normal and peaceful, more often had a long labor lasting more than twenty hours, with complications and sometimes even serious difficulties. Now, wait a minute, you say, isn't that counterintuitive? You'd think that the women with serene dreams would be the calm ones who would sail through labor, wouldn't you? It happens, though, that in pregnancy, a woman's level of the hormone progesterone is higher than normal. This may have a dampening effect on her conscious experience of emotions. So in a normal waking state, a pregnant woman may not fully experience the fear and anxiety that are inevitable in anyone facing childbirth. The researchers theorized that the women with the troubled dreams were releasing their fears and anxieties about childbirth in their sleep, bringing them to the surface, into consciousness, and confronting them.[11] The women who didn't experience fearful dreams, on the other hand, may actually have been repressing or denying their emotions even further. Since they never dealt with their fears, these fears became somaticized, or physically expressed, in various dysfunctions and problems during the anxiously anticipated event of childbirth.

In other words, disturbing dreams function as a sort of pressure release, or safety valve. The pregnant women who were perhaps in a more receptive mood, with all the progesterone coursing through their systems and calming them down, were able to deal effectively with the terror that came to them in their dreams.

Some scientists believe that unless disturbing emotions—emotions surrounding unacknowledged problems or issues in your life—are released into consciousness through your dreams, they stay stored in the body. There they decrease the function of the immune system and increase your susceptibility to any number of diseases, including cancer.[12] Cases have shown that the images in dreams can even symbolize the type of cancer a person may have and indicate its location.[12] In one case, a woman repeatedly dreamed of a dog tearing at her stomach. Two months later she was diagnosed with stomach cancer, and she died three months after that. In another case, a man complained of dreams in which coals were burning his larynx or a medicine man was sticking hypodermic needles into his neck. Ultimately, this man developed thyroid cancer.[13] In another, a woman with breast cancer dreamed that her head was shaven and the word "cancer" was written across the top of it. She reported waking up from that dream certain that her cancer had spread to her brain, even though she had no symptoms indicating that this had happened. Yet soon afterward her self-diagnosis was confirmed.[13] Another patient, with gallbladder cancer, dreamed that his entire body exploded and shattered into a thousand pieces. It was soon discovered that his cancer had spread throughout his body.

Cases of strange and prophetic dreams preceding the onset of physical illness abound in the scientific literature. One man, a heavy smoker, had dreams of being back in the army and taking cover during a military action in the hollow of a large tree. As he huddled there, bullets from a machine gun tore into the tree and cut through the lower left side of his chest. Later, he was found to have a small tumor in the lower lobe of his left lung, right where the bullet had hit him.[14]

Other cases include that of a young woman who dreamed her stomach burst open after she ate pizza. She ended up with an ulcer.[15] Another woman dreamed she was lying on the ground when the earth began to give way and form a cavity beneath her, in which she began to suffocate. Two months later she developed tuberculosis, which is characterized by cavitylike lesions in the lungs and difficulty breathing.[16] Yet another woman was troubled for more than a year by dreams that someone was holding a lighted candle to her left leg.[17] She thought she had a mental illness and sought out psychiatric help. The psychiatrist listened to her repeatedly describe this dream and sent her to a doctor, who ordered an X-ray of the woman's leg. It revealed that she had osteomyelitis, a severe inflammation and infection of the bone, in her left leg.

How can dreams like this be possible? Studies show that through dreams, the internal organs give us news either that they're not working well or that they're working just fine. Scientists claim that during sleep the cells of the body send signals by way of chemicals and other codes to a part of the unconscious mind.[14] These signals then provide the basis of dreams warning of impending disease. But there's more to it than that.

Scientific evidence shows that the physiology of the body actually changes while we dream. During sleep, our organs behave in the same way they do when we are awake and under stress. For some people, dreaming can be stressful. Some people undergo marked changes in pulse, blood pressure, and respiration.[18] Adrenal steroids, which are a measure of stress, have been shown to rise during the dream period in these people.[19] This isn't surprising, because during the dream state we're actually reliving stressful events and emotions in our lives and trying to find solutions for them. In other words, we're doing some unconscious and intuitive problem-solving.

Most interestingly, the body changes that take place during dreams have been found to be in exactly the organ systems that are most stressed while we're awake and active. One scientific study looked at a group of people, some of whom had ulcers and some of whom did not. Tubes were inserted through their mouths down into their stomachs, and they were observed while they slept. Guess when the ulcer patients released the most stomach acid? During dream periods.[20] The non-ulcer patients, meanwhile, didn't show any increase in stomach acid. In their dreams, the ulcer patients may have been reliving their problems and trying to find solutions to them. And as they experienced their problems in the dream state, they activated the same organs that were affected by stress during the day.[20]

To put it simply: if you don't pay attention to your emotional life and you can't hear your intuition speaking to you about it in your dreams as it does when you're awake, you run the risk of your emotional problems showing up symbolically and symptomatically in your body. They may make themselves known in your dreams before they become apparent in your waking life.

An interesting case illustrates this very phenomenon. A man dreamed about a rat gnawing at the right upper side of his abdomen. During the day, he had some acute indigestion and a sour stomach, but he felt better when he followed the dietary recommendations he'd read about in a health magazine. A little while later, however, he again dreamed that a rat was gnawing at his stomach. After this second dream, he noticed a deep pressure and tenderness in the very area where the rat attacked him. He went to the doctor and, sure enough, was found to have an intestinal ulcer in that very spot.[18]

It's easy to imagine a man like this experiencing a certain kind of stress during the day. He might have been in an intensely competitive work situation, or maybe he was upset about problems on the job. It's possible he was having right upper abdominal pain during the day but was ignoring it because he needed to stay competitive and productive at work. But his brain kept the pain just below the surface of his consciousness. In fact, he felt there was nothing wrong with him whatsoever, and he was able to work quite efficiently. But at night he could not repress the truth. He had dreams of what was going on with him at work, and all of a sudden, during his dreams, he felt a rat gnawing at his stomach.

When we dream at night, we gain access to emotional wishes we need to attend to. We also gain access to how these emotions are expressed through symptoms in specific organs. The organs that will eventually develop illness when we're awake are the ones that are most susceptible to stress while we dream. In fact, some scientists believe that you can predict an illness based on which organs are activated during the dream state. They believe that the symptoms of diseases such as ulcers, ulcerative colitis, asthma, high blood pressure, thyroid disease, and rheumatoid arthritis will be expressed symbolically in dreams at night much sooner than any symptoms will become apparent in the waking state.[21]

So in other words, if one of your organs is susceptible to specific stress or specific emotions, your body may indicate that weakness before it becomes a physical problem through symbols in the dream state. If you don't pay attention to the emotional issues that persist in your dreams, and if you're not aware of the symptoms that are symbolized in your dreams, illness can occur in your body in that organ. In fact, the dream period itself is like a mini-illness, because during that time you can activate the organs involved and have a sort of dress rehearsal of illness before your illness actually occurs.

What about a person without an illness? you ask. Everyone has a target system, a system likely to be affected by specific emotional issues, a weak link in the chain. Even if you're not ill, that organ or link will show the greatest activity during the dream state. My nurse friend with the recurring dream probably had a weak link somewhere that was undergoing stress during her dream experience. If she hadn't acted on the intuition coming to her about her emotional life, she might soon have noticed some sort of metaphorical rattle in her dreams coming from that organ or body system. And if she had ignored that, she could have ended up dropping a transmission.

Dreams are part of our intuitive guidance system, which knows what emotional issues in our lives need to be addressed. The body symptoms we exhibit in our dreams all have a correlative in our emotional lives. If we don't address the issues in our emotional lives and make the requisite changes in our lives, these issues might set the scene for disease in specific organs of our bodies. Dreams are like open windows through which we can focus and see images of our emotions, of what our intuition is trying to tell us, without the gauzy curtains and distractions of life during the day getting in the way. Dreams send us images we can work with to make changes in our lives before it's too late.

Actual cases have shown that once the physical and emotional trouble signaled in some of these dreams goes away, the dreams disappear. That was the case with the man with the rat eating his stomach. After surgery for his ulcer, he reported never having the dream again. When I first started having problems with my spine, I had dreams that I was walking down the stairs in my house and all of the steps were giving way beneath me. Workmen needed to nail every board into place, fusing that staircase together to keep it from collapsing. When I had spinal surgery, that's exactly what it was like: several vertebrae were fused together to keep my spine from collapsing onto my spinal cord. After the vertebrae had successfully fused, I never had that dream about the crumbling staircase again, thanks not only to the surgery but also, as you'll see, to important decisions I made affecting my emotional situation. Because I had changed something that needed attention in my life, my intuition didn't need to lecture me about it anymore.

DREAM SYMBOLS AND THE LANGUAGE OF DREAMS

Our dreams often seem to be a morass of nonsensical images. How do we make sense of the bizarre happenings that take place while our bodies are asleep but our brains are working overtime and intuition is feeding us vital information about things we've been ignoring in our lives? How do we learn to understand the language of intuition as it speaks to us through our dreams?

Through the ages, various symbols and images have been accepted as representing specific objects and specific states of being, including body states, in dreams. Long before Freud, for instance, it was thought that a house in dreams represented the body.[2] Separate organs are frequently regarded as individual rooms in that house. An entrance hall, for instance, might be the mouth. A staircase, as in my dreams, might be the spine, or it could be the throat or esophagus. Ceilings covered with spiders are often believed to be a metaphor for headaches and migraines, while a blazing furnace or a bellows has to do with asthma or respiratory problems. Women, during ovulation, frequently dream of boulders smashing through windows (eggs being released by the ovaries) or about being in a house where the walls are coming down (the uterine lining sloughing off during menstruation).[8] Then there is the ever-popular upright column or pillar, which in best Freudian tradition is of course believed to represent the male phallus.[2]

Here are some of the most frequently appearing dream symbols and the body organ or the physical state they are thought to represent:

Symbol	Body Organ/State
House	Whole body
Rooms or parts of house	Separate organs
Entrance hall	Mouth
Staircase	Throat, esophagus, or spine
Ceiling with spiders	Headache
Blazing furnace	Lungs, breathing
Hollow boxes or basket	Heart
Round bag-shaped object	Bladder
Upright stick or pillar	Male genitals

More than two thousand years ago the Chinese observed that certain types of dreams were related to health or disease in certain organs or organ systems. Dreams of terror, for example, seemed to be related to problems in the heart. Dreams of suffocation denoted the lungs, while dreams of water obviously indicated the kidneys or bladder. Many of these observations are still accepted today.[22]

Affected Organ	Dream Content
Heart	Terror. Anxiety at the moment of waking. Usually short dreams involving horrible death. Fire, blazes.
Lungs	Dreams of suffocation, crowding, and fleeing. White objects. Cruel killing of people. Objects made of metal.
Digestive tract	Enjoyment or disgust of food. Lack or abundance of food or drink. Putting up buildings or walls. Hills, marshes.
Kidneys and bladder	Ships, boats, drowning people; walks and excursions; lying in water; back and waist split apart.

As tempting as it would be to say that all dreams can be deciphered on the basis of these established symbols, they're at best only guidelines to an understanding of the intuition of our dreams. They don't hold true across the board. Each of us has unusual experiences that we may interpret symbolically in different ways. For example, my father was a carpenter, so a lot of my dreams have to do with houses and construction equipment. Women have more dreams about houses than men do. Snakes in women's dreams are supposed to symbolize the erotic, but if a depressed person dreams about a snake, it could represent a rope or a noose. For someone else, a snake might represent a road or a path that person might need to follow.

In the past, Freudian interpretations of symbols have dominated our approach to dreams. That's like putting on Freud's eyeglasses and then looking at life through his life experiences, his brain and his body. But his experiences aren't necessarily valid for others, and sometimes something you see in your dreams may be exactly what it appears to be, nothing more and nothing less, with no hidden meaning. This isn't what Freud thought at first. He once famously wrote, in discussing the issue of a pipe appearing in a patient's dreams: "This is not a pipe."[2] He frequently saw penises as prominent themes in dreams, represented by various symbols. Well, I don't know about you, but while male genitalia show up in my dreams occasionally, they hardly do so consistently. I guess Freud eventually got the point, because later he modified his theory and admitted that "sometimes a cigar is just a cigar."

Moreover, modern life has introduced elements and objects into dreams that didn't exist in Freud's day, much less two thousand years ago in China. We have to find a new understanding for these symbols in our dreams. Usually, their meaning may be very specific to the person who's dreaming them. I began having problems with my neck in a period when I was trying to do two things at once—working on my Ph.D. and going to medical school at the same time. In addition, I would ride my bike twenty to forty miles a day and run seven miles a night. You could say I was running around in overdrive. During this same period I'd have dreams about contact lenses. I would dream that my soft lenses swelled up to twice their size, making them really hard to insert into my eyes. I'd always manage to get them in but only with a lot of difficulty. During the day, I had trouble balancing the two different doctorates and all the exercise, but I always managed to pull it off. Since I'd studied a lot of psychiatry and was interested in the brain, I tried to apply all the Freudian stuff about imagery and came up with the idea that the contact lens dream had to do with my changing self-image as my career was changing.

I struggled to finish my Ph.D. and also to run around the hospital in med school. Then I woke up one morning to realize that I couldn't feel parts of my hands and had trouble moving some of my fingers. An MRI showed that two disks in my spine had fallen out of alignment in my neck. The disks were pressing on my spinal cord, causing the numbness and partial paralysis. To avoid surgery, I opted for conservative treatment, which included osteopathic manipulation, acupuncture, and psychotherapy. I also decided not to pursue a neurology residency, as I'd been planning. (As if I hadn't had enough going on already!) The disks diminished in size and began to retreat into their proper location and alignment in the spine. And presto! The contact lens dreams stopped.

Of course, at that point, I hadn't made the connection between the dreams, the disks, and the emotional pattern in my life that needed to be corrected. I moved to Maine and began a psychiatric residency. Three years later, though, I found I was bored and began to look around for more challenge and stimulation. I began to think about trying to do two things at once again, and planned a double residency in both neurology and psychiatry. I made plans to move to Chicago to do this. And my neck pain and hand numbness started up again.

So did the contact lens dreams. This time the contacts were so big it was impossible to put them in. Then one day I sneezed, and two additional disks slipped out of my spine. I had to be rushed to the hospital because I couldn't move my left hand and was beginning to lose sensation in my legs. The enlarged disks in my neck were sitting on the spinal cord and causing the paralysis. This time I had to have surgery.

The day after the operation, I had my last contact lens dream. In the dream I was just about to put in a lens when it disintegrated in my hand, shattering into a million pieces. I woke up in a cold sweat, with the strong feeling that the dream was significant. But I still didn't get it. I thought I needed new contact lenses! I even had a friend make an appointment with the ophthalmologist. A few weeks later I got the report from my operation. And suddenly I did get it. The report stated that several pieces of disk fragments had been removed from the surface of my spinal cord. In other words, one of my disks had shattered. And what shape are spinal disks? Approximately the same convex shape as a contact lens.

Now I understood the language of the image in my dream. And I understood that my intuition had been warning me, through my dreams and through my body memories, the memories of back pain associated with difficult periods in my life, that trying to do two different, conflicting things at once might not be a good idea. In fact, it could make something in me snap. What had been going on with me?

My head got an idea that it wanted to do something—pursue neurology and move to Chicago—while my heart and the rest of my body had an opposing view: stay in Maine and do psychiatry. So my head was going one way, to Chicago, and my body was going the other way, to Maine. And what was the area in between that snapped? My neck.

My dreams were telling me that unless I changed what I was doing and why I was doing it, I was going to cause myself significant harm. I now have one disk left. That disk is at T3-T4, right near my heart. If that disk blows, I will literally have to have a thoracic surgeon and a neurosurgeon take me to the operating room, break open my ribs, push open the lungs, and pull out the disks with a pair of tweezers. So it's imperative that I understand now what my dreams have told me (and when I haven't listened to them, what my body has screamed at me): that I must choose my heart's and my body's path to stay alive, instead of running back and forth between my head and my heart.

Neither the ancient Chinese nor Freud, of course, had ever heard of contact lenses, so their lists of symbols weren't helpful in interpreting my dreams. Moreover, somebody else might have used a different dream image to represent the spinal disks. However, anyone can relate to something like my lens dreams. All of us have had dreams that warned us, that have made us wake up in a cold sweat, wondering what they meant. We knew they were important, but we didn't understand their images. Only, perhaps, after telling a friend, who helped us to understand, did we begin to get insights into what emotional situations we really needed to attend to and what parts of our bodies would be in peril if we failed to confront those emotional situations.

A lot of the language of intuition in dreams is unique to each individual. That means that all of us have to learn to decipher the ways in which our dreams communicate to us specifically what we need to change in our emotional lives and what parts of our bodies may be in trouble if we don't act.

Scientific evidence from a fascinating study in the 1930s supports the idea that dream imagery is related to our body functions and body states. On the West Coast, a researcher would ask women to describe their dreams.[23] On the basis of the dream content, the researcher would predict what phase of the menstrual cycle each woman was in. The doctor would figure out what the woman's ovaries and uterus were doing based solely on the content of her dreams. The women's Pap smears were then sent to a physician on the East Coast, who would examine the smears and determine exactly what phase of the menstrual cycle each woman was in. In nearly every case, the prediction and the actual determination matched. Before ovulation, the women's dreams involved activities in the outer world. But during menstruation, the dreams were almost uniformly inner-directed—of staying at home, taking care of the house, nesting. The psychological content of the dreams mirrored what was going on in the woman's body.

If you pay attention to the information coming to you through your dreams, you can get direct access to the state of your body. You can also get access to the state of your emotions and what you want to do in your life, often in very powerful ways. I once did a reading for a woman who I intuited had some sort of serious blood deficiency. I didn't know specifically what it was, but I knew it was related in some way to her family and to a sense of loss. I asked her whether she'd had any strange dreams she could describe to me. At first she insisted, as so many people do, that she never had dreams. So I let it go for a while, and we talked about other things. After she had relaxed, I asked again, "Are you sure you don't have dreams? Just tell me anything." I had to ask three more times before she finally admitted that yes, she did have a single recurring dream she wanted to tell me about. She dreamed of flying through the sky and meeting her cousin, who had died of lymphoma, a type of cancer of the white blood cells. In the dream, the woman hugged her cousin as they floated in the sky. And as they embraced, she felt her cousin's lymphoma pass through her own body.

It turned out that this woman had a blood condition of her own that severely depleted her white blood cell count. But the amazing thing was, *she had developed this condition six months after her cousin died!* It was as though she had developed a sympathetic form of her cousin's blood ailment out of the sense of loss she felt over her cousin's death. Her dream told her this in the form of very forceful and dramatic imagery. And once she understood that and accepted it, she was able to begin to work with the intuitive knowledge this dream had given her to improve both her physical condition and the quality of her life.

THREE

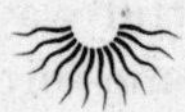

East Side, West Side, All Around the Brain

We think of the brain as the seat of intellect and intelligence. But intellect and intelligence represent only *half* of the brain's potential. Too often we forget about intuition, the other capacity our brains make available to us.

The character of the Scarecrow in *The Wizard of Oz* is typical of most of us in his idea of what constitutes a brain. If he only had a brain, he could calculate Einsteinian equations in his head and rattle off Shakespeare's sonnets word for word. What he is actually expressing in these wishes is a desire for a *left brain,* the part of the brain most important to intellect and rational thought. Because indeed, he already clearly possessed some sort of brainpower, as the Wizard well knew, although the Scarecrow himself didn't recognize it. If he was able to help Dorothy through her trials in the Land of Oz, it was because he had access to intuition, a capacity to which the *right brain* is more attuned.

Intuition is less accessible to some people than to others because most of us, unlike the Scarecrow, are heavily left brain–oriented. We live in a world that emphasizes the intellectual and, like the Scarecrow, overlooks the intuitive.

We rely on the left brain, with its close attunement to the outer world and to logic, to order most of our actions and control our responses to events in our lives. Meanwhile we neglect and discount the other half of the brain, a half that's more inwardly oriented and gives us our greatest capacity for intuition.

In the cineplex of our minds, the Battle of the Brains is an ongoing feature. Yet if we can learn to call off the tug-of-war, come to a meeting of these opposing yet equally indispensable minds, and integrate them with all the other parts of the brain, we can change the production and create the possibility for intuition to play a greater, more positive role in our lives.

Two Brains in One

We all have a single brain in our heads, but it's split into two different personas. The left half, or left hemisphere of the brain, is the seat of logic. It's sequential, rational, linear, fact-based, and focused on the external world. It constantly searches for value in the information it receives. Its strengths are speech and language, and it's usually thought of as the masculine half of the brain. The right hemisphere, on the other hand, is more irrational, receptive, visual, and gestalt-oriented.[1] It's interested in beauty and aesthetics. Its focus is on emotions and the state of the body, and it's generally designated the feminine half. The left brain is out in the world, or yang, and the right brain is more inward, or yin.

Some people are left-hemisphere dominant, and some are right-hemisphere dominant. Women, on the whole, have greater access to the right brain and a greater ability to move back and forth between the two hemispheres simultaneously.[2] Men, as a general rule, are apt to use one hemisphere or the other but not both at once; they tend to stay more in the left hemisphere.[2]

I went to a concert with a friend and her family one evening. Afterward the local symphony conductor gave a short talk about the importance of music education. He spoke fascinatingly about how music appeals to our right-brain emotions and how it helps people appreciate beauty and understand life. He also mentioned research which showed that studying music or learning to play a musical instrument helped people develop better science and math skills. My friend and I were enthralled.

When the conductor finished, the audience gave him a standing ovation. My friend turned to her husband, usually a very sensitive man, who was still sitting and hadn't joined in the ovation. "Wasn't that the most amazing talk?" she said. Her husband shrugged. "I really didn't get much out of it," he said. "I thought it was pretty vague. I mean, what was his point?" My friend was astonished. "I don't believe you!" she cried. "It was wonderful." Her husband shrugged again. "I didn't see that it had much value," he repeated.

And I thought to myself, Wow, a right brain and a left brain are having a discussion right next to me in the bleachers.

My friend's reaction to the music lecture was quintessentially right-brain. (In fact, I'd be willing to bet most women in America feel as if they've had that discussion in the bleachers.) She wanted to loll in the experience and get her husband to join in her feelings: That was so wonderful. Didn't you think what he had to say was beautiful? Her husband, on the other hand, was thoroughly left-brain in his response. He couldn't share in her feelings because he wanted logic, specifics, value, and, most of all, a point: I didn't get it. It was too general. What was he trying to say?

The right hemisphere, considered more free-wheeling and creative, is generally thought to be the half of the brain most receptive to intuition.[3] That's why, given women's better access to the right brain, "women's intuition" makes a lot of sense. Because our culture, like most people in it, is left-hemisphere dominant, it tends to neglect, belittle, or even dismiss intuition. Those who are left-brain dominant tend to think intuition and people who believe in it are a little wacky. On the other hand, those who are right-hemisphere dominant think the left-brainers are a bunch of unimaginative stuffed shirts. Yet when it comes to understanding what intuition has to tell us, one brain is as essential as the other. Just as the brain needs both its halves to function with maximum efficiency, you need both your right brain and your left brain, indeed, your *whole* brain and all of its parts, to tap into your intuition most effectively.

INSIDE THE BRAIN

The central command post of the intuition network—the brain—is a multipart, multilayered, and multifunctional organ. You can picture it in two different ways. First, imagine it as an avocado. The rind is the cortex, an outer layer of cells that function like computers and do all our thinking. The green meat is like wires that connect all the different areas of the brain, helping them talk to each other and share information and make associations. The pit inside is the deep part of the brain. It contains the deep structures, like the unconscious, and the nuclei that help fire up the cortex.

Another way to picture the different areas of the brain is to think of the brain as a car. The hood is the frontal lobe, which controls social comportment. It rules and regulates and inhibits; it tells you don't do that, don't touch that, don't act that way. It's like having a parent, a high school principal, and the nun who runs your Sunday school in your head all at once. At the back of the car, the trunk is the visual part of your brain, a sort of video camera, telling you how to interpret what you see. The fenders are the temporal lobes. Some people have temporal lobes impressive as a 1950s Cadillac's fenders, stretching down the entire side of the brain. These lobes are important for interpreting what we see and hear, for creating memories, and for expressing emotions. The temporal lobes are also vital to intuition.

If you open the hood and look inside the car engine, you'll see that it's got layers of wires interconnecting the car's many parts—its locks, windows, lights, and many other components. The longer you live, the more wires your brain develops to connect its front with its back and the sides with each other. These internal wires make associations between what we see (the back fender), what we hear, and how we feel (the side fenders), and what we should and shouldn't do about all this (the hood).

In addition, the brain is split in two down the middle. The right half of the brain controls the left side of the body, and vice versa. The two halves are connected by a pathway of nerve fibers called the corpus callosum, which is like a series of telephone lines that allow the two hemispheres to communicate with each other. This communication is critical, because each of the hemispheres performs a markedly different and distinct function. While each of these functions has its own value and significance, only when they work together do you get the most out of what your intuition is telling you.

Form and Detail

If I asked you to draw a house, your right brain would take care of the form, the outer shape. It would draw the outline of the building and its roof. The left brain would then take over to fill in the details. It would draw the doors and windows, the doorknobs and window sashes, the chimney, the smoke curling out into the sky, and any other specifics you wanted to include in the picture.

The right brain thinks in terms of gestalt, or overall form.[1] It can take nothing more than the shape or outline of something, and deduce what it is. Look at the following outline of a word. Can you tell what it is?

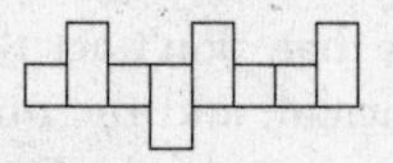

If your right brain is dominant, chances are you've already figured it out. If, however, you're left-hemisphere dominant, like most people, you probably need to have your left brain primed with a clue: It's the name of an animal. Now can you read it?

Once the left hemisphere has been primed, most people can read the word immediately: elephant.

If you were able to decipher the word from just the configuration of the letters, you probably have a right hemisphere the size of Iowa, maybe even Texas. When I perform this experiment in a course or lecture, two people out of two hundred might be able to read the word without priming. What this means is that they were able to make a correct determination on the basis of very few facts. Remember the definition of intuition in Chapter One: the ability to make a correct determination on the basis of inadequate data.

Of course, the right hemisphere isn't always infallible. I remember once driving behind a car on the highway and noticing a bumper sticker in Gothic lettering. I was too far away to read it, but the general outlines, the curves and humps, made me think, Hey, those people go to Holy Cross! Well, when I pulled up alongside them, it turned out the bumper sticker didn't say Holy Cross at all; it said Grateful Dead. Okay, so I was way off. Still, my right brain had taken a guess based on insufficient data. That time it was wrong, but lots of other times it's right. Most right-hemisphere people actually read that way. The right hemisphere forms a guess, an approximation based on the shape of a word; then the left hemisphere fills in the details. Some dyslexics don't read letter by letter; they look at the shape and match it to a word. When people have strokes in their left brain and become aphasic, meaning that the brain's language center has burned out, they can regain some ability to read on the basis of these same general principles. An aphasic could never read words printed in full capital letters because such words have no shape that could be interpreted by the right hemisphere. "ELEPHANT," for example, would look like a solid blob. But they would be able to elicit "elephant" from the outline pattern above. It's much like the pattern recognition we talked about earlier.

The right hemisphere may be able to decipher a form or gestalt, or receive an insight through intuition, but it needs the left hemisphere to add details so that both hemispheres can work together to reach a conclusion. Remember the nurses who "knew" that their patients were in trouble or distress even though they exhibited no obvious signs or symptoms? When challenged by the doctors, the nurses began to cast about for external data to support their intuitive conclusions. Unable to come up with them, they were usually unable to convince the doctors that steps needed to be taken on behalf of the patients. So those nurses lacked two things that are vital to intuition: confidence in what their right hemispheres were intuitively telling them, and the support of the left hemisphere to communicate and explain that information to others. You may get a gut sense in your right hemisphere—"Something's wrong here"—but then you have to start looking around for left-brain facts on which to base a rational argument; otherwise you won't be able to assert the validity of the intuitive information.

The two hemispheres complement each other. The right brain provides the intuition while the left gives it expression and communicates the intuition to the individual and to others. Without input from the left brain, the right brain's messages to you can be gibberish. When I first started doing readings, I remember saying of a person with a liver ailment, "Oh, his liver, it's just spread out in pieces all over the place in his abdomen." It turned out the man had had a liver transplant, and his body was rejecting it. I was getting great right-brain visuals of the problem, but I was basically unable to articulate what I was intuiting. This, of course, was of no use to the client. He needed to understand precisely what was going on and why. Why was his body doing that to him? What aspect of his emotional life was associated with this rejection? Only when I brought my left hemisphere on-line to explain and communicate in a logical and linear way what my intuition was telling me did I become an effective intuitive. A lot of psychics are very good at receiving right-brain intuitive information, but they are then unable to articulate it effectively through the left brain. They talk on and on about what they're feeling, but they lack the ability to analyze or interpret these feelings for the benefit of clients. But right-brain intuition that's unanchored in the words of the left hemisphere is like someone who wants to be the conductor of a symphony without knowing how to read or write music. Intuition without grounding in the world is helpful to no one.

At the same time, being left-hemisphere dominant—logical, analytical, organized—doesn't mean that you aren't or can't be intuitive. We're all intuitive. Even that calculator-wielding engineer who looks as though he wouldn't have an imaginative or intuitive bone in his body could surprise you with his intuitive abilities. Who's more buttoned-down and organized than a business executive, for example? Yet research has shown that the best business executives use more right-hemisphere thinking processes than left.[4] You know all those elaborate decision-making and management models that are constantly being developed and taught in business schools? It turns out that the best managers ignore them! They prefer to read facial expressions, tone of voice, and gestures in assessing people and situations and arriving at decisions. They're using their right, not their left, hemispheres.

I know a woman who is what I call a house intuitive. She can read houses, walk into one and know instinctively—intuitively—where objects belong in them, where things look and function best. She practices the Asian art of fêng shui, which maintains that how your home is arranged can affect your life and your sense of balance and harmony.

This woman wouldn't fit most people's image of an intuitive. She's extremely detail-oriented, logical, and organized—all left-brain characteristics. In fact, I didn't consider her intuitive myself at first. Inwardly I sort of scoffed at her elaborate advice for arranging my furniture according to invisible fields of electromagnetic energy that affected different areas of my life. Still, I followed most of it. Along the southern exposure of my house, for instance, I arranged items having to do with my career; along the western side I focused on love and partnership and so on. But I ignored her advice about the area where I should focus on health. Oh, it's no big deal, I thought, not really believing in her system.

Then came Christmas, and I cheerfully hung lights in all my windows, a series of strings running continuously from the career and prosperity area across the health area, which I had ignored, and on to the travel and adventure area. What do you suppose happened? The next morning I got up to discover that the brand-new strings of lights in the health area had inexplicably burned out. Not only that, but they had also blown out two fuses and filled my house with an acrid smell of burning wires! Now where do I have recurring problems in my life? With my health. My now controlled sleep disorder is actually a form of electrical problem where my brain is either on or off, just like the lights.

You won't be surprised to hear that I became an instant convert to fêng shui and to believing that this woman was indeed a real intuitive despite her very obvious left-hemisphere characteristics. Her *right* brain provided her with the insights and the overall sense of how a house should be arranged. She was like the interior decorator who sweeps in with a grandiose vision: "Oh, this will be beautiful! We'll make it Early American with a dash of Santa Fe." Her *left* brain filled in the details as to how this could actually be accomplished, like the decorator's partner who follows behind with instructions for the workmen: "Hang that picture there. Move the couch over here. The red rug goes in front of the fireplace."

Left over Right

Ideally the two hemispheres should work in tandem, but they usually don't. The left brain tends to lord it over the right, like the president or Congress, running things and making laws. The right hemisphere acts like the electorate, which is there to be governed. The reasons for the left hemisphere's dominance, however, aren't just cultural. In fact, numerous studies suggest that the cultural bias may well proceed from a biological basis. Studies were performed on individuals whose brains were clipped, or cut, along the callosum, the central nervous pathway connecting the two hemispheres. Their findings are remarkable and very meaningful. They explain a lot about why people so often squelch or ignore their intuition.

When an individual's brain is clipped, the right and left hemispheres cannot communicate. Each acts independently and has separate experiences. Yet researchers have found that when the hemispheres are given these different experiences, the left hemisphere will always have the dominant perception. What's more, it will also actively deny the perception of the right brain, the part that's more concerned with intuition![5]

For example, say you present a right brain with a copy of *Playboy* (put it in a person's left hand). At the same time, you give the left hemisphere a *National Geographic* (put it in the right hand). The person will emotionally respond to the *Playboy* and will begin to turn red, but then he will ignore all of this and will say, "Aren't these pictures of Africa simply breathtaking?" His left hemisphere will ignore and deny the experience of the right.

Amazingly, this will be true even if you give the left hemisphere no experience of its own. Once again, say you give the *Playboy* magazine to the right hemisphere. This time you give nothing to the left. As before, the person will respond with his right brain and begin to laugh and turn red. If you ask him why he's blushing and snickering, however, he'll either be unable to answer and will say nothing or the left hemisphere will confabulate—will make something up that has nothing to do with the experience of the right hemisphere—and in fact will deny its perception rather than admit, or submit to, the truth of the right brain.

This is remarkable because it's exactly what happens in our world. We ignore the right brain's emotions most of the time. What's the value of admitting to anger or pain? we ask. What good does admitting to pain and anger do? Sometimes it's more convenient and less complicated to ignore these difficult emotions. In the same way, we ignore the intuition of the right brain as well. Our left hemisphere–centered society tends to deny the experience and perspective of the right hemisphere. The left side tends to dominate at every turn. Consider the music lecture I discussed at the opening of this chapter. The conductor's remarks on the beauty and value of music were very wise and moving. Yet notice that he threw in the information about music helping people do better in math and science. It wasn't enough that music be appreciated for itself as something of intrinsic value; most people can see value in right-hemisphere emotions and intuition only if they can somehow be made to serve the rational left brain. Patricia Benner, who did the nurse study, suggested that people might more readily accept intuition if it's called pattern recognition instead. In other words, you need to give it a label that's acceptable to the left hemisphere and thus more palatable to a wider audience.

The left hemisphere is more sure of itself than the right. Even in situations where it's performing poorly, it tends to control behavior.[5] The left hemisphere will take a stab at naming something even if the object or situation is unclear. It makes errors of *co*mmission. I call this "seldom right but never in doubt." The right brain, in contrast, makes errors of *o*mission, losing the opportunity to win by hesitating to shoot the puck. It tends to hang back, survey the scene, act cautiously, be less dominant. We see errors of commission more often in men than in women. Men are more aggressive about asserting themselves, more likely to charge ahead even though they don't know whether they're right or wrong. Most women, though, are more cautious and reluctant to take a chance, for fear they might be wrong.[6] A lot of this changes later in life, as we'll see in other chapters.

When it comes to getting the correct answer in the least amount of time, the right hemisphere has the advantage. The left hemisphere proceeds along a long and arduous series of logical steps, while the right hemisphere proceeds by trial and error and just hunch.[1] This latter method, of course, is more intuitive. If you give the right hemisphere a test, it won't get the easiest questions right and the hardest ones wrong. In fact, it may often be the other way around. The left hemisphere will exhibit a sequential advancement in obtaining correct answers; but as the questions become harder, it drops out, and the right hemisphere takes over. This is the essence of intuition, a correct determination not based on logical steps. It's the boy and girl who've just taken an exam. When they compare notes afterward, the boy, who used his left hemisphere throughout, will ask the girl with wonderment how she got a particularly tricky question right. And the girl, who ranged into her right hemisphere when the going got rough, will shrug and say, "I don't know."

The right hemisphere, however, is more submissive and receptive than the left. One scientist noted something interesting when he was driving with his wife in England.[7] Sitting on the right-hand side at the steering wheel, with his wife in the passenger seat on his left, he found that he was far more receptive to his wife's conversation, including her directions and instructions on his driving, than he was at home in the United States, where she sat on his right. In England she was talking into his left ear and to his *right* brain and was much more easily able to persuade him of her points. In England he did whatever she wanted. Back home, however, he was back in the driver's seat in every sense. In America, where his wife spoke into his right ear to his *left* brain, he was far more resistant to her suggestions. His left brain could assert control over the situation. He didn't listen to his wife anymore. No wonder men always want to do the driving in the United States!

Persuasion, in other words, is easier if the right hemisphere is activated. This is why educational and instructional audiotapes are usually played to the left ear.

The right hemisphere is emotional, while the left hemisphere is very fact-based. And because it tries to deny the experience of the right, it's actually uncomfortable with emotion. It may avoid emotion-activating material because it doesn't want to listen to it. And intuition is always telling us things we don't want to hear.

THE PATHOLOGY OF SUPERIORITY

You may think I'm engaging in paradox by bringing up the word "superiority" in conjunction with this right brain–left brain discussion after saying that both hemispheres are essential to intuition. In some individuals, however, one hemisphere or the other is superior or better developed, and this results in certain cases that physicians classify under the term "the pathology of superiority."

While in most people the left hemisphere is superior or dominant, some people's brains develop differently. If you have a small left brain, you may have difficulty reading or writing (dyslexia). At the same time, though, you may well have superior capabilities associated with your right brain. If the development of one hemisphere is delayed, the other side may be larger or have some capabilities that it otherwise might not have had. This is commonly seen in the brains of people with autism, who frequently have savant characteristics.[8] In these people's brains, there might be a small wartlike area where the cells never developed correctly. Nearby areas, however, might have exaggerated development. Some scientists believe this explains why such people have specific areas of genius, such as an extraordinary ability to calculate numbers or an exceptional memory for dates, yet are unable to put this genius into context for practical use. They may be able to tell you that Abraham Lincoln brushed his teeth on Friday morning, June 13, 1862, but they don't know who Abraham Lincoln was or why he was important.

If you look at my brain, you'll see that my left hemisphere is about as big as an acorn (an exaggeration, but you get the point). My right hemisphere, though, is huge. I'm dyslexic, but I make up for it with intuition. So you could say that the pathology, or the abnormal function that developed in my left hemisphere, created superior capabilities in my right hemisphere.[8] In fact, many dyslexics have superior right-hemisphere talents, spatial skills that counteract their disadvantage in language. Some of them don't fit very well into a linguistic society, but if they lived in a society where language didn't exist, they wouldn't have a disability at all.

If you looked at the flip side of this, you could even say that some people with very dominant left brains are actually "righthemispherexic," or underdeveloped on the right. (Most of these people are men, I'm afraid. Haven't you noticed that most intuitives are women?) There is, in fact, a group of people who are alexithymic. This means that there is a relative disconnection between their emotions and their capacity to name them. The phone lines between their right and left brains are down. These people have a profound difficulty, because although they may feel an emotion, struggle as they may, they're unable to express it. In fact, this small group of people may represent the one segment of the population that may indeed have exceptional difficulty gaining access to intuition.

On the other hand, people with excessive crossover between their hemispheres have other problems. Take someone with attention deficit disorder, or ADD. These people have a lot of lines running back and forth between the right and left brain. At the same time, their frontal lobes are wired differently. As a result, their frontal lobes have difficulty telling them what's important and what isn't. A left hemisphere–dominant man probably has frontal lobes like Arnold Schwarzenegger, telling him not to pay attention to most of what comes out of the right hemisphere. But a person with ADD is more apt to have a frontal lobe like Barney Fife, the deputy on the old *Andy Griffith Show*.[9] Not too intimidating, in short, and pretty indecisive. It will let literally a whole switchboard of information come flooding in, without weeding out the calls that are irrelevant. Although a lot of people with ADD have an enhanced capacity for intuition, they're not able to order it and pull out only the salient facts and features. This, once again, is where the left hemisphere comes in.

Staying too much in one hemisphere can also have troublesome consequences. Some studies suggest that madness or schizophrenia may be the result of a hyperactive left hemisphere.[10] One researcher demonstrated that schizophrenics actually use the right hemisphere for verbal tasks, suggesting that the left hemisphere is dysfunctional, not operating properly.[10] He also noted that these people tend to look to the right much more frequently than to the left, which he believed indicates that the left hemisphere is hyperactive, causing the dysfunction. This is really remarkably counterintuitive, because it demonstrates that staying too much in the left hemisphere could lead to emotional instability, even though the *right* hemisphere is the seat of emotion! Clearly, staying away from emotion, segregating emotion from our lives, is not only unproductive, it may even lead to madness!

People who are overly left-hemisphere are overly analytical, overly conforming, conscientious, rigid, and perfectionistic.[9] They have difficulty relaxing. If you're too much into your left hemisphere, you could be prone to obsessive-compulsive disorder, a syndrome wherein an individual has recurrent, persistent thoughts or feels compelled to perform some act repeatedly to allay anxiety, such as washing hands, checking and rechecking locks, or counting household items. On the other hand, relying too much on the right brain can cause you to be hysterical, excessively emotional, rarely analytical, excitable, mostly unstable, and overactive. People who are excessively reliant on the left hemisphere have a tendency to look upward to the right; those too much into the right hemisphere look upward to the left.

Statistically, women have a larger callosum than men, meaning that they have more connections, more telephone lines, between their two brains and thus are able to move more freely between them.[11] A woman may have as many as five lines on her phone, while a man has only one. When he's on the phone in the left hemisphere, that line is busy and the right hemisphere can't get through. If he's emptying out the dishwasher, you can't ask him how he feels about the beauty of the streets with the snow falling outside. He can't talk about his feelings, because he's busy with the left-brain details of getting the dishes stacked and organized. A woman, though, can literally be talking on one line about her feelings, be emptying the dishwasher on the second line, pick up her child and comfort him on the third, worry—Oh, no, am I gaining weight?—on the fourth, and on the fifth wonder, Do we have enough money to go out Friday night?

Something called turning behavior can help determine whether a person is more right brain or left brain–oriented.[12] Would you like to know whether your new love interest is a good prospect and a hopeful match for you? Try this in the restaurant on your first date. Have him or her walk over and get you a fork off another table and watch which way he or she turns to head back. Most right-handed women will walk up to the table, pick up the fork, and turn to the left. This shows that although they are mostly lateralized to the left hemisphere, they still, by virtue of being women, have ready access to their right hemisphere. Most right-handed men will walk to the table and turn to the right to come back. These guys are strongly lateralized to the left, with a big left hemisphere and a narrow callosum, meaning they can't easily get access to the right hemisphere. They're a bit like a left hemisphere on a stick. They're probably great conversationalists, but they may not make the most ideal, understanding mate. Ambidextrous women will turn either way. Most left-handed men, however, turn to the left. That's because left-handed people have 11 percent more fibers in the callosum. That means the left-handed man turning to the left will have greater capacity to use both sides of his brain than most men do. You might want to call that one back.... Then again, he'd have more capacity to be intuitive and to read your mind, so you might need to think about it first.

The important thing to remember, though, is that neither hemisphere is preferable to or "better" than the other, just as men aren't better than women or vice versa. A certain school of thought holds that because intuition comes from the right hemisphere, we should just get out of our left hemispheres and chuck them altogether. But then you'd end up with a right hemisphere on a stick, all emotion and intuition but not able to talk about it or put it into an intelligent framework. That's as bad as the left hemisphere denying the value of the right. It's like thinking that men are what's wrong with the world, and if only women could run things all our problems would be solved. That isn't so, because women have a "man" inside them, since they, too, have a left hemisphere. The key is to find a balance between the two sides, to bring them into harmony with each other.

Intuition and the Wise Mind

I have a behavioral therapy group session every week with a number of women who have borderline personality disorder. This is a condition of severe depression. Individuals with this disorder are so overwhelmed by emotion that they can't think or behave in a socially appropriate manner. They literally become paralyzed by their emotions and their intuition. They are stuck in the "emotional mind"—that is, in the right hemisphere. In fact, you could say they're hyper–right hemisphere.

One day a member of the group posed a challenging question. "What if your intuition is telling you, 'I want to die. My life is over'?" she demanded. "Why can't I just go with it? You're supposed to go with your gut, your intuition."

She had a point, except that she wasn't balancing with her left side. She was totally in the emotional mind. Being too much in the right hemisphere isn't good. You may be intuitive, but you're not getting the point; you're not balanced with the rational mind, the left hemisphere.

We psychiatrists teach these people about the "wise mind." Think of three circles on a page: the left circle is the mental or rational mind, the left brain; the right circle is the emotional mind, or right brain; and the circle in the middle, linking the other two, is the wise mind, truly a unity of both minds.[13]

Wise mind works in intuition as well. It's a balance of the right and left hemispheres. This balance is demonstrably beneficial. It's been shown that true geniuses have a more fluid partnership between the two hemispheres than most people, a greater ability to switch rapidly and smoothly between the two.[14] They demonstrate flexibility, as opposed to the rigid hemispheric reaction most people exhibit to a problem. Gifted children identify sounds equally through both ears, meaning that they have no hemispheric preference. A child of average intelligence most frequently shows a predisposition for the right ear, or the left brain.

Even though we may be dominant in one hemisphere or the other, the brain actually oscillates between the two hemispheres all the time.[15] The hemispheres cycle in and out of dominance, perhaps somewhat on the order of a dolphin's brain. When dolphins sleep, one of their brain hemispheres always stays awake. Two hours later the hemispheres switch, and the one that was awake goes to sleep while the other takes over the watch. Our brains switch, too, the way we shift from foot to foot when we're standing for a long time. Every ninety to one hundred minutes, one hemisphere will be up, or more active, while the other goes down. It's the same as when we sleep and we go in and out of the dream cycle, to which the right hemisphere is important. This is significant for people who believe they just don't have access to their right hemisphere. In fact, they do. There may be times during the day when they're cycling in and out of that capacity but are simply unaware of it. If they could learn to become aware of it, they could widen their doors of perception.

The hemispheres also cycle in concert with other bodily rhythms. Although language ability is primarily left hemisphere, it exists in the right hemisphere as well, especially in women. Studies have shown that the left brain is primed for mostly positive words such as "joy," "happiness," "love," and "cheer," while the right hemisphere picks up negative-toned words. It's been found that before ovulation, most women's ability to hear words occurs chiefly in the left hemisphere, or the right ear.[16] After ovulation, however, the right brain picks up the tempo. Now the women hear more words such as "grief," "anger," and "depression." This is more than an explanation for PMS. What's happening is that the brain is allowing women to hear things they don't usually want to hear. As they turn inward premenstrually, they may actually be getting more access to matters they need to hear about but ignore during the rest of their cycle. Might this be a part of intuition? You may think so after hearing this story. A friend of mine had a patient whose husband insisted that whenever she was premenstrual, she would get a sense that she should go back to school, that she needed to change her career. After her period started, she would give up these career plans and just want to serve her husband. It's not surprising that her husband had brought her in to the OB-GYN with the order to "fix her" because she had PMS. He didn't like the intuitions she was getting about what to do with her life.

It's clear that our doors of perception can, in fact, be widened. This has been demonstrated by certain psychiatric therapies. It has been found that left hemisphere–dominant individuals are more successfully treated psychiatrically by using a behavioral therapy that employs the right brain.[17] This makes a lot of sense, because if we're dominant in a given area, we can also use that dominance to defend against what we don't want to know or face. Right-hemisphere people can come fairly unwound when they get overly emotional. The best way to deal with them then is to batten them down and teach them to gain more access to the left brain, to be sensible, logical, linguistically oriented. On the other hand, have you ever been in an argument with someone who's very left hemisphere–based, very logical and sequential? Trying to beat such a person with words is useless, like doing dueling banjos with Roy Clark. You can't take control. The best thing to do is to throw the person off-balance by approaching him or her from the unexpected angle. This accomplishes two objectives. First, it sneaks you in under the wire, past their defenses. Second, it compels the person to learn to use his other, relatively underdeveloped function. So someone who is very left hemisphere–dominant but needs to learn to deal with his emotions is better healed with imagery. Someone who's more emotional, on the other hand, is better off talking about her anxieties, using the verbal process.[17]

In our left hemisphere–dominant society, therefore, there's something to be said for learning intuition. If we really want to heal our lives, psychotherapy, or simply talking about our problems, may not be sufficient, because it keeps us in the left hemisphere. Since intuition requires us to gain access to the right hemisphere and, as we're about to see, to the body, it may in fact have an actively healing effect.

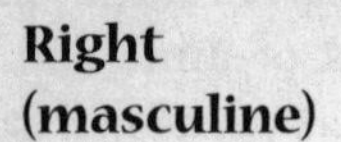
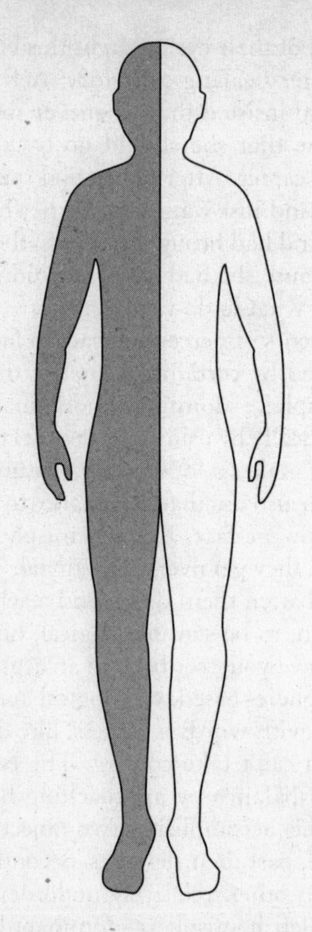

Ancient data suggest that the right side of the body symbolizes masculine function and the left side of the body symbolizes feminine function.

THE BRAIN AND THE BODY

Our left brain–right brain split doesn't stop at the brain and end with logic versus emotions. It shows up in our bodies as well.

We know that the left brain controls the right side of the body and the right brain controls the left side. If the left brain is considered masculine and dominant, and the right feminine and receptive, then the right side of the body is also masculine, while the left side is feminine (see the accompanying figure). Studies of hermaphrodites, people who have a split sexuality and are half male and half female, bear this out. In true hermaphrodites, the right side of the body usually harbors male sexual organs, while the left side has the female organs.[18] And, not surprisingly, the male testis usually develops first: there's that left brain asserting its dominance again! The first one out of the barn is the bull. This is what happens in normal people, too. One study of men, who are usually left brain–dominant, determined that the right testis is frequently higher and heavier than the left.[19] Moreover, the right testis usually develops first. In women, however, it has been found that the *left* ovary generally develops first.[20] This is understandable as well, since the ovary corresponds to the feminine, yin, receptive nature of the right hemisphere. There are women who have extra nipples, which usually appear on the right side.[21] Similarly, breast hypertrophy, or breasts that grow too large, and difficulties with lactation, usually occur on the right.

Significant connections also exist between the brain's hemispheres and various body organs. The thyroid, as we'll discuss in greater detail in a later chapter, is an organ that's associated with communication or expression and asserting oneself in the outer world. Communication, of course, is language. Which side of the brain, then, do you think would have greater control over the thyroid? Just as you'd expect, tests on laboratory rats have shown that the left side of the brain, having to do with expression and communication in the outer world, controls the thyroid more than the right.[22] Ovaries, a symbol of femininity, however, are more dependent on the right side of the brain, the feminine side. Tests have shown that causing damage to the right hemisphere disrupts ovarian function in rats.[23] We have to extrapolate from these tests to humans, but again, these results make sense because the right brain is the feminine, receptive half.

Because the right and left hemispheres have different connections with the body, the memories encoded in our brains will be expressed in different fashion in the body depending upon which half of the brain is involved. Diseases occur differently in the body on different sides. Take bowel cancer. Amazing as it may seem, most men have bowel cancer on the left side and most women on the right. I noticed this myself once when I was working on the surgery floor at a hospital. I thought I was crazy until I pulled a surgeon over and asked him whether I was just imagining that most of the women coming in had colon cancer on the right side. "No, it's not your imagination," he told me. "We don't know why this is, but it's true." My own theory—and that's all it is, since I don't have data to support it—is this: Bowels have to do with unexpressed feelings about a relationship, and it makes sense that men might have unresolved issues involving the women in their lives, so they get bowel cancer on the left, or feminine, side. The opposite happens to women.

Breast cancer offers another striking example of the right-left split. Studies have shown that most right-handed women get cancer in their left breasts in the premenopausal years. Postmenopausally, they get it in their right breasts.[21] In left-handed women, the exact opposite occurs. What does this mean?

In the premenopausal group, there's more left-side breast cancer. There's also more breast cancer among women who give and give and give and are prone to martyrdom. Could it be that these women have overactive responsibility glands in their left, or feminine-side, breasts? The left side of the body, the feminine, which means the right side of the brain, has to do with nurturing, taking in, the receptive function. So it might be that these women, having patterns of overactive responsibility and being martyrs in relationships and not getting enough nurturance themselves, may set the scene for cancer in the left breast. Imagine a woman—we'll call her Cynthia—who spent her whole life focusing on her family. She wanted a big family, because she liked the feeling of being needed by a lot of children. Her whole life was packing lunches, folding socks, putting underwear away in drawers. Everyone came to her for everything. Cynthia was also the pillar of the community. A normal Thursday for her was baking brownies for her daughter's Girl Scout troop, preparing a covered dish for the church social on Saturday, driving the car pool to soccer games, and helping her children with their homework. She noticed, however, that she was always exhausted, never had time for herself, and worried about what her life would be like when her children were grown and gone. Cynthia's life is characterized by overactive responsibility, hypernurturance, and martyrdom. We also see no receptive function; Cynthia never allows others to do anything for her. But the critical thing is that she knows something is amiss, not quite right with her world. Once you sense that, the cows are out of the barn. On some level, Cynthia knows that she could change her life and get more back for what she's giving, and she knows that part of her life needs to grow in that direction. This growth is really important, because her receptive function has gone fallow. If it doesn't grow, cancer may grow in its place to signal that change needs to happen in her life.

After menopause, the cancer switches to the right side for another logical reason.[21] There are many women who, after menopause, go out into the world and try to accomplish everything they had put on hold and sacrificed during their childbearing years. Now the situation has reversed itself. The issue is no longer about being receptive; it's about having a voracious appetite and wanting to make up for lost time, but going about this in an unbalanced fashion. Now the breast cancer appears on the right side, left hemisphere, because these women are ambivalent about being out in the outer world.

Let's go back to Cynthia. A biopsy on her left breast was positive for cancer. She had a mastectomy and went into therapy. She is now past menopause and her children are twelve, fourteen, and fifteen. She decided to return to school and complete her bachelor's degree in nursing. Now she has evening classes and homework to do at night. Meanwhile, her husband says, Aren't you going to help with the church supper? Her children want to know who's going to bake brownies. Cynthia is feeling torn. Perhaps the degree could wait, she thinks. But then she says, "No, this is my time." In the end, her cancer recurs, this time in her right breast.

Although both hemispheres have connections to the body, the right hemisphere is more connected to the body overall, and especially to body pain and organ function, an important part of the intuition network.[24] The right brain's increased connection to the body is a double-edged sword. It can increase our capacity to feel our pain and the pain of others, but it can also increase our capacity for intuition and medical intuition. Studies suggest that pain is more lateralized to the right hemisphere, meaning that the right brain has more capacity to feel it.[24] One type of intuition, clairsentience—the ability to feel other people's pain and physical states in one's own body—is also known as mothers' intuition. Some mothers have a capacity to feel in their own bodies what's going on physically with their children; obviously, this has an evolutionary basis in the need for a mother to have an intuitive sense of what her baby needs when its body feels pain. It could be one reason why the right hemisphere and emotions have a connection with the body. On the other hand, however, women, with their right-brain capacity, are more likely to have what is called a somatiform disorder. This is a state of emotional distress accompanied by an inability to talk about that distress, which is then transferred in the form of pain to the body.

Another group of people with enhanced right brain–body connections are people with so-called conversion disorders. These people are unable to express a wish or emotion in the outer world—that is, with their left brain. So they express it unconsciously through some kind of functional loss in the left side of the body. In reality, there's nothing physically wrong with them, but because they are unable to work through and talk about an emotion, that emotion gets symbolically transformed into a loss of bodily function, usually neurological. They might literally go blind, usually in the left eye, be unable to move the left arm or a leg, or even feel a lack of sensation on the entire left side of the body. Even though these people have enhanced right-brain intuition, they can't express it and they can't figure out its importance by using their left brains. They are completely in their right-brain emotions. As a result, the emotions from the right brain get shunted down into their bodies. Some scientists believe this is the essence of what causes all illness. *The inability to talk about emotions that you feel intensely will usually get transformed into a symbolic language of symptoms and eventual illness in your body.*

Ultimately, a lot of people who are stuck in the left hemisphere are also losing a lot of *their* intuition as well. Not only are they not experiencing all the emotions and hunches in their right hemisphere, but they're also relatively disconnected from their bodies. They may not be feeling bodily pain, but they're also not feeling as much pleasure.

Of course, a lot of people, including doctors, think that not feeling the body's pain is a desirable thing. But I disagree. It's important for you to be able to feel pain in your body, because it's telling you about something that needs to be changed in your life. Pain can be a gift. A woman came up to me at a conference once and said, "I don't want to cause pain to my body anymore. I want to heal everything that's wrong with my life right now so I can heal it once and forever." All I could say to her was "That's not going to happen unless you die right now." Symptoms occur in your body, or in your dreams, to tell you that something needs to be changed.

Pain is a warning signal, like the light that goes on in your car to alert you that you're low on gas. Now, isn't it a *pain* when that light goes on? It means you've got to look for a gas station and stop and fill your tank. You might actually have to readjust your course. The right hemisphere has a very low threshold at which that light will go on. The left hemisphere, however, has the capacity to deny the experience of that light, so that you *could* run out of gas. In the short run, there's a beauty to the left hemisphere's ability to deny. To get through a battle, the soldier can deny pain. But ultimately that pain is there for a reason; it's telling him his leg has been shot off and he's going to bleed to death unless he gets help. At all times, the right hemisphere is feeling pain from your body for a reason and bringing that pain to your consciousness. That's important. That's the whole point of intuition, to tell you where in your life there is pain and when something needs to be changed.

But, you ask, how can I get my left brain to stop denying the pain that my right brain is feeling? It's a matter of awareness. This is where "wise mind" comes in again. Say you're a doctor and you're with a patient when all at once a warning light goes on. You get a pain in your stomach that signals that you have another ulcer coming on. If you are a somatiform person, truly in your right brain, who feels emotions intensely, who stays in the pain and can't name it, then you'll become immobilized by it. But of course you can't become immobilized, because you're a doctor and you're with a patient. You can't interrupt yourself in the middle of a sentence and say, "Oh, sorry, I can't see you now. My warning light has come on, and I can't stay one moment longer. I must stop everything now and analyze the emotional situations in my life that might be contributing to my illness." That would be crazy. Luckily, your left brain kicks in, saying, "You know, this isn't important. Just keep going." Denying, in other words. But in fact, it *is* important.

At this point you need to come to a committee decision. As in wise mind, you have to accept your emotions and your feelings as important. You have to acknowledge the painful emotions and the pain in your body. Then you have to use the left hemisphere not to deny but to prioritize. When the right hemisphere cries, "My stomach hurts!" the left responds, "Okay, that's good to know, but let's finish seeing this patient first, then call up your therapist, finish up the day, and then think about what emotions in your life need to be attended to." The two hemispheres work together. The right brain notices the pain; the left brain validates it, sets priorities, and devises a plan. If the hemispheres don't work together, the body screams louder.

The physical consequences of a failure of the two brains to work together have been demonstrated by actual cases. One study psychoanalyzed twelve cases of individuals, each of whose left hemisphere had been cut off from communicating with the right hemisphere about emotions and memories in the body. Some individuals underwent a commissurotomy, a severing of the corpus callosum to correct seizures in the brain's hemispheres. The study found that all these people had few dreams, and their speech lacked emotion.[25] The researchers reported *the same effects* in people with certain types of diseases, such as thyroid disease, high blood pressure, and coronary artery disease, in that these people had few dreams and had difficulty talking about emotions. The study concluded that patients with these types of diseases have what is called a functional commissurotomy, meaning that the left brain is functionally incapable of communicating with the right brain, and they can't talk about emotions in the right hemisphere or feelings in the body. In other words, these people might have been more prone to developing diseases because their capacity for rational thought, in the left brain, was cut off from the emotions and intuition of the right brain. In other words, there you are, seeing your patient and suddenly getting a stomachache. Your left hemisphere says, "Forget it. Keep going. You've got patients to see." When the right hemisphere protests, the left hemisphere ignores it: "This is nothing. You're just hungry. Leave it alone." And so the right hemisphere decides to turn up the brightness of its warning light. What starts out as a small irritation on your stomach wall on Monday is the size of a canker sore a week later, as big as a quarter the next week, and the week after that you have a bleed and get four units of blood in the emergency room. The longer you go on ignoring your body's intuition telling you things need to be changed, the more serious the illness will become.

Moreover, the people in this study—both those whose brains had been clipped and those with the various diseases—were found to have fewer *dreams* and less capacity for *intuition*. In truth, we can't know whether or not they actually dreamed; we can only know that they didn't remember their dreams. This may well mean that their left hemispheres were telling them to forget their dreams, that they weren't important. It was functionally disconnecting itself from the right hemisphere. This may well be an act of will. These people are ignoring their warning lights, ignoring intuition in their lives. It's not that they can't express what their right hemispheres are feeling; it's that they don't want to. They don't even want to listen to it, because it would mean they'd have to change something. So the right hemisphere is telling them something's wrong, but the left hemisphere denies it. The right hemisphere screams louder, and the left hemisphere denies louder. Then it backs up into the body, and the body screams "Illness."

These can be the very real physical consequences of disconnecting from your intuition.

The Temporal Lobe

The right hemisphere is thought to be the intuitive receiver, but we may actually be able to pinpoint a specific area of the brain through which intuition is powerfully transmitted. The temporal lobe serves as the heart of the intuition network and sends us intuitive thoughts and feelings through its connection to other centers in the brain and the body.

Temporal lobe function is important to both visual and auditory experiences, what we see and hear, as well as to dreams and intense emotions. It also assigns meaning and significance to our experiences.[26] It tells us how we feel about something and what we ought to do about it.

The temporal lobe also plays a vital role in memory formation, one of the critical elements of the intuition network. It contains the hippocampus, which helps form verbal memory (memories in the brain) and plays an important role in dreaming, and the amygdala, which constructs memories you can't put into words, which is known as body memory.

Some investigators believe the temporal lobe is sensitive to low electromagnetic energy frequencies,[27] the currency in which intuitive information is believed to be transmitted and received. The temporal lobe neurons fire when they come into contact with low-frequency electromagnetic energy that can penetrate brain tissue.

It has been noted that particularly intuitive people undergo changes in the temporal lobe. This is most dramatically seen in people with temporal lobe epilepsy, a condition in which the temporal lobe hyperfunctions or actually seizes. These individuals have altered memory function, including repeated déjà vu, and experience dreamlike states of consciousness, time distortions, out-of-body experiences, the sensing of presence, internal hearing, complex visions, anxiety, panic, and feelings of doom.[28] I had one patient with temporal lobe epilepsy who regularly saw angels who came to visit him while he worked in his garden. He actually saw and heard them. If they began to talk to him about something he didn't want to hear, he would tell them to go away because he was busy gardening. Another patient is a woman with temporal lobe seizures who always sees "home movies," visual memories before her eyes. It's literally a laser show of experiences she remembers from when she was seven years old.

People with temporal lobe epilepsy are also believed to have greatly increased intuitive capacities.

A physician friend of mine was making his rounds at the hospital one morning. On the chart a nurse had noted that one patient with temporal lobe epilepsy had startled her in the night by suddenly sitting up in bed and announcing, "My father is about to die." The nurse had asked whether the father had been ill or aging. The patient had replied that his father was only in his fifties and hadn't been ill. But he was about to die, the young man had repeated.

The doctor didn't know what to make of this report. Then, later that morning, an unsettling call came into the nurses' station. The caller was a relative of the epileptic patient. The night before, he reported somberly, that young man's father had suddenly and unexpectedly passed away.

In foreseeing his father's death, the patient had experienced a precognitive event, an intuitive experience that allowed him to know something would happen before it actually did happen.

Most people don't acknowledge that this kind of event can ever take place. It represents a frightening phenomenon that falls outside their normal frame of reference. In fact, when the event I've just described was presented to one of the hospital physicians for his opinion, he flatly rejected the idea that it had occurred. "Since it is impossible for anyone to know the future before it happens," he said, "this event could not possibly have occurred." Maybe this doctor was "temporal lobe–challenged" himself. More likely, since the event didn't fit within his day-to-day conceptual framework, it was simply frightening for him to accept that certain people may have the capacity to understand things before they happen. This would mean that the world is not as controllable or controlled as most of us get used to believing that it is. It would mean that intuition is a capability that all of us may have, since we all have a temporal lobe that allows us to gain access to information that would help us make necessary changes in our lives.

It's important to understand that intuitive experiences are not just a form of temporal lobe epilepsy. People with intuitive experiences who have normal temporal lobe function and no seizure disorder share many of the phenomena experienced by temporal lobe epileptics, from déjà vu to visions, prophetic dreams, and out-of-body experiences. There's also a marked similarity between the daily timing of temporal lobe seizures and intuitive experiences. Most temporal lobe seizures occur between 10:00 and 11:00 P.M. and between 2:00 and 4:00 A.M.[29] When do individuals who report intuitive experiences such as knowing that a family member is going to die receive their insights? *Between 10:00 and 11:00 P.M. and between 2:00 and 4:00 A.M.* Remember my friend Mildred, who had nightly "visitors" whom she tried to chase out of her room? She had those experiences between 10:00 and 11:00 P.M. We all have microseizures, or microspikes, in our temporal lobes at night when we dream. The most hidden information comes to us in the darkness of the night.[30]

Our lives would be very different without temporal lobes and their vital role in memories, dreams, and intuition. The frontal lobes are the seat of judgment, planning, and morality, the part of the brain we spend most of our time developing. Studies have shown that monkeys whose frontal lobes were destroyed continued to live and to interact with their group, albeit in altered fashion. But when both temporal lobes were removed, the monkeys died.[31]

Without the temporal lobe, we can't interpret what's emotionally important to us; we can't determine whether or not an experience or emotion is relevant, how we feel about it, and what we're going to do about it. We simply can't remember a single thing, and we have no access to intuition, either. Without temporal lobes, all you can do is live in the moment. This is dramatically demonstrated by the famous case of H.M., whose temporal lobes were removed because of a seizure disorder.[32] After the operation, he lost the ability to form new memories. His remote memories, formed before the operation, remained intact, since they had been laid down all over his brain. But new memories have to go through the hippocampus, which is in the temporal lobe. Without his temporal lobes, H.M. has no recollection of anything that has happened to him since the surgery. He can't even remember eating lunch. Five minutes after he's eaten and the tray has been carried away, he'll ask his nurse, "When's lunch?" He truly lives only in the moment and can never learn anything new.

In another series of experiments, scientists removed the amygdala from the temporal lobe of some test monkeys' brains.[31] Beforehand, the monkeys had been able to recognize that the men in the white lab coats coming into their cage to put electrodes in their heads weren't the Welcome Wagon people. They would recognize that this was an emotionally significant moment ("Hmm, all my friends are disappearing; I don't think this guy is good for me"), and they would feel appropriately threatened and would get angry and spit at the experimenters. But once their temporal lobes were cut up, their behavior changed dramatically. Instead of being appropriately fearful of dangerous situations and responding accordingly, the monkeys did not react from fear. They lost the capacity to distinguish fear from safety, trust from mistrust. All at once they didn't know how they felt about this guy in the white coat. Instead of appropriately hissing and trying to bite him and defend themselves, they began to behave as though he were either something to love or something to eat. Rather than perceiving the experimenter as a predator and acting appropriately, the monkeys would think he was a potential source of nourishment and attempt to mouth him or try to consume inanimate objects around him. In addition, the monkeys appeared to perceive the investigator as an object to be enamored with and would want to copulate with him. The monkeys became passive in the face of physical threat and danger.[31]

Eating and having sex. Does this ring any bells? In our society, what do so many people who are confused, who don't know how they're feeling or what to do about anything, do instead? We eat, and we have sex. Our temporal lobes may be intact, but we sometimes walk around disconnected from them, not listening to the wisdom coming from them, telling us what's emotionally relevant and how they should respond. Like the monkeys, we become passive. One of the leading causes of depression, especially in women, is passivity—helplessness and hopelessness.

The monkeys had been detached from the intuition centers of their brains. Previously they had taken one look at the researchers and known intuitively, "This guy isn't right for me." Afterward, they couldn't tell. They thought, "Well, I'll have sex with him, or maybe I'll go to dinner with him." Just like so many women. Even though warning bells go off in our heads telling us that this guy reminds us of the last three guys we dated in disastrous relationships, we go out with him anyway. We accept his dinner invitation, we spend the night with him, and eventually we're even likely to marry the guy!

The researchers who conducted these tests called the monkeys' affliction psychic blindness. I think that's perfect. Psychically, these monkeys are blind to the world. They don't know how they feel about what they see, and as a result they don't know how to respond appropriately. Even though they can see, and hear, and move everything in their bodies, they are totally helpless and hopeless.

One of the major causes of disease is learned helplessness and hopelessness.[33] We see a lot of this in American women, who just don't care, don't know how they feel, don't know what to do. They're like Gomer Pyle's girlfriend, Lou Ann. He'd say, "What do you want to do tonight?" and she'd invariably reply, "I don't know." These women never know what to do, especially in threatening situations. Instead of responding to inner wisdom and intuition, and acting appropriately in a situation with reference to how they feel, they are forever looking for advice and guidance from other people. This may not always be the wisest course. Would it be wise for the monkey to ask the research predator if it's safe for him to get out of the cage? I don't think so. But this is no different from the woman who ignores her gut and asks the boyfriend who has just beaten her three times, "Do you think it's safe? Can I trust you?"

Intuition is a way of getting access to how we feel about something, why we feel that way, and what actions we should take as a result. If you can't live fully, in a way, without the temporal lobe, then in a way, you really can't live fully if you're disconnected from your intuition.

Furthermore, the amygdala and temporal lobe are important in learning how to modify what we feel is threatening or rewarding. This is very important, because this is a major role of intuition. This role is confronting beliefs, stored in our brains and our bodies, that no longer serve us. Intuition is facing these beliefs and then considering changing them. If you were afraid of heights, but you were offered a million-dollar-a-year job in the field of your dreams on the top floor of the Empire State Building, what would you do? Would you have to turn down the job? No, you could appeal to the part of your brain, the intuitive center, that's important for memories and emotions, and learn how to modify your fear of heights. So can we modify many of our attitudes. Many men and women go through life thinking wrongly that one type of person of the opposite sex is loving and another type threatening. For example, many women unerringly pick the wrong type of man in the early part of their lives because somewhere in their brains and in their bodies they've encoded a series of memories about what was rewarding and what was threatening, and they got the two mixed up, as in a shell game. If they keep choosing Mr. Right who turns out to be Mr. Wrong, they may not figure out with their brains why their relationships keep failing. Their bodies, however, will create symptoms and illness to let them know in a bigger way that something is just not right. That it is, in fact, very wrong.

Big Weeds or Small Flowers?

The brain is intricately wired to give us full and continuous access to intuition as part of the intuition network. We're still lagging, however, in making the necessary societal and individual change in how we perceive this important tool for our health and well-being.

An unusual physical condition offers an interesting metaphor for how the left brain dominates us culturally. In some individuals, for unknown reasons, one entire side of the body develops faster and grows much larger than the other. You won't be surprised that the exaggerated growth is on the left hemisphere's side—the right side.

I've always been intrigued by the choice of name for this condition, however. It's called hemihypertrophy, or overgrowth.[34] I read a lot into that word choice. Its focus and emphasis are on the overgrown side, the side that's pushing out of the barn. People don't focus on what's lagging behind, the growth of the right brain. I'd be more inclined to call this condition hemi-*atrophy*, or stunted growth of the right brain. I'd look at the fact that one side is not growing enough. To me, the bias toward the overgrown and dominant side is the equivalent of walking into the garden and saying, "Gee, these weeds are too big." It would be much wiser to say, "My flowers need to be bigger."

This is the point of intuition: to give you a whole new perception, a way of seeing that does not focus on the obvious but discerns what is hard to see. Intuition helps you look beyond the dominating weeds to search for ways to make the flowers grow.

FOUR

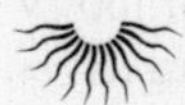

Remembrance of Things Past: Memories in the Brain and the Body

Memory is one of the most powerful forces in our lives. Everybody has a first memory, a hazy recollection of a moment in earliest childhood, like a frozen snapshot, grown blurred with time, that can be retrieved at will from a drawer of the mind. This is a conscious memory stored in the brain. But we all have other memories, too, of which we're usually not consciously aware. They not only linger in the deeper recesses of the brain but are also sequestered in our bodies. We have physicalized memories, laid down in a systematic organization in our tissues and our organs, a record of something that has happened and affected us in ways we may never have completely grasped or grappled with. Medical intuitives read the memories that are stored in our brains and our bodies.

Do you get a headache whenever a certain co-worker approaches you? Or a stomachache whenever you go home for the holidays? Have you wondered why this happens to you? I know a woman who's afraid to ride in elevators. As soon as she hears the doors slide shut behind her and the elevator bells go off, her heart begins to race, her palms begin to sweat. She's filled with a nameless anxiety and dread. After being attacked in an elevator as a child, she repressed most of her conscious, brain memory of that traumatic event. But her body remembers, and every time she gets on an elevator it relives the trauma with which she has never entirely come to grips.

From the moment we're born, or perhaps even earlier, starting in the womb, we begin to collect memories. This record of our past experiences, of significant and emotional events in our lives, builds and shapes our personalities. It therefore also inevitably affects how we shape our futures and the ways in which we organize and arrange our lives. It determines the kinds of jobs we choose, the kinds of partners we pick, the goals we set for ourselves, and even what we perceive to be enjoyable or painful.

Memories are our records of wisdom and trauma, stored in the warehouses of both our brains and our bodies. Certain memories can predispose us to health or disease. They are part of our intuition network, and they are constantly sending us signals, warnings, and information about our lives and what is happening to us. Through intuition, we can learn to understand the language of our brain and body memories as they speak to us about what is wrong in our lives and what we can do to change it.

MEMORY AND EMOTION

One theory about the way memory functions holds that all memory is not completely preserved and that forgetting things means that those memories have been lost from storage. Another theory holds that nothing that we experience is ever truly lost. Everything we see, every gum wrapper, every hole in the road, is stored somewhere in the brain. The fact that we don't remember every one of these things only means that we have lost the route of associations that would enable us to remember them. It's like losing a pair of earrings. They don't cease to exist because you lost them, but you can't figure out where they're hiding, so you can't get to them. Once a memory is created, you never lose it; you just can't find it under the bed among all the dirty socks and other objects.

It's generally believed that our memories are laid down all over the brain and that our capacity to retrieve them involves certain neuroconnections, which are like telephone lines in the brain. Forgetting represents a disconnection of some of these lines. In other words, if you don't use a memory, the brain simply cuts off the telephone line to it. Or think of it as a credit card that you haven't used for six months, so the bank cancels it. You can't use it to retrieve money from the ATM anymore, but you still have the credit card itself, right there in your wallet.

It's fair to say that we don't remember most of life. The things we do remember, the memories we retain a connection to, are those that have an emotional charge to them. You're not likely to remember a bottle cap you saw on the ground at the county fair when you were six years old. If, however, you slipped on that bottle cap, fell, broke your arm, cried in the ambulance all the way to the emergency room, and then had to walk around wearing a cast for six weeks—*that* you would remember.

Memory, in other words, is the experience of an emotion encoded and empatterned in our brains and our bodies. Some of the memories are pleasant and good; some are upsetting and bad. A memory that is unusually happy or pleasant, and not particularly stressful, is usually encoded mostly by way of the hippocampus in the temporal lobe, which helps record verbal memory, or memory that can be talked about. When an experience is painful or traumatizing, however, the hippocampus is unable to encode it because it's suppressed by stress hormones released by the brain and body. That's when the amygdala, another area in the temporal lobe, steps in and takes over, encoding the experience as a nonverbal memory, or one that can't be expressed easily in words. The memory is stored in body memory. You may not consciously recollect it, but it still lives in your brain and the tissues of your body.

This is how the brain works when you lay down a memory. As you live a certain experience, the brain records it in the visual area and the auditory area, taking in the sights and the sounds of what is occurring. It also records what you're feeling in the body-sense area. These are all primary sensory areas of the brain. Later, when you evoke that memory, all three areas come on-line. You get a hologram in your mind of your wedding day, for instance. You see the people milling around at the reception, you hear the music, you feel your shoes pinching your feet, and you hear your train sweeping against the floor. It's a memory without trauma that you talk about easily and often and with great enjoyment.

But now let's say you go for a walk one day down a country road. Your feet are crunching on the pebbles, you smell the lilacs in the air and feel the breeze against your arms and face. You're feeling strong and carefree when suddenly out of the bushes beside the road charges a huge dog, snarling and baring his fangs. You see his great teeth, you hear him barking, you feel the gooseflesh. Terrified and panic-stricken, you run as fast as you can to get away from the dog.

That evening at dinner your husband asks you how you enjoyed your walk. "Oh, it was fine," you say. You don't really want to mention the incident with the dog, so you don't talk about it. In a sense, you've already begun to forget it, because it was unpleasant and frightening and therefore something you don't want to confront again. This is very similar to what happens after you have a bad dream or nightmare. If it's a particularly frightening dream, and you don't wake up and tell someone about it immediately, then it's not laid down in verbal memory. It stays in body memory, however, and you might walk around for an hour or two feeling extremely shaken from the experience of the dream, even though you can't really recall it. Like a bad dream, your emotionally charged encounter with the dog is encoded in your body memory. What you have done, however, is to dissociate it from your conscious memory, mentally split it off or isolate it as painful and unacceptable.

This is what we do with trauma. We act out the line from the Barbra Streisand song: "What's too painful to remember, we simply choose to forget." To the degree that we do this, however, with memories that it is *important for us to face,* we will experience the consequences in our emotional state, our physical state, or the state of our organs and their relative health or disease.

Dissociation and Disease

The most dramatic examples of memory dissociation and its consequences can be found in cases of multiple personality disorder. Most popularly known through the movie *The Three Faces of Eve* and the television miniseries *Sybil,* multiple personality disorder is a major dissociative disorder in which two or more distinct personalities share an individual body. You have a single brain and a single body, but a number of different personalities, each of which has its own separate memory bank. Moreover, one of these personalities might have a certain disease while the others do not.[1]

Studies of people with multiple personality disorder have found that certain personalities have migraine headaches while the others do not. Or one personality will have allergies and drug reactions while the others don't. One personality will be right-handed, while another is left-handed.[1] One study used careful eye measurements of a multiple personality patient to determine that one personality had better eyesight than another.[2] A diagnosis of multiple personality disorder is often controversial, and the possibility of faking is always present. But in another study, scientists asked some people to pretend they were changing into different personalities and then measured their eyeballs. They found that the eyes didn't change the way they did in the multiple personality cases.[2]

In another case, one of the personalities was a child with exotropia, or walleye, an outward turning of the eye that's seen often in children but rarely in adults. When the person switched into an adult personality, the walleye disappeared. Researchers in another instance measured the skin temperature, respiration, heart rate, and skin conductance of the different personalities in a multiple personality patient. In each personality the measurements were different. The same was true in a study in which scientists studied the evoke potential of multiple personalities. This is a brain wave test that shows how people respond to stimuli in the outside environment. Over four days, the evoke potential varied consistently, in the same pattern, from personality to personality.[1,3]

What all this shows is that in these people, as their personalities changed—in other words, as their memories changed—so did their responses to the outer world, and so did their bodies, their health histories, and their diseases. Clearly, their memories were not just in the brain but also in the body—and empatterned differently depending upon which personality was in control.

A patient with multiple personality disorder dissociates parts of his personality, parts of his life, from consciousness. In his case, this dissociation is so severe that another whole personality is formed to deal with the extremely painful experiences or memories of trauma he is cutting off. Then the personality that's carrying the traumatic memories develops disease.

But in fact, most of us do the same sort of dissociating in a much less extreme fashion. I did a reading once on a person who had just gone off to college. On the first day of classes, she went to her first class but found she couldn't walk into the room. For some reason she was terrified. Her hands started shaking, her palms got sweaty, and she felt a nameless dread. She forced herself to go in and sit down all the same. When class was over, she ran back to the dorm and started vomiting.

She didn't know what was going on. She had talked about her problem with a psychiatrist, but it hadn't helped. When I did her reading, I saw irritation in her stomach and the beginning of an ulcerative formation.

When I read her emotional life, I saw that earlier in her life, this client had had a very strict upbringing. Some rupture arose between her parents, and she was sent away to a very restrictive school. There she had a lot of unpleasant experiences, from being rapped on the knuckles for misbehaving to being barred from lunch for not noticing that the collar of her uniform was askew. I could envision the client being so unhappy that she was holding her stomach and not eating at all. I could see her sitting at a table in the cafeteria and pushing the tray away. I saw her lying on her bed a lot, away from the other children who were playing outdoors. She lost a lot of weight and became very ill.

Eventually I saw her returning home. Her parents had reunited for the sake of her health. The client's stomachaches went away, and she began to eat again. For the rest of her childhood, she really didn't think much about this brief episode when she was separated from her parents. Her parents were still in the habit of disappearing behind closed doors for heated discussions, but she was sheltered from what was happening. She believed that her parents were happy and that the family was secure and content. She put her boarding school experience behind her. Until she went away to college.

Walking into her first college classroom evoked in her body and in her stomach the same fears she had experienced as a child at boarding school. Her body memories of that time began to act up. She began to get nausea and to throw up, and she didn't know why.

If we ignore our emotions or our memories from the past, our bodies will express them all the more forcefully. If we don't pay attention to the rattle in a car, it will get louder and louder, and eventually the transmission will fall out. We're paralyzed until we deal with the emotions that are playing out in our bodies' symptoms, trying to get our attention. Medical intuitives are not the only ones who can read the emotions in a person's life and how they're encoded in the tissues of the person's body. Every one of us can start to learn the intuitive language of our own body that tells us which aspect of our lives requires our attention.

When we dissociate memories and emotions and put them out of our consciousness, they go into our bodies, via the autonomic nervous system, the system of telephone wires that connect emotions with organ function. We can see this happen quite literally in people with a psychiatric condition called conversion disorder. A patient was brought into the hospital once with complete paralysis on the left side of her body. An examination showed that there was nothing physically wrong with her, but she couldn't walk and was unable to move anything on her left side. We learned that both her parents had died within the last few years, and she had experienced several other deaths in the family as well. She wasn't able to talk about this or deal with it, however. Half of her life, half of her family, was now gone, and she was at a loss about how to move forward. As a result, half of her body was lost, not felt, and she was literally paralyzed and unable to walk forward. She couldn't cope with the enormity of the emotion she was experiencing, so she split off the unacceptable ideas at the root of it. Since she couldn't talk about it, it had gone into her body and become symbolized by her physical problems.

Some scientists believe that disease is a temporary dissociative episode, a disruption of our normally integrated functions. In a multiple personality, only one personality gets a disease, the personality that harbors the memories or emotions that are being banished from consciousness. Imagine, for instance, that a patient with multiple personality disorder is caught in the middle of a horrendous fight between her mother and her sister. The sister has an accident, goes into the hospital, and begs the multiple personality patient to come and visit her. But the mother warns that she'll be disowned if she so much as goes near the hospital where her sister is waiting for her. In this terrible dilemma, the patient splits off the painful emotions and banishes them to her alternate personality. Now she can go to see her sister in the hospital without worrying about her mother's reaction. But the other personality, aware of how infuriated the mother will be, worries and gets sick.

Something similar happens to most people. Most of us have only one personality, it's true, but we will incur disease in the body organs associated with the emotions that we have split off. We won't know why, but that's when we must use our intuition. Investigations into multiple personality disorder have helped scientists recognize that feelings occur in multiple levels of the mind, most of which we're not aware of. And part of that mind is in the body. I had a colleague who treated a dramatic case of a woman who had suffered from multiple personality disorder for years. She had developed a severe infection in her left arm that could not be cured. Ultimately the arm had to be amputated. Incredibly, after the amputation, the patient no longer suffered from multiple personality disorder! The doctor who took care of her wondered whether painful memories that had perhaps been encoded in that limb had been causing her to fragment into multiple personalities. Was it possible that once that limb was removed, she would no longer

Emotional Center	Organ System	Physical Dysfunction	Emotional Power	Emotional Vulnerability
1	Physical body support	Chronic spinal problems	Mistrust	Trust
			Independence	Dependence
	Whole spine	Sciatica	Standing alone	Belonging in group
	Blood	Scoliosis		
	Immune system	Rectal problems	Resourcefulness	Helplessness
		Chronic fatigue	Fearlessness	Fearfulness
		Fibromyalgia	Ability to cope	Adaptability
		Autoimmune disease		
		Arthritis		
		Skin problems		
2	Uterus	Ob-Gyn problems	*Drives:*	
	Ovaries		Active	Passive
	Vagina	Prostate and testicular disorders	Uninhibited	Inhibited
	Cervix		Direct	Indirect
	Prostate		Go-getter	Receptive
	Testes	Pelvic and lower back pain	Shameless	Shameful
	Penis			
	Bladder	Sexual potency	*Relationships:*	
	Pelvis	Fertility	Independent	Dependent
	Large intestine	Urinary problems	Needed by others	Needs others
	Lower back		Takes more	Gives more
			Good boundaries	Poor boundaries
			Assertive	Submissive
			Protects others	Needs protection
			Opposes	Cooperates
3	Abdomen	Gastric problems	Adequacy	Inadequacy
	Upper intestines	Duodenal ulcers	Skills	Inferiority
	Liver	Colon and intestinal problems	Making it work	Giving up
	Gallbladder			
	Lower esophagus		Responsibility	Irresponsibility
	Stomach	Ulcerative colitis	Caught in the middle	Addiction
	Kidney			
	Pancreas	Crohn's disease	Aggressiveness	Defensiveness
	Adrenal glands	Heartburn	Threat	Escape
	Spleen	Gastritis	Intimidation	Avoidance
	Middle spine	Diabetes	Territoriality	Restraint
		Constipation and diarrhea	Boundaries	Limitations
		Anorexia	Competitive	Noncompetitive
		Bulimia	Win	Lose or concede
		Hepatitis	Gain	Loss

4	Heart	Coronary artery	*Emotional*	
	Lungs	disease	*expression:*	
	Blood vessels	Myocardial	Passion	Love
	Shoulders	infarction	Anger	Resentment
	Breasts	Arrhythmias	Joy	Serenity and peace
	Diaphragm	Chest pain	Stoicism	Emotional
	Upper esophagus	Hypertension		effusiveness
		Asthma	Courage	Anxiety
		Lung cancer	Bereavement	Depression
		Pneumonia	Loss	Abandonment
		Upper back		
		problems	*Partnership:*	
		Breast disease,	Isolation	Intimacy
		including	Giving help	Taking help
		cancer	Giving	Accepting
			Fathering	Mothering
			Martyrdom	Nurturance
				Forgiveness
5	Thyroid	Graves' disease	*Communication:*	
	Neck vertebrae	Hypothyroidism	Expression	Comprehension
	Throat	Bronchitis	Speaking	Listening
	Mouth	Laryngitis		
	Teeth and gums	Mouth ulcers	*Timing:*	
		Cervical disk	Pushing forward	Waiting
		disease		
		TMJ (temporo-	*Will:*	
		mandibular	Willful	Compliant
		joint)		
6	Brain	Brain tumor or	*Perception:*	
	Eyes	hemorrhage	Clarity	Ambiguity
	Ears	Stroke	Focused	Unfocused
	Nose	Neurological	Unreceptive	Receptive
	Pineal gland	disturbances		
		Blindness	*Thought:*	
		Deafness	Wisdom	Ignorance
		Ménière's disease	Rationality	Irrationality
		Dizziness	Linearity	Nonlinearity
		Tinnitus	Rigidity	Flexibility
		Parkinson's		
		disease	*Morality:*	
		Learning	Conservative	Liberal
		disorders	Law-abiding	Risk-taking
			Critical	Available for
				feedback
			Repressive	Uninhibited
7	Any organ	Developmental	Clear sense of	Undefined life
	system	disorders	life purpose	purpose
		Genetic disorders	I create my life	The heavens direct
		Multiple sclerosis		my life
		Amyotrophic	I can influence	Things happen the
		lateral sclerosis	events in my	way they should
		Multiple system	life	
		abnormalities	Attachment	Detachment
		Any life-		
		threatening		
		illness or		
		accident that		
		serves as a		
		wake-up call		

be susceptible to those particular memories? We may never know. The patient is fine now, although it's conceivable that she could have a recurrence of her disorder at some point. I am not suggesting that we should simply saw off the diseased part of someone's body to remove memories that may be stored in it. That would be like saying that if the woman who had stomach pains and ulcers associated with going to college could just have her stomach removed, she'd be fine. This story does illustrate, however, that once something changes in your body, your emotions might in fact improve. And conversely, if your emotions heal, a more healthful body may also result.

Cases of multiple personality disorder show that if we can heal those parts of our personalities that are unhealthy—negative perceptions of memories and present emotions in our lives—then, if we are having physical problems or disease, we can change our body state to one of health. We can change from the personality with the disease to the personality that is disease-free. Since symptoms and feelings develop in our bodies constantly as part of our intuition network, we need to learn to connect emotions to body states in a lifelong process. Medical intuition is the process of consciously connecting emotions to body states. Physical symptoms let us know when our emotional life is not working well, what we need to change, and what's working fine.

True multiple personalities can't do this. The various areas of their intuition network are completely segregated from one another, residing in different personalities, so that they can't communicate on how to change their lives to achieve health. But most of us don't have this problem. Through conscious attention to intuition, we can learn how to use all parts of our brains and our bodies to get a unified understanding of what's going on in our lives and what we should change and adapt, instead of constantly reliving the traumas of the past.

The Black Hole of Trauma

A famous study raised rats in boxes where they regularly received electric shocks from birth. It sounds awful, but for the rats it was just home sweet home. It's not unlike life for a great many people who grow up in an atmosphere of trauma. The rats grew up with the shocks, and after they reached adult rathood, so to speak, they were allowed to leave their boxes and were given the opportunity to move to other boxes, where they would receive no electric shocks. Well, they all chose to return to their original boxes, and the memory of life amid electric shocks.

The rats were happier reliving their known distress than trying out unknown possible future health. They had learned that helplessness was the only way of life. It was the song they lived by, the beat they marched to. In their boxes with the electric shock, they were in control. They thought, "Hey, I can control this. I've lived all my life with getting shocked." In the same way, many of us have lived all our lives with being overburdened at work or being unhappy in an unfulfilling relationship. We can handle that, because it's familiar. The prospect of changing jobs, though, or striking out on our own, leaving the bum and possibly being alone, is downright terrifying. It's easier to stay where we are.

Unfortunately for the rats, however, their helplessness ultimately affected their immunity. They got used to the idea that the world wasn't safe, that they would continually be shocked. Even though they had learned to tolerate this emotionally, their bodies would not physically tolerate it. Body intuition and body memories always win. Eventually our minds block out the number of shocks we feel. But the body keeps score. With each shock our white cells and immunity slip lower and lower. Over time, the rats' immune systems broke down, letting in all kinds of disease. They had become the physical incarnation of the rats' belief that they were constantly vulnerable to attack from the outside world.[4]

Like the rats, most of us tend to relive past trauma over and over. We fall into the black hole of trauma. Past memories increase physiological arousal—that is, they prepare us physically and emotionally for additional shocks. It's as if we're bracing ourselves for the other shoe to drop, except that there are simply more and more shoes. At the time of the trauma in the past, we secreted the stress hormones cortisol and norepinephrine. These get us revved up for the next attack. As a result, we're more and more receptive and prepared for attack. And guess what? We actually attract further attacks! When we recall that traumatic memory, the brain and the body release these hormones again and again. What that means is that when we find ourselves in an environment that evokes a traumatic memory, we interpret it as being stressful and traumatic, *just like the past.* Our bodies experience it as if a real trauma were occurring, even though it's only a memory, only like a bad dream. The body is shaking as though we've been having nightmares all night, even though we're only reliving a pattern encoded in the brain. As a result, we'll re-create traumas in the present and the future.

I have a tendency to drive too fast. I used to get a lot of tickets and points for speeding. Once, I was late for my own birthday party and hurrying to catch the ferry to the restaurant. I was going 53 in a 35-mile-an-hour zone. The policeman who stopped me asked me if I had turned my speedometer upside down. I got a $116 ticket. Just a few days later I turned right on a red light without stopping, and another policeman caught me. Two days later I came down with a severe cold. Now every time I see a car that just has a ski rack on the roof and no flashing lights—and you see a lot of those in Maine, where I live and practice—my heart starts to pound, my hands get sweaty, and my foot goes straight for the brake. I'm overly interpreting my environment as traumatic, based on my memory of past experiences. I'm fearful of getting stopped and ticketed. Reacting as I do, I'm also once again releasing cortisol and norepinephrine, and actually strengthening the memory of a trauma. It's like a needle that gets stuck in a record groove and keeps going around and around, making the groove deeper and deeper. A stressful memory registers in my body as though I were getting a ticket, even though there's no police car. My immunity dips down, and soon I get a cold.

A friend of mine was unhappy in her job but was afraid to go out and look for another one. The stress of her job had registered in her body as diverticulitis. Every time she went on vacation, she would relax and promise herself that when she got back, she wouldn't let the job affect her, that she'd take care of herself first, before worrying about everyone else in the office. Without fail, though, the day before she went back to work, she'd start getting intestinal pains as her chronic diverticulitis acted up. Every time she went back to the office, she anticipated trauma as it had happened to her in the past. She experienced increased physiological arousal and released the same stress hormones that would have been released if the trauma were actually occurring. Consequently, her diverticulitis now acts up even before she gets back to work. And it takes less and less irritation to cause a diverticulitis attack. She is always going back to the same place, to the black hole of addiction and trauma. Little did she know that she was acting like the rats in the box with the shocks.

Energy Leaks and Memory Maturation

Imagine that every one of us is a set of encyclopedias. In the present perhaps your life has reached volume 17. But something back in volume 2, in the past, is still affecting you, causing ulcers or some other illness. You have to go back and figure out what this ulcer is all about. Its cause could be five volumes back or four volumes, or it could be in the current volume. The stomachache you have today may be due to your boss yelling at you this morning, but it may also be due to the fact that your mother yelled at you every morning in volume 2.

Trauma in the form of experiences such as child abuse, military combat, man-made or natural disasters, witnessing violence, or even lesser emotional and mental traumas increases levels of dissociation. This means that certain emotions and memories are split off; they lie in the body tissue or areas of the brain we can't talk about. If not dealt with properly, they can create disease in the body.

The important point—and this gets a little complicated—is that it's not the memory itself, not the actual trauma of the past, that causes our problems in the present. What the memory means to us is what is important—as is the way we react to what that memory evokes. In other words, it's not the boarding school that caused your problems, it's that you *perceive* college as being the same as boarding school. You could have an absolute angel of a professor, the class you're taking could be wonderful, you can go get lunch any time you want, but your body is perceiving the current experience as being just as traumatizing and stressful as the former experience.[5]

This has been demonstrated scientifically. In one study women who were to have mammograms were questioned about events in their lives over the previous five to eight years. Researchers discovered that they were able to predict which women would be found to have cancer on the basis of the answers they gave to those questions. Those women who had experienced a severe life event—living through a natural disaster, perhaps, or the loss of a loved one or the loss of a job—in the last five to eight years were consistently more likely to be diagnosed with cancer. Even if a woman had had trauma in her early life, *it was not that event that triggered her problem*. She did not come down with cancer because she had been a victim of incest and had never had the capacity for love. It was because of the way she reacted to the more recent crisis.

The researchers looked at the differences between the women who approached their crises actively and those who disengaged from them.[6] Disengaging is a minor form of dissociating, separating conscious reality from our feelings about it. They compared women who had formed an action list, a series of steps for dealing with the problem, with those who didn't, and they compared women who got support from others in dealing with their problem with those who didn't. Which strategies do you think increased a woman's chance of getting breast cancer? Amazingly, it was the *activist* strategies.[6]

You might think that the activist approach of really grappling with your problem is what I've been advocating. But these women were faced with severe and unavoidable life events—death, permanent loss, inescapable stress. There was no changing what had happened to them. Their strategies might have been acceptable in other settings, but not here. They had to face the question of when to hold them and when to fold them. In the act of trying to fight something unavoidable, the activist women were actually just reliving this inescapable event over and over, making the trauma groove deeper and deeper. You can't bring dead people back; you can't relive your childhood. Some things are simply irreversible. It may not seem fair, but no one said that life has to be fair. Look at the birds at the feeder sometime and watch the big, powerful bluejay with his long beak and cap swoop in and elbow out the little sparrows. The birds don't start squawking, "Hey, hey, hey! You better get in line, bubba!" They just go back in there. This is the way of nature, and the best thing to do is to accept it. In fact, this is called radical acceptance. Without this capacity, the activist women were using up physical and emotional resources that could have protected or healed their bodies instead. The researchers actually concluded that the women's behavior *caused* their breast cancer.

We want to pay attention to body memories and figure out what emotions are related to the body symptoms we're experiencing. You want to focus on those memories, however, so that you can transform them, acknowledge them, deal with them, and then release them and move forward. If you're forever focused mentally on some trauma or emotion that occurred in the past, you're losing energy to the past and sapping healing energy from the present.[7] Your lightbulb in the present will only be operating on a level of 60 or 70 watts instead of 100. In medicine this is called the steal syndrome. Cancer cells have been shown to "steal" energy from adjacent normal tissue.[8] So if you're repetitively reliving and reexperiencing a traumatizing memory, two things happen: you begin to see the pattern of that memory everywhere and re-create it in the present, and it causes the area in your body that carries the metaphor for the trauma to steal energy from other areas that are normal and to reinforce the disease in that area.

In psychiatry we no longer focus exclusively on the past; we teach our patients how to deal with the present. We teach memory maturation. This consists of four steps: (1) locating the traumatic experience in the past and differentiating it from current reality; (2) focusing on living in the present without feeling or behaving according to irrelevant demands belonging to the past; (3) decreasing hyperarousal by means of meditation, relaxation response, and exercise; and (4) decreasing intrusive reliving and stopping traumatic black hole cycles.

The brain has its own mechanism for decreasing the influence of painful memories. As you lay down new memories that contradict the old one and help you reframe it, the neuroconnection to the old painful memory is weakened. It becomes the credit card you stop using. In the meantime you use other, new credit cards more frequently. Think of the story of the pianist David Helfgott in the movie *Shine*. His father tyrannized and abused him while professing to love him, forming a traumatic childhood memory and helping set the scene for a mental breakdown. But after the boy left home, he had a lot of other experiences of people being loving to him, including various teachers and mentors and his eventual wife. Their love was expressed differently, and had a healing effect. David never lost the memory of his father, but he was perhaps able to change the way he interpreted that memory, because it was being replaced by memories of other people showing him love in a different way. As the neuroconnections to those memories strengthened, the old ones weakened.

An illustration of how this works can be found in an eye study performed on monkeys. Researchers put patches over the monkeys' right eyes to force the left eyes to do all the work. Over the period that the right eyes were patched, the neuroconnections that helped those eyes function became retracted, or pulled back. When the patches were removed, the monkeys were functionally blind in their right eyes, unable to see clearly. The neuroconnections to their left eyes were strong, but the right ones had been weakened simply due to lack of use.

Memories work the same way. There's no reason to believe that you are ruined or trapped for life if you have a bad memory. If you don't constantly reinforce the trauma, it will weaken. We all know people who go around talking, almost with pride, about their terrible allergies, for instance, and telling the story over and over of how they ate something that made them swell up so badly that they nearly *died*. They keep looking out of the same eye and reinforcing it. Consequently, they're not using the other eye, the one that can see all those times that they *didn't* swell up and were absolutely healthy.

We can all learn, forget, and change our behavior. We can all put the past aside and learn to live in the present. Our brain and body memories can help us do that.

MEMORIES IN THE BODY

How do we know that memories exist in the body?

We might have a hard time believing that there's a mind in the uterus, as some physicians say,[7] or that every part or area of the body is associated with its own specific emotions. In fact, however, scientific studies not only support such theories but clearly demonstrate that the body is the repository of actual physicalized memories of events and emotions that have befallen us and that continue to affect us in the present.

The idea that the body can speak of our emotions even while the tongue remains silent reaches back to antiquity. In the third century B.C., the Greek warrior Antiochus fell in love with his stepmother, Stratonice. This was a forbidden love, and Antiochus strove to suppress and conceal it. Soon, however, he fell ill and slipped to the verge of death. None of the many physicians who were called in to examine him could find the source of his illness. His anxious father then called in the renowned physician Erisostratos. When he, too, could find no physical disease, Erisostratos surmised that the problem was in Antiochus's mind. He understood that the mind and the body are linked.[8]

As people came to visit the sick youth, the physician observed Antiochus's physiological reactions. He studied his face and his body movements to see how they reflected "the inclination of his soul." And he noticed that anytime the stepmother, Stratonice, came into the room, Antiochus would stammer and break into a sweat. He would be overcome with heart palpitations, helplessness, stupor, and pallor. "His soul," the physician reported, "was taken by storm."[8]

Erisostratos assumed that the memories and emotions of his passion were encoded in Antiochus's autonomic nervous system, and when he was unable to talk about that passion or express it openly, the autonomic nervous system channeled it into his body, which expressed it for him in the form of symptoms and illness.

Galen of Pergamum, the father of modern medicine, witnessed a similar phenomenon in the case of a woman suffering from insomnia. He found her to be suffering from fever, restlessness, and a reluctance to answer questions, and diagnosed her as having "melancholia, dependent on black bile." In plain English, she was depressed because she was angry and couldn't talk about it. Over the course of two days, Galen noticed that whenever anyone came to see the woman and began to talk about a certain hero named Pylades and his dalliances with other women, the patient's pulse would become irregular, and she would become violently agitated. The physician concluded that the woman was in love with Pylades but couldn't talk about it. This caused changes in her body hormones, which in turn caused changes in her immune system, creating her illness. Her body, in short, was talking about the matter her tongue couldn't voice, and expressing it in terms of heartsickness.[8]

This affliction is familiar from the pages of great literature as well. In his fourteenth-century masterpiece *The Decameron,* the Italian writer Giovanni Boccaccio tells the tale of a young nobleman who falls in love with a servant girl. Seeking to hide his unacceptable passion, he falls ill. His physician stands by his bedside and takes his pulse whenever anyone comes into the room. When the servant girl enters, the nobleman's pulse races. Unable to talk about his love, he had tried to suppress it, but his body cried out the truth. His heart, like that of Antiochus, carried the memory of his love and expressed it when his tongue would not.[8]

We all experience something like this on a more mundane everyday level. Haven't you ever noticed how your body changes when you hear a song that evokes certain memories? Lots of couples think of a certain song as "their" song. Whenever they hear it, they become flushed and feel a rush of physical warmth. This is a real body memory; the song is evoking a memory that's particularly pleasant.

The same thing happens with body memories of an unpleasant experience. I was attacked once, years ago. To this day, if anyone walks up behind me, I literally jump. This is my body reacting, pure and simple. It's not my brain telling me, "You have to jump now—someone's behind you." Long before my brain has registered a presence, I've left my skin behind.

A nurse once told me about a woman with multiple personality disorder who had been abused by her father. Only one personality, the nurse said, knew about the abuse. Whenever this personality emerged, burn marks would appear on the woman's arms. When she flashed out of that personality, the burn marks would go away. This sounds far-fetched, but in fact it's borne out by scientific findings and case studies.

Researchers described one case of a married woman who had a severe problem with hives. Dermatologists will tell you that the skin is closely tied in to the brain and has an extensive autonomic nervous system, a series of nerves that receive input from the brain. This particular woman's skin would break out in large hives during periods of a certain type of stress, usually when she was around someone very domineering. Most of her problem involved her mother-in-law, with whom she had a difficult relationship.[9] Her very first experience with her mother-in-law had been so traumatic that she had broken out in what Chinese medicine calls blood heat. It was as though her blood literally boiled over, and she broke out in huge hives. Yet this relationship with her mother-in-law was never fully released and processed. It continued to torment her on many levels. Whenever she had a memory involving her mother-in-law, she would break out in hives.[9] If she went to the mailbox and found a letter from her mother-in-law, she would break into hives. And when she talked about her mother-in-law in the psychiatrist's office, the psychiatrist would watch the boils form on her skin right in front of him.

Bodily changes occur to us when we have certain experiences, and they will come to the surface when we remember or relive those experiences, consciously or unconsciously. Another case published in a distinguished medical journal tells of a woman who was regularly beaten by her husband. As her sons grew up, they prevented their father from beating their mother. He then began to attack her with words. Whenever he unleashed a barrage of verbal abuse, the woman developed so-called psychogenic purpura.[10] These real bruises and black-and-blue marks would appear on her skin in the very places where she had previously received bruises from her husband's beatings. Now they were appearing even though her husband never physically laid a finger on her! A psychiatrist watched the bruises appear on the woman's arms right before his eyes when she talked about the verbal abuse. It doesn't require much of a leap to see that the physicalized body memories of the earlier beatings were asserting themselves as the present trauma of verbal abuse recalled her past experiences.

In order to prove that thoughts, memories, and emotions are capable of creating changes in our bodies, a number of researchers have conducted studies using hypnosis. In one study, a group of men and women were hypnotized and asked to imagine blisters forming on their hands.[11] Only a few of the subjects were able to raise actual blisters on their skin. At first, the researchers believed that this indicated that some of the subjects had greater powers of visualization than the others. Then, however, they noted that one woman was able to raise blisters on the back of her left hand only, and always in the same place.

When they questioned her later, they learned that the area where the blisters formed coincided exactly with an area of her hand that she had burned six years earlier with hot grease. Those people who had never burned or injured their hands were unable to raise any blisters under hypnosis. The researchers concluded that hypnotic suggestion was bringing an actual encoded memory to the surface, that the patient was reliving an experience both *mentally* and *bodily.*[11]

A sleepwalking case illustrates the same concept. It describes a man who experienced such frequent and dangerous bouts of sleepwalking that he had to be restrained. To prevent him from sleepwalking, his wrists and arms were bound with rope and tied behind his back. On one occasion he struggled to release himself from the bonds, causing welts on his wrists. Nearly a decade later he continued to have sleepwalking episodes, and in them, he occasionally relived the experience of struggling to loose himself from the ropes. He would sleepwalk holding his arms behind his back and making movements as though he were struggling to free himself, even though his arms were not tied. And as he struggled, deep weals would form on his wrists in the pattern of rope marks.[9]

Well, all right, you say, you've shown that memories are in the skin, but you've already told us the skin receives a lot of brain input. What about other areas of the body? Here's an example of memories in the ankle and the forehead. It's the case of a woman who had vivid memories of being injured and buried in rubble after a bomb explosion during World War II.[9] Years later, when she remembered and talked about this experience, her left ankle and the left side of her forehead swelled visibly. These were the parts of her body that had been injured when the bomb exploded. Another woman appeared to have memory in her ribs. At the age of thirty-five she recalled a riding accident when she was ten, in which she fractured the ribs on her right side. As she recalled the memory, she developed a line of hemorrhages down the length of the tenth rib on her right side.

Doctors observed another woman on more than thirty occasions as she talked about her father having beaten her when she was a child. As she spoke about her memories, the doctors watched her body speak as well: the body memories of her trauma emerged right in front of them. When the woman spoke about her father having fractured her wrist, that wrist began to swell. When she remembered him striking her left shoulder with a whip, she developed linear red marks on her skin that lasted for twenty minutes or more. She also had memory in her arm. As she recalled how her father had beaten her with a stick, red marks appeared on her arm, bearing an elaborate pattern that matched the carvings on the stick he had wielded.[9]

Memory is everywhere in our bodies. There's a memory in the skin, the breast, the cervix, the uterus, the prostate, the stomach, and the heart. The memories stored in these organs can have a real and functional effect not just on our emotional development but on our physical development as well. Changes in emotions, which means the memories we form, have been shown to affect the development of sexual traits and characteristics, especially in women. Since nerve pathways exist between the emotional brain, the brain important for memory, and the hypothalamus, which provides hormone function, then memories can affect our hormonal development. Researchers describe the case of a young girl from a troubled home. At the age of fifteen she was considerably smaller than normal in overall size, which indicated a lack of growth hormone. In addition, she was completely lacking in any secondary sex characteristics—breast development, body hair, and the like. This is highly unusual, as most girls begin to develop some secondary sex characteristics as early as seven or eight. The young woman was removed from her home and the adverse environment in which she had been raised. Six weeks later her breasts had developed and she had grown an inch in height. By age sixteen she had grown four more inches and showed substantial breast and pubic hair development. Once she was removed from her memories of trauma, her personality and her body were free to grow.[12]

If we change our emotions and memories, can we develop emotionally and physically later in life as well? A remarkable study would seem to indicate that the answer is yes. Scientists theorized that certain emotions occurring during certain stages of our lives can arrest our development. We can control blood circulation to various areas of the body through hypnosis. Migraine sufferers, for instance, can learn through hypnosis to shunt blood to certain areas to relieve the pain of their headaches. Might it not, then, be possible, researchers wondered, to increase breast size in women by shunting blood and hormones their way? Experiments were performed on twelve women of varying ages, including some postmenopausal women, over a period of twelve weeks. Under hypnosis, the women were sent back to the age of twelve and told to place their hands on their breasts and imagine them getting bigger. As the researchers watched, the women's hands actually rose from their chests. At the end of the study the women showed a statistically significant average increase in total circumference of 2.11 inches! This was an increase in breast size itself, not an expansion of the chest or an expansion due to weight gain. In fact, none of the women gained weight (some actually lost), and their overall contours became more feminine, meaning that their waists became smaller and the circumference of their chests below the breasts decreased by an average of five-eighths of an inch.[13]

Significantly, though, two of the subjects dropped out of the study midway for emotional reasons. Clearly, this kind of experiment is not for the faint of heart. If you send people back to the age of twelve and ask them to relive what was happening to them at that period in their lives, you're likely to bring back and expose emotional scars from that period as well. In fact, at least three other studies were conducted along the same lines, and in each instance, a number of subjects were reported to have dropped out for emotional reasons, which the researchers essentially ignored or belittled. Yet this is important information that appears to indicate a side effect of the treatment.[13]

The success of the hypnotic breast augmentation indicates that memories stored in the women's breasts may have repressed or stunted their growth. Emotional changes in their lives may have caused physical changes in their bodies. Yet when they adopted a more positive approach to the memories through hypnosis, they were able to change their body states. Many studies have similarly shown that we can alter the state of our bodies through self-hypnosis. If this is true, then we should be able to change that body state to one of health if we listen to and understand the signals the body is sending to us, telling us what memories from the past and the present are stored there.

Carrying Other People's Memories and Scars

It's easy to see how we carry the memories of our own experiences in our bodies. It takes a bit more of a leap to see and accept that we carry memories from other people as well. Strange as this sounds, it is demonstrably true.

The noted researcher Salvatore Minuchin conducted a notable study on what he called enmeshed family systems, families in which all the members function together almost as one being and one body. He described troubled families in which one member, frequently one child, becomes the repository of all the family trauma, which is symbolized by disease in this family member's body.[14]

Minuchin demonstrated that behavioral events that occur in a family can be physically measured in the bloodstreams of the family members. He placed a set of parents in a room, where they argued and bickered while their two daughters watched through a one-way mirror. One of the daughters was a brittle diabetic—one whose sugar cannot be balanced with insulin—who had visited hospital emergency rooms dozens of times in the course of a year. As this daughter watched her parents argue, she experienced a rise in her level of plasma free fatty acids (FFA), a biochemical indicator of emotional arousal or excitement. After some time, the daughters were called into the room with the parents. As soon as the girls came in, the parents stopped fighting with each other but began to vie for the emotional support of the diabetic daughter. Then the family's FFA was measured once again.[14]

Dramatically, the parents' levels had decreased to normal, as had the other daughter's. The FFA of the brittle diabetic daughter, however, remained greatly elevated, indicating that she was still highly stressed. It was apparent that this daughter deflected conflict from the others and served as a receptacle for the stress physiologically of the entire family. This stress expressed itself through her disease, diabetes. It was as if her body kept score in the arguments between her mother and father, and she carried the scars of trauma for the whole family.

Much has been written as well about telesomatic events, or instances in which one person can feel, in his or her own body, something that is happening or has happened to another person. In Minuchin's case, the daughter was in the room with her family, feeling what they were feeling. But many cases describe events where individuals *separated by great distances* feel identical sensations in their bodies. One woman was writing a letter to her daughter, who was away at college. In the middle of a sentence, she abruptly felt such a strong burning sensation in her right hand that she had to drop the pen. Within an hour, she received a telephone call from her daughter, who reported that she had severely burned her right hand with acid in the chemistry lab. The accident had occurred at the precise time when the mother was writing her a letter.[15]

I had a very similar haunting experience with my mother when I was hit by a truck while jogging. At the moment when I was getting ready to cross the bridge in Oregon where I was struck, my mother and father were attending a meeting of the historical society in their hometown all the way across the country on the East Coast. All at once, in the middle of the meeting, my mother stood up and said, "Ed, something's just happened to Mona Lisa." We know this happened, because it's right there in the historical society minutes. What's even more remarkable is the time, which is noted in the minutes, too. My mother's outburst occurred at the moment of impact, as her daughter was being hurled down a concrete escarpment 3,000 miles away.

Mother's intuition, which is particularly strong, stems from the mother-baby connection, the oneness a mother and child experience during the nine months of pregnancy. It's very common for pregnant women to have cravings that don't make any sense until after they've given birth to their children. When my mother was carrying me, she couldn't stand the smell of meat. Guess what? I was a vegetarian for many years. Pregnant women often have dreams about their babies' health. Their doctors take these dreams very, very seriously, because they don't want to get sued. Dreams, of course, are a part of the intuition network, and the doctors know there's a connection to the baby through the placenta and the umbilical cord.

After the baby's born, the physical umbilical cord is cut, but the emotional umbilical cord remains. Mothers always somehow know when something is not quite right with Johnny. This intuition drives millions of pediatricians crazy. But its validity is undeniable. And these incidents occur not just when Johnny's in the room with her but also when he's in the next room or 3,000 miles away on the other side of the continent.

Close connections of this sort also exist between twins and other siblings as well as husbands and wives. In fact, scientists assert that experiences of an intuitive nature about another person are increased by a physical or emotional or empathic connection to that person. Science has documented many other stories of telesomatic events. One woman told of experiencing numbness in her arm when her husband's arm was badly smashed on the job.[16] We've all heard stories of wives or fiancées or mothers knowing instantly when a soldier or a relative has been killed at war.

Clearly there is a human apparatus or technology, an intuition network, that makes such experiences possible. And clearly, therefore, a person with empathy and caring, like a medical intuitive, can make these same sorts of connections. I once did a reading of a woman whom I was finding very difficult to grasp. I was able to pick out some of the emotional concerns in her life, but I couldn't find anything significant in her body. As I was doing the reading, though, I found myself growing increasingly uncomfortable, feeling hot and flushed. I had to take off my sweater and get up and adjust the thermostat in the room. I noted, however, that it was set at a normal temperature. I got back on the phone and said to the woman, "I must be coming down with a cold, because I feel as though I have an incredible fever." And the moment I spoke those words I realized that this was precisely the woman's problem. She was suffering from fevers. I had picked up the memory from her life in my own body. And as soon as she confirmed it, the heat I was feeling dissipated.

We can take this phenomenon one step further. Science has puzzled over people with stigmata, the wounds of Jesus Christ, appearing on their hands and feet and the side of the body, and the marks of the crown of thorns on the head. We know that people have circuitry in their brains that can create ongoing changes in their bodies during times of stress. We can also create changes by will or through imagination. A famous experiment showed that a person can increase the temperature of his right hand by imagining it touching a hot stove. At the same time, he can lower the temperature of his left hand by imagining that it is holding an ice cube.[16]

This would indicate that by imagining and connecting empathically with someone, either in the brain or through whatever intuitive aperture you possess, your body can make a change that symbolizes the memories and the scars you are sensing from the other person. In the above reading, it's possible that my body felt that it was burning up because I was having an empathic feeling for the woman with the fevers. Therefore a mystic, whose empathy with God is so great, and who spends so much time trying to feel the pain of Christ and to experience it fully, may be able to call forth in her own body that pain as it was lived by Christ. And this may, as a result, be symbolized by the changes in her skin—the stigmata.[17]

Whether we call it a telesomatic event or empathy, an emotional umbilical cord does exist between people, and we pick up messages from one another. Some people are able to become more skilled at this than others, and they call this ability medical intuition. Some people have a somewhat greater innate capacity for intuition than others, in the same way that some people have innate musical ability while others do not. But most people have the ability to acquire more skill at anything they set their minds to learning. This is as true of intuition as it is of playing the piano.

Scars of Past Lives

Some people, including some medical intuitives, believe that we have all lived past lives and that our present bodies are still experiencing painful events that occurred to us during those lives. They believe our bodies are carrying the memories and scars of past traumas and that we have returned in our present lives to deal with those traumas once and for all.

I've had experiences of my own where I've seen the past lives of the people I'm reading. For instance, I did a reading of a woman I saw as being involved professionally in a highly structured and rigid organization, which I sensed was no longer right for her. She no longer felt that she fit in; membership in this organization was no longer fulfilling to her, and she needed to express herself more fully in the world and discover a new path for herself. The woman agreed with everything I had said, and then she revealed that she was in the military. She had repeatedly asked for transfers and new assignments in an effort to find her place within the army structure, but nothing had worked or quieted her restlessness.

In her body, I saw her as having a problem in her neck. I saw a huge red area on the left side of her neck. I couldn't figure out what it was. I didn't know whether it was her thyroid or simply inflammation or something else. She laughed when I told her this. That, she informed me, was a birthmark, a huge port-wine stain on the left side of her neck that traveled up into her face. As soon as she started to tell me this, I began to get pictures of her in battle in another time, being stabbed in the neck with a sword and spurting blood. But I did not tell her this. It would have made no sense for me to do so, for several reasons. First, the pictures I get are very much like scenes from a movie. They're disconnected from the present and don't have any meaning in the here and now. I believed it was more important for this woman to know that her ability to express herself fully in the military, *in this life,* was being stunted.

Knowing that she had been stabbed in battle in a past life is certainly interesting, and it might help explain why she joined the military. But this kind of understanding had nothing to do with helping her to heal her life in the present. You can't go back and talk to those people on the battlefield. They're gone, and there's nothing you can do about what happened to you in the eighteenth century. Churning through past lives could even have an effect very much like the one we saw in the women with breast cancer who tried to address an inescapable stress by marshaling their forces against it. What can you do about a past life? You can't do anything about it. You can't go back and say, "I'm not going into that battle, because I'm going to get stabbed in the neck and have a port-wine stain in a future life." You can *reframe* it, like any other memory, in terms of what importance or relevance it has in your life, but you can't cut it out or remove it. Dealing with the present and changing what needs to be changed in our lives *today* is the purpose of using our intuition to read our brains' and our bodies' signals and memories.

Health or Disease?

Memories are one of the cornerstones of the intuition network. Certain memories, as we've seen, can predispose us to health or disease. These memories reveal themselves in specific body symptoms, which we'll explore in greater detail in Part Two of this book. We can learn to use our intuition to get in touch with what those body symptoms mean, and to understand why and how our bodies talk to us when we're in a certain emotional situation or state.

Understanding that memories are stored both in our brains and in our bodies, and changing our perspective on them and the way we react to them in the outer world and in our inner world, can help determine whether we will enjoy health or endure disease.

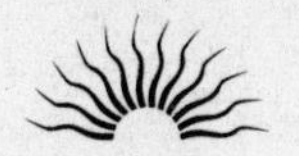

Part Two

The Inner Voice: The Language of Intuition

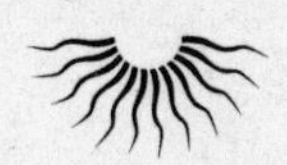

FIVE

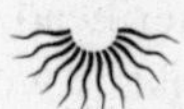

Body Language: The Meaning of Health and Disease

"Why me?"

It's the first question we ask when illness strikes. At a loss to understand what's happening to us, we let the questions fly. Why did this happen to me? Why now? Why can't I get better? Who can help me? Illness seems random, inexplicable, and the answers of science still limited and unsatisfying.

In truth, however, these questions *can* be answered. In many cases, the situations that set the scene for an illness can be traced and understood. Finding them means tapping into the intuition network. It means learning the language of your body and what it seeks to tell you through the memories and emotions collected and stored in all your organs over the course of a lifetime.

When we succumb to disease, our overwhelming instinct is to seek a medical cure, relief of the physical symptoms that are causing us pain and discomfort. At the very least, we want escape from that pain. All too often, however, we end up merely numbing the pain, ignoring the symptoms, and, as a result, silencing the very voice that is trying to help us find a way out of the situation that underlies our present distress.

I once treated a woman whose case I've come to view as a powerful example of this kind of escapism. She was a widow in her seventies whose daughter brought her to the hospital because she was suffering from weakness in her legs and had repeatedly fallen during the past few days. Several doctors, including a rheumatologist and a neurologist, had examined her and had been unable to find anything physically wrong. They suspected a conversion disorder, a psychological problem that manifests itself as a loss of physical function—that is to say, they thought it was all in her head.

I was called in to do a psychiatric workup. The woman was calmly sitting in a chair, showing no signs of disturbance or anxiety over her inability to walk. She insisted that she was not depressed, that pain was no longer a problem. She simply was unable to do anything for herself and needed total care. Her daughter told me privately, however, that for the last few weeks, her mother had been withdrawn, shown little appetite, and been given to bouts of crying. These were all clear signs of depression.

Her chart indicated that she had chronic pain and fibromyalgia and had also developed diabetes. Two years earlier she had been brought to the hospital after taking an overdose of a diabetes medication and falling into a coma. When she came to, she had writhed in pain from her fibromyalgia and declared, "I can't handle it anymore." She demanded and received painkillers. In fact, I was stunned to see that she had been on a potent painkiller *for the last six years.* She had been taking the drug so long that she was addicted to it. Her chronic pain, however, was hardly being dealt with if she was on around-the-clock painkillers. Moreover, she wasn't confronting the problems that lay behind the chronic pain.

I ran a few psychological tests and determined that she did indeed have a mild to moderate dementia and had problems remembering. She was also slightly delirious from all the painkillers. We were going to have to slowly get her off the painkillers in order to determine what was really wrong with her. The nurses began to cut back on the pills. The next day I was called in urgently to see her. The nurses reported that the patient was delirious and having hallucinatory conversations with pets and people who were nowhere present.

I went into her room. She was sitting up in bed alone. There wasn't another soul in the vicinity.

"How are you, Mrs. Brown?" I asked pleasantly. She answered just as pleasantly. "Oh, I'm fine, Doctor. I was just about to have lunch." Then she stopped, glanced sharply to her left, and then looked back at me apologetically. "Excuse me, Doctor, just a second." She turned to her left again and spoke into thin air, addressing her daughter, the one who had reported to me the previous day that her mother was depressed and lonely.

"I am sick and tired of you," Mrs. Brown declared in sharp tones. "I'm sick and tired of the fact that you are trying to control my life. You say you're trying to help me, but you're controlling my life. I will not have you interrupting this conversation with this doctor, and I'm going to ask you to stop it right now. You are not going to rule my life anymore." She turned back to me with a sheepish smile. "I'm so sorry, Doctor," she said. "My daughter is very, very rude."

It was a startling scene—and an extraordinarily revealing one. Obviously the patient had a profound psychological conflict with her daughter, and most likely, by extension, with herself. She had been unable to articulate or even to confront her feelings about her daughter's behavior, her overdependence on her family, and her emotions had been shunted into her body in the form of a conversion disorder that had robbed her of locomotion and normal physical function. It was highly probable, however, that the unacknowledged conflict of dependency also underlay the patient's earlier problems with chronic pain. Yet she had so feared listening to what her body was telling her that *for six years* she had drowned out its voice—and the voice of her intuition—by loading herself with medication, masking the memories and the emotions in her body and numbing the pain that was a steady warning signal that something was wrong in her life. She had ignored the rattle in her bodily engine until at last her transmission fell out, and she was literally unable to move.

When we cut back her medication, something happened. The numbness began to recede, and the pain, the memories, and the emotions began to resurface. In the slight delirium caused by withdrawal from her medication, the patient was able to speak freely, without inhibition. At long last she was able to talk about what was really upsetting her. With luck, emotional support, and time, perhaps she could begin to work it out and thereby work her way out of her physical situation as well.

Simply drugging the symptoms of illness is not only ultimately ineffective, it can be truly counterproductive. Health and disease are ways through which our bodies speak to us, telling us what's right and wrong in our lives, what's good and should be preserved and strengthened, and what's bad and needs to be reevaluated and adjusted.

BODY TALK

How many times have you uttered phrases like the following: "I feel it in my bones," "I know it in my gut," "My heart is full," "That makes my blood boil"?

We all say these things without thinking. They're phrases so time-worn they've become clichés, but they show that we listen to the messages our bodies speak to us. What we think and feel and see and hear is affecting our body organs constantly. Some event or person or emotion can make your blood boil, and the boiling can literally appear on your skin in the form of hives, as happened to the woman with mother-in-law problems. That was the language of her body, reporting on an emotional problem that was affecting both her emotional life and her physical health.

Some popular books have appeared in recent years about animals and how you can learn to understand the language they speak. You can learn "cat" and "dog" and how to communicate with your pets on their own level, to read the signals of their behavior and actions so that you will understand what they're trying to tell you and how to respond to their needs and wants. If you can learn "cat," then you can certainly learn "body." You can learn to understand the language your own body uses to communicate to you the needs and wants you are fulfilling or failing to fulfill. I'm talking not just about physical needs but about emotional needs as well, because the language of our bodies is actually part of the larger language of intuition and the soul, part of the intuition network, broadcasting vital information about our lives as a whole.

Our bodies speak to us every day in every way, through their own vocabulary of symptoms tied to emotions and memories from the past and the present. We can learn to read those symptoms in the same way we learn to read signals in relationships or other areas of our lives. It's like the boss and his secretary who are having problems they never discuss. They go along for months and months, and everything seems fine on the surface. The secretary may call in sick for half a week; she comes back, and they go along again. But then she calls in sick for a week, and it's obvious she's not sick. Again they ignore it when she returns. After the third time, however, the secretary quits because she feels her boss won't address the problems and she feels she can't address them herself. Hopefully, both boss and secretary will learn from this episode that they have to pay attention to the signals of conflict before it's too late to do anything about the fundamental issue.

Everyone has issues in his or her life about which the body speaks most loudly. Based on my experiences, I now consider myself fluent in several body dialects. I speak fluent immunologicalese. I know the language of my white cells, when they've had it and are about to snap. I can actually feel my white blood count going down as a cold or bronchitis comes on. I am also fluent in the dialect of "disk." When I get numbness in my hands, I can read the quality, intensity, and frequency of it as signifying that various things are going on in my life. And I pay close attention whenever my disks start talking in any way. Recently, for the first time in years, I dreamed about contact lenses. It was the old dream, that I was trying to get the lenses into my eyes, and they were huge. I just about managed to get them in, but it was very tough. I woke up in a fright. What on earth did that mean? I didn't think it signified a problem with my neck, as it had in the past, when swollen contact lens dreams had to do with swollen disks in my spine. The emotion related to this dream had to do with learning how to express myself and what I do in the world confidently, freely, and at the right time. This time I had no pain in my neck. I wondered whether I had recently made the right decision about a job, but that seemed all right to me as well. Then I went in for surgery on my nose, to repair an old injury. I had to go into the operating room without my contacts. The next day, when I tried to put my contacts in, I wasn't able to, because my eyes were nearly swollen shut. Of course, *that* was the meaning of the dream! So I didn't try to force the lenses into my eyes. I was relieved to know that the language in this case wasn't signaling a problem in my spine, but it was vitally important that the dream made me sit up, take notice, and take stock once again of all that was happening in my life.

If your body wants to get your attention, it's not going to speak a language you can't understand. It will use symbols and symptoms that are somehow familiar to you. You may also find you can communicate more clearly with certain parts of your body than with others. I have lots of communication with my spine but not so much with my pelvis. A colleague at work is intimately familiar with the language of her bowels. When she feels a burning sensation in her bowels, she knows it has something to do with her assuming responsibility that is not hers.

The language of each individual's body has its own unique dialect, and you have to learn the specific symbolism and symptoms of your own body. At the same time, certain universal symbols apply to everyone. Almost from the beginning of time, people have noted that certain emotions appear to be attached to certain organs or areas of the body while other emotions affect the body more generally. As we go through life, amassing experiences, feeling emotions, and creating and storing memories, the language of our bodies develops and evolves.

THE EMOTIONAL DIMENSION

Everything that we see, hear, or feel has an emotional dimension to it. Everything in life is tinged with love or joy, anger or sadness, fear or shame, and so on. Depending upon your own experiences, you have a pattern of seeing certain things in certain ways. This pattern helps to shape your personality and affects how you live your life, what choices you make in relationships, careers, and everything else. It's a pattern encoded in memory in both your brain and your body.

Certain emotions are more strongly empatterned in memories than others. These emotions are also not localizable; they don't correspond to specific organ systems but can be stored anywhere in the body. One such emotion is fear. We all know the feeling of fear. When we see or hear something frightening the image is encoded and travels to the amygdala in the brain, which applies an emotional response and tags the experience, giving it a label that says "fear." The amygdala then sends the signal of the fearful memory to the hypothalamus, which is the master switch plate for the body. The hypothalamus empatterns the fear in certain *body responses.* Certain hormones go up or down, your blood pressure goes up or down, your heart rate changes, your immune system changes. Fear, in other words, doesn't just affect your emotional behavior; it also causes changes in the way your organs behave.

Some people are afraid of elevators; some people are afraid of snakes. Other people are afraid to speak in public, or they have agoraphobia and are afraid to go outside. Fear goes directly to the body and stimulates a fight or flight attitude. So you try to escape from the podium and giving that speech, you try to run away from that man who looks like your ex-husband, or you try to run from the kind of love you've found painful in the past. Once you experience something as frightening, your brain and body never forget it, even if you don't remember it consciously. The amygdala has recorded the body memories.[1] As a result, whatever fears you have will always affect your behavioral patterns and your unconscious plans. You may not even be aware of some of the fears you have, but they may be changing your organ behavior and body behavior all the same.

You can reframe your memories and work your way around your fear, but the fear itself will be there your whole life. I did a reading of a woman whom I saw as having a lump in her throat. I didn't see it as a tumor or mass, but it was a clear lump. I told her that I felt she had fears related to expression and that these were lifelong fears, symbolized by this lump in her throat. I was surprised when she became very angry with me. "I don't have a fear of speaking," she said indignantly. "I used to, but I don't anymore. I've overcome it, and in fact I now teach people how to communicate and get over their fear." She admitted that she had a lump in her throat, but she insisted that it was a tumor, even though various CT scans and MRIs had failed to diagnose a tumor of any kind. She could not accept that the lump was associated with her fear of expression and communication. A year and a half later this woman called me again. She had been working intensively with a new therapist. She told me she now realized that when she felt a lump in her throat, it was the way her body experienced the emotions of fear and anxiety. These emotions were not all in her head, they were also in her throat—in her body. Whenever she felt that lump, she now understood that her body was telling her she had something important to express, something that might not always be well received, but that it was vital to her health, creativity, and vitality to pursue. The lump in her throat was the warning sign that she needed to be well prepared for any external lumps or blockades to her ideas.

Once a fear is within you, however, it's always there. You can take a so-called counterphobic approach to it and confront the fear. For example, I'm afraid of heights. This is a fear that's empatterned, as anybody with a fear of heights can tell you. Once you get up high somewhere, you heart races, your knees tremble, your palms sweat. The autonomic nervous system, your visceral brain, is transferring the fear to your amygdala, and the amygdala is waking up all the body memories. I went on a hike up the Blue Skyline Trail outside Boston and joined a group of people rappelling down the mountain. I remember looking over the edge and watching these figures flying down the side of the mountain attached to ropes that looked about the size and strength of dental floss. My body kept speaking to me, saying, "Fear fear fear fear fear," through my shaking knees, sweating palms, and dry mouth. The instructor came over and asked me if I was ready to try it. My brain said, "Let's go to McDonald's instead," but my mouth said, "Yes." And so I went down the cliff with my heart in my throat. I "overcame" my fear. But I didn't get rid of it.

You can't excise or purge a fear, because it's empatterned in your brain and your body. Trying to do that is like trying to stop little boys from hitting each other. In moments of stress, a fear or phobia will come out. You can learn to work around a phobia, but only after you have come to understand and accept that it is always there and always has the potential to affect your life and your body.

Anxiety is very closely aligned with fear, but it is in fact a very different emotion. Fear is usually about one thing; it's tied to a single specific stimulus or object. Anxiety is a fear of everything. Anxiety has more to do with thoughts, whereas fear has to do with feelings. A person with anxiety has a sort of gerbil wheel in her head, where she thinks, "If this, then this, then this," and she keeps going around and around endlessly with her thoughts. Fear and anxiety also have different patterns in the brain and the body, because different kinds of memories and a different kind of chemistry are associated with each one.

Another significant emotion affecting the brain and the body is depression, which is closely aligned with grief and sadness. Depression is one of the strongest emotions in the intuition network, and learning the language of it can be extremely useful. Certain studies show that when you're depressed, an area in the brain called the cingulate gyrus, which is part of your limbic system, or your headquarters for feelings, initially goes through a phase when it's very fired up. It crackles away like popcorn in the microwave, telling you that something needs to be addressed. You may be agitated, or you may be angry; you are, in any case, experiencing an emotion with great intensity.

This will go on for some time. Eventually, however, if the depression continues and deepens, this area actually burns out. Now your cingulate gyrus goes to sleep. The initial message your brain was sending gets repressed because you have not heeded it. Your frontal lobe also burns down, until you're unable to get in touch with the emotion or talk about it.

This is similar to what happens in people with obsessive-compulsive disorder. The same area of the brain is hyperactive, causing them to check things constantly or to wash their hands every few minutes. This kind of behavior is driven by a desire to soothe an emotion—fear—which has been repressed. Eventually the behavior gets out of hand, because the patient can't cover up his fear. He repeats the behavior so many times that it becomes hard-wired and uncontrollable. His body is expressing an emotion that his brain can't talk about. This occurs in many other situations as well. Say Johnny is a nervous three-year-old who keeps putting his thumb in his mouth. Initially, if you ask him why he's sucking his thumb, he'll be able to tell you that it's because his daddy left home, because he's hungry, or because his parents are arguing. You'll know, then, that his body is communicating an emotion, that every time Johnny puts his thumb in his mouth, he's anxious. Thirty-five years later, John is at work and he notices that he's always putting his hand in his mouth. *But he won't know why*. By this time, however, the behavior has taken on a life of its own, and it has become disconnected from the emotion that spawned it.

What happens when you're chronically depressed? Your body starts to express the emotion that your depression was initially trying to signal you. You might not be able to talk about it, but your body talks instead. Your sleep is disturbed; you lose your appetite. You release excess cortisol, a stress hormone, and this suppresses your immune system. Your body becomes defenseless, so you might get pneumonia or even cancer. Many studies have shown that unresolved grief and depression are related to specific cancers.[2] Which organ is affected by cancer will depend on what situation you're going to be around—family, job, or a relationship. It also depends upon your own innate vulnerability and your past feelings, experiences, and memories. It's true for everyone, though, that if you don't fully process and release what you're sad about, you could change the function of your body in significant ways. The woman I described at the beginning of this chapter was clearly depressed, yet hadn't been able to talk about her situation. Unable to talk about her depression, it got converted into her body, so that she quite literally got paralyzed by her sadness. The emotional paralysis became physical paralysis, and her legs and body literally could not move.

Another client, Melissa, was able to break out of her paralyzed emotional state and her overdependence on her family by focusing her full attention on her depression. While her solution is not for everyone, I think the kind of clarity of intent to heal herself that she mustered is instructive. Melissa checked herself into a hospital for five days and scheduled intensive therapy for herself and group therapy with her family. She discussed with her therapist how to take steps to restructure her life and gain independence from her family. She decided to try a course of antidepressants under the close supervision of her physician to jump-start her body and mind out of the physical effects in which the depression had mired her. She also worked with a social worker, who got her a volunteer job as a reader for the elderly in a local nursing home. This took her out of her usual routine and gave her a sense that she could help other people. She also had a consultation with a dietitian, who helped her see how to change the way she ate. When Melissa was depressed, she ate more, which made her gain weight, which made her more depressed.

The Positive Emotions

Joy, passion, love, and happiness are what our society calls positive emotions. These emotions signal us that we're on the right path. Physiologically, positive emotions are not localizable in the body in the same way that negative emotions like anger and hostility are. When we feel these positive emotions genuinely—that is, when we don't use them falsely to varnish grief, sadness, anger, or shame, and as long as we don't suffer from inflationary or manic delusions—we can generally trust that our lives are in balance. We need to work to acknowledge the whole gamut of emotions that affect our lives, however; an overabundance of either side of the emotional spectrum is not healthy. Women who hide anger, sadness, or grief behind a brave, stoic, or ever-cheerful face have been shown in the medical literature to have a higher incidence of breast cancer. They try to stay in the joy lane of the highway of life instead of paying attention to the congestion or accidents or roadblocks that come before them and maneuvering their car skillfully around them. In a comparative fourth emotional center issue, men who get heart attacks are frequently described in case studies as having overexpressed but unresolved hostility—they are stuck in a rut in the other emotional lane. These men and women are allowing themselves to experience only a limited polarity of their emotional potential. Neither is creating health.

Body Mechanics

How do emotions get transformed into symptoms in the body? When we're under stress, or feeling certain stressful emotions, our brains release the hormone cortisol. Chronic stress or any chronic emotion—anger, hostility, fear, or sadness—is an important factor that will cause the body's adrenal glands to start to express those emotions in symptoms mediated by cortisol. Chronically elevated levels of cortisol are known to change the behavior of certain organs. The arteries begin to get stiff and hardened (arteriosclerosis). Hostility, a specific form of anger, is an emotion that's associated with hardening of the arteries.[3] Chronically elevated cortisol has also been related to cancer.[2] The cancer can affect various organs depending on what situations or settings the emotions occur in.

The immune system, however, requires adequate levels of cortisol to function properly. This means that we need a certain amount of stress or stimulation in our lives to function efficiently and to feel alive. Otherwise we go to sleep. What constitutes an adequate level varies from person to person. I went to the gym one day with a friend, ostensibly to relax and get rid of some stress. My friend worked out on the treadmill while glancing at the television set every once in a while. I was going 100 miles an hour on the stationary bicycle while at the same time reading the newspaper, listening to music on my headphones, and watching TV. Even while relaxing, I still needed three times as much stimulus as she to keep going.

Excessive cortisol, however, can rev up the immune system dangerously.[4] Say you have a fear, but you ignore it and ignore your body telling you to stay away from that cliff. In fact, you purposely head for every metaphorical cliff you see. You take jobs that aren't good for you; you repeatedly date people who treat you badly. You're constantly living on the edge of the cliff of fear and ignoring your body's language of fear—trembling knees, racing heart, and sweaty palms. You have a cold all the time, and you're not listening to your body saying, "I'm stressed." So your body begins to interpret the whole world, not just the cliff, as something to be feared. It secretes more cortisol and begins to make immune cells and molecules against all the dangers out there, real and imagined, reacting as though the outer world were a giant petri dish of bacteria. You wind up making immune cells against everything. This is what happens with people who get chronic colds, chronic bronchitis, or chronic fatigue. Ultimately, because they're making so many excess antibodies, the antibodies turn against the body itself. The result is autoimmune disease, such as rheumatoid arthritis, lupus, or vasculitis.

Alternatively, after living so constantly near the metaphorical cliff, you become emotionally and physically tired of the struggle. Your body can't keep producing armor and weapons against the world it fears as being inescapably threatening. It eventually can't produce cortisol and immune cells in wartime amounts. The levels of these go down, and you become chronically depressed. Your body minerals become exhausted from constantly waging this war against an enemy that is mostly in your mind and your body-mind's traumatic memories. Ironically, the exhaustion of fighting an imagined war leaves you defenseless. Having exhausted your ammunition and dropped all your bombs, you're now a sitting duck for a *real* enemy that can invade your environment and attack you. You've unwittingly set the scene for infections and possibly tumors.

One way or another, when certain stressful or traumatic emotions or memories live in us, and we fail to deal with them, they find ways of making their presence known. Body symptoms become the language that tells us we need to change something.

Emotions and Illness

For more than two thousand years humans have observed that certain emotions appear to be related to certain organs in the body.[5] In Chinese medicine, for instance, the heart is equated with fire, and its associated emotions are joy and happiness. The liver and gallbladder are equated with wood and are related to the emotions of frustration and anger. The lungs and large intestine are equated with metal and have to do with worry and grief. The spleen and stomach are associated with earth and with overthinking, overworrying, or ruminating. Is it just a coincidence that cows, the original ruminators, have an auxiliary stomach?

In the early 1980s the medical intuitive Louise Hay theorized that certain illnesses are related to certain emotions.[6] Many of her theories have been upheld by scientific studies. For instance, she maintained that being accident-prone was related to a certain emotional pattern: being unable to speak up for onself, being in rebellion against authority, and believing in violence. Several studies have in fact shown that accidents, especially in children and families, are related to impulsiveness and resentment of authority. Hay related AIDS to a sense of defenselessness and hopelessness. The literature shows that a feeling of hopelessness and inescapable stress, a lack of a sense of security and safety in the world, is related to a breakdown of the immune system. Hay also believed that lower back problems may be related to emotions involving money and a fear of losing financial support. Guess what? A wide range of studies suggests that people who suffer from lower back pain also have emotional struggles related to their employment or work.[7] Lower back pain, in fact, is one of the leading causes of workmen's disability. Hay thought that Parkinson's disease was associated with fear and an intense desire to control everything and everyone. Studies have supported this link, showing that patients who develop Parkinson's disease have a lifelong pattern of believing that it's their obligation to uphold standards of morality and to champion them to their families and society.[8] The many studies that support Hay's theories, in fact, are gratifying proof that intuition—the information that comes to an intuitive or to an individual about certain emotions and their relation to physical illness—can be supported by scientific research.

Louise Hay's system is at bottom elegantly simple. Hay essentially looked at each organ system, observed its function, and correlated that with an emotional experience in our lives. Thus she sees illness in the bowel, which releases waste, as having to do with issues of letting go of the old and what's no longer needed. Problems in the breast, the source of nourishment, have to do with a failure to nourish oneself and always taking care of others first. Blood problems, including poor circulation and anemia, have to do with a lack of joy in life.

Much of Hay's system overlaps with Chinese medicine.[9,5] The Chinese have also observed that problems in a given organ are related to an emotional behavior or condition that mirrors the organ's function. Problems in the small intestine, which sorts out the nutrients that come into the digestive system, are related to issues of "sorting out" in the patient's life. People who think too much, ruminate too much, have stomach problems. Seeing this takes not much more than simple common sense. And intuition is common sense at its most basic level.

Other, independent scientific studies have also indicated that certain emotional and psychological patterns are associated with diseases in specific organs. For example, early sexual abuse can set the scene for chronic pelvic pain in women,[10] and childhood sexual abuse is associated with ailments in the genitals or urinary tract. Women who stay in a relationship that's not nurturing or supportive have been shown to have an increased risk of breast cancer.[11] Hostility has been correlated with increased risk of heart attack.[12]

Other studies have shown that gastrointestinal disorders, asthma, Parkinson's disease, Grave's disease, multiple sclerosis, infertility, heart disease, and many other illnesses also have distinct emotional counterparts. The data can be inconsistent, however, and many individuals who suffer from these illnesses don't exhibit the typical emotional characteristics that the research claims they should. As I said earlier, your body's language is uniquely yours. You need to decipher the way in which your individual body communicates past and present emotional experiences through feeling, sensation, pain, and disease.

THE BODY'S EMOTIONAL CENTERS

Eastern philosophies and religions have described an anatomical structure of seven emotional centers in the body. Each of these centers encompasses a particular group of organs and is associated with a given set of emotions. These emotional centers, or hubs, also reflect and symbolize our emotional and psychological development from birth to death. The subsequent chapters of this section are organized along the lines of these emotional centers and their associated emotions and illnesses. You will need to view the universal rules in light of your specific situation, but you can use them as a springboard to help you find the key to your own intuitive guidance system.

Each emotional center is characterized by a set of contrasting emotions. One of these emotions expresses itself in terms of power, or assertiveness, and makes us appear more powerful and strong in the outer world (yang). The other emotion can be perceived as vulnerability, but it actually endows us with power and strength in the inner world (yin). Thus we would have fearlessness (power) versus fearfulness (vulnerability), assertiveness versus submissiveness, willfulness versus compliance, and so on. In each center, we can determine whether most of our strength and health is connected to the power side or the vulnerability side. We need a balance of both for optimum health. If you have a great imbalance between the two, or only one or the other, then the scientific literature suggests that you're setting the scene for greater susceptibility to illness in the organs of that emotional center.

The first center contains the emotions that affect body structure, your physical framework, including the skeletal system, the blood, and the immune system. Metaphorically this center also has to do with the framework of your life, that which gives you the structure of your identity, starting with family and branching out to church, work, and various other organizations and institutions. The issues that affect this body area have to do with feelings of independence versus dependence, capability versus helplessness, hopefulness versus hopelessness, fearlessness versus fearfulness, and trust versus mistrust.

The second emotional center is in the pelvis. Of its two parts, one part has to do with our drives—what sends us out into the world in search of fulfillment. These drives include sex, money, and creativity or fertility. Issues associated with these drives also have to do with holding on or letting go, being able to separate from the family of origin. The memories and behavior patterns that affect organs here have to do with following a drive to go after what you want versus feeling guilty about going after what you want. The other part of this second emotional center has to do with relationships, the capacity to be an individuated, solitary person set against the ability to be in an intimate relationship with someone outside of your family. The organs affected by memories and behavioral patterns in this emotional center are the lower gastrointestinal tract, the bladder and urinary tract, the lower back, and the reproductive organs.

The third center is in the middle abdomen and gastrointestinal tract, covering the intestines, stomach, pancreas, kidneys, spleen, liver, and gallbladder. It's associated with emotional issues and patterns of behavior relating to choosing a role in society, acquiring and harnessing the skills for that role, and becoming competent in that line of work.

The chest area houses the fourth emotional center, which encompasses the heart, the lungs, and the breasts. This region has to do with emotional expression, with love and passion. It also has to do with partnership and the extent of intimacy and emotional expression we're able to establish in marriage and love relationships. Where the relationship issue in the second emotional center has to do with the ability to maintain your individuality within a relationship, the partnership issue of the fourth emotional center has to do with allowing yourself to become one with the other person. The issues related to this center have to do with love, hostility, intimacy, martyrdom, and nurturance, which is a form of emotional expression for many women.

The fifth center is in the thyroid, neck vertebrae, teeth, mouth, and gums. This area is concerned with communication and expression and with asserting one's will in the outer world.

The area around the head, including the brain, eyes, ears, and nose, is the sixth center, associated with matters related to perception, including paranoia, and knowledge and wisdom versus ignorance.

The final energy center encompasses the muscles, connective tissues, and genes. The emotions and behavioral patterns tied to this center have to do with a sense of purpose in life and a sense of connection to God or the divine, versus feeling existential and alone. Other issues revolve around feelings of unlimited possibility in the world as opposed to a sense of despair and predestination.

Your Personality and Your Health

Doctors and scientists have long known that people with certain temperaments are more prone to certain diseases than to others. For example, much has been written about the male type A personality, which is prone to heart disease.[13] The heart is associated with emotions and passion—hate versus love, hostility versus empathy—in Chinese medicine and in Louise Hay's system. Type A individuals experience extreme emotion, in the form of rage and hostility, and they have difficulty expressing joy and passion. The scientific literature shows that excessive hostility, with its concomitant deficiency in joy, is associated with excess levels of cholesterol and sudden death from heart attacks.[12] What situations and memories set the scene for an individual to express emotion chiefly through rage and hostility and to have difficulty experiencing love and passion? If the person with this problem could find the answer to that question and understand it, he could create better health. The excess cholesterol is his heart's way of crying out, "Warning, warning! This is not the way I want to be. Surely there's another way of being."

Each of our emotional centers corresponds to a certain universal set of emotions. But also housed in each center are specific memories of each person's specific, individual life experiences. Each emotional center corresponds to a stage of psychological and emotional development. As you grow through life, these emotional centers are formed in a continuous building process that progresses from past to present to future to the end of life. The nature of the centers and their significance to your health is determined in much the same way that your personality is formed by the experiences you have in your life. Depending on what happens to you at each stage of your development, the organs of the emotional center corresponding to that stage may be affected in very specific ways, and the memories of those experiences are laid down to affect the developmental stages and emotional areas that come later.

For instance, the first emotional center has to do with the framework and the base of support that we receive in the family. Within the structure of the family, where our basic needs as children are met, we learn to trust and to feel safe, or we fail to learn trust and come to feel that the world will never be a safe place. We learn how to help ourselves, or we learn to be helpless. This has been noted by neurologists and psychologists in the past. This is the "us" stage, when the child is still undifferentiated from the mother or others and has no true sense of self. What we get in this first stage of development is critical to our future and will affect everything that happens to us in later stages and how our bodies will speak to us. Think of life as a Monopoly game. We all start out in the same place on the board, with the same amount of money. But what if, on your very first throw of the dice, you have to go to jail and pay a $200 fine? It's safe to say that you won't thereafter feel very safe on the board of life. What's more, you've already lost some of your money—that is, the resources you had to start with. Your further play along the board of life will be hampered because of your earliest experiences. The memories of this experience are then encoded in your brain and your body, in the tissues of your organs, and they will remain there to return to the surface if and when events recalling these early experiences occur later in your life. They will also affect what happens to you in each subsequent stage of your life. Suppose a tiny child is the only person to survive a flood in which his entire family dies. You can easily see that this person's approach to the next turn around the board of life is going to be different from that of people whose families loved and supported them; he's going to be more hesitant, take fewer risks. His ability to form relationships with others, in the second stage, will be affected, as will the organs in the second emotional center, and so on up the line.

The second emotional center is double-sided. The first side is related to what drives us in life and to holding on versus letting go. This is where we begin to differentiate ourselves from others; we go from "us" to "you versus me versus us." Early neurologists and psychologists have noted that a child learns when to hold on to his parents and when to let go and walk away at the same time that bowel development occurs. They noted that issues involving holding on or letting go, impulsiveness versus inhibition, often affect people who also have bowel and bladder problems. The other side of this emotional center has to do with relationships—the capacity to be an autonomous individual versus the capacity to be in a relationship with another person outside the family. We now focus on the opposite sex and struggles for power and position. This is a tough stage for many women, who have difficulty distinguishing "you" and "me" from "us." Neurologists, psychiatrists, and OB-GYNs have long noted that these issues are related to health or disease in the sex organs.

In the third center, the child is old enough to go out and play or go to school. He sees things in terms of "me against the world." This is the phase where, having given up on understanding sex, we throw ourselves into our work. Here, psychiatrists have noted, we experience a conflict between initiative and guilt and between industry and inferiority.

The fourth emotional center—in the heart, lungs, and breasts—revolves around the paradigm of "You and I are one." Having spent our lives trying to learn to be individuals in the outer world, we now turn around and head back into oneness with another or others. But we still retain a sense of autonomy, so that if one person leaves, be it a spouse or partner or child, we are still left with an "I" that can stand alone. Psychiatrists describe this stage as "intimacy versus isolation."

The fifth emotional center, in the neck and mouth, involves communication, expression, and asserting one's will. "I will" is its mantra. Psychiatrists describe it in terms of "generativity versus stagnation."

In the sixth center, in the head and organs of perception, we have reached the stage where, like Descartes, we say, "I think, therefore I am."

Finally, in the seventh emotional center, we're dealing with the whole body. At this stage, we should be able to say, "God and I are one," and we understand that all of life has a given purpose. We also understand, after a lifetime of learning about the function of family and relationships, that ultimately each of us is alone in the world.

In this fashion, our society attaches certain meanings to certain organs, which are then overlaid by our personal experience, to give each organ a meaning that's specific to each of us as an individual. As you explore these connections, you can begin to see how your personality, the person you become as you move through life, is intertwined with your health and what happens to you physically. What happens to you at each stage affects the memories you form, modifies the way you develop further, and influences the health of every organ in your body.

As you examine your life and health in terms of the organs and emotional centers presented in this book, you can take stock of your powers and vulnerabilities in each area to help you determine how best you can cope with and adapt to improve your life and health. Reflect on the associations that the case studies and client readings bring up for you. See if any of the emotional patterns you read about feel familiar. As you do this, you will be getting in touch with your mind-body intuition network.

Think again of your life as a set of encyclopedias. We all hope to amass a full set of volumes as we proceed through life, but sometimes we miss one volume or another. When I was growing up in the 1960s, you used to be able to buy encyclopedias in the supermarket, one volume a week. But if you went away on vacation, you might miss a volume, and it might never become available again. Then you had to fill in the gaps left by the missing volume using other means or sources. Or imagine that you are taking trigonometry in high school. Your family has just moved to a new home, and you've missed the first three weeks of school—the critical weeks when the foundation for the entire trig course was laid. Now you have to acquire the missing information as best you can and catch up with the rest of the class. You can do that, but you'll always be missing that solid foundation, as would someone who missed out on the strong sense of safety and security that underlies the first emotional center.

This is what happens to us in life; we're strong in some emotional centers, weak in others. I'm very strong in the third emotional center, for instance. I have a cast-iron stomach and a solid sense of self-esteem and responsibility. I'm sure of my roles as a physician, scientist, and medical intuitive, and I have been sure of myself and my life's purpose and profession since the age of seven. I've worked hard to acquire skill and competence in these roles. My problems are mostly in my bones, or my first emotional center, because I've never had a firm sense of support in the world. I think the people I love and count on will disappear at any moment. I don't want to depend on anyone, and it's difficult for me to accept help. In fact, I could even say that in a sense I grew from the top down, as in a pattern that Joan Borysenko, the noted biological psychologist, calls "reverse shaman." From earliest childhood, even though I felt alone in the world, alone in my family, and separate from others on the earth (first emotional center), I've felt a strong connection to things in the heavens (seventh emotional center). I've always talked to God and have seen him everywhere—in the wind and the trees and all around me. And because I was taught that God made everything, including the trees, then I believe I must be part of the trees and that we are all a part of God. I've also always been good at "I think, therefore I am" (sixth emotional center). My mother says I used to spend hours in the playpen, just sitting and thinking. She also says I was very willful (fifth emotional center) from the start, so obviously I have no problem with "I will"—except that I perhaps overdid it. When I start getting into trouble is when we get down below the waist.

Most people, though, grow from the first emotional center upward. And what we're aiming for, as we move through life, is a *balance* in each stage. In each energy center we all experience both strength and weakness—*power* and *vulnerability*. It's important that we experience *both* of these, in balanced measure. Being too vulnerable in an energy center obviously creates problems. Being too powerful or strong, however, means that you have no room to grow and develop in that area of your life. You'll become pinched and pained, like a child with shoes that don't provide any growing room. The type A personality, with all of its *powerful* rage and hostility and its insufficient *vulnerability* in terms of love and nurturance, is prone to sudden death from heart attack. But the type D personality—who has a marked tendency toward martyrdom, has a hard time expressing emotion, and isolates himself from others—is also prone to heart disease.[13] What both need is a balance, an ability to feel emotions fully, express them fully, and then release them fully. We need both the yin of vulnerability and the yang of power in all the organs of our bodies in order for them to function optimally.

In addition, we all do two things in our continuing effort to become whole. We *cope* and we *adapt*. We have to find the right combination of these two actions to make our lives work as smoothly as possible. *Coping* is the ability to change or manipulate our environment in our own interests, so that it will serve us better. *Adapting* is changing ourselves to fit into our environment and improve our lives. It's fairly easy to see that in our society, women adapt more readily than men, who are more inclined to cope. Generally, with some exceptions, women are like Camelot's Guinevere, understanding the strength of being able to depend on someone in a relationship and to be vulnerable. But they have difficulty with power and assertiveness. In contrast, men are like Lancelot, more comfortable with power and assertiveness and changing the world than with allowing themselves to be vulnerable and to need others in a relationship. Too much success and satisfaction can be enervating and weakening, however, while some deprivation can help drive us to develop strength.

Accepting Your Role in Your Own Health

Once, after attending a lecture on medical intuition, I was invited onstage with several other medical professionals to talk about intuition and health. In the middle of the discussion, a member of the audience got up and insisted, quite heatedly, that we were all blaming the victim, with our theories that illness was related to memories in the body and how people dealt with their emotions. This man himself suffered from chronic fatigue, and he resented the implication, he said, that he had somehow brought it upon himself.

Although at first I was taken aback by his assertions, I could see his point. Let's look at it from the purely scientific, mainstream medical perspective. Suppose you're a middle-aged, overweight man who smokes and whose father died of a heart attack. In addition, you fight a lot with your wife, who claims you have a chip on your shoulder and are always angry about something. One day you have sudden chest pains. Given your family history, this scares the daylights out of you, and you waste no time getting to a doctor and asking what's going on. You tell the doctor you're willing to do whatever is necessary to lower your own risk of having a heart attack. Now, the doctor knows all the scientific data: he knows that cigarette smoking contributes to heart attacks; he knows what obesity does; he knows what having a certain set of genes does; he knows all this has been implicated in the risk of heart attacks and heart disease. He has no trouble telling you about those risks. He tells you you should eat less, lower your weight, lower your cholesterol, and quit smoking. There's nothing, he says, you can do about your genes.

Recently this same doctor read an article in a medical journal that cited numerous studies noting the association between hostility, high cholesterol, and heart attacks. But perhaps he doesn't tell you about this. Like most doctors, he is afraid you'll feel he's blaming you for your condition. You might continue your cycle of conflict but make the dietary and lifestyle changes and still have a disabling heart attack. Perhaps your doctor does tell you about the article, however. You then do some additional reading about this correlation between anger and heart disease, and you learn some healthful ways to release your anger, perhaps through exercise or meditation. By doing so, you might save your life.

In a third possible scenario, your doctor might tell you of the anger–heart disease correlation and you might decide he's blaming you for your condition and disregard the information and his advice. This does occur in our culture. A patient may feel responsible for being overweight or for smoking cigarettes, but might well perceive himself as being unjustly blamed if the doctor asks him whether he knows how to express his anger fully and release it and whether he is aware that not attending to this emotion hurts his health. To some patients, certain data bear the stigma of "assigning blame," while other data do not. Ironically, a patient may have had repeated fights and arguments with loved ones over the very issue of his anger and hostility, yet he may never have addressed the emotions directly or known how to attempt to understand and redirect the emotions in appropriate ways.

For a doctor to deny a patient indisputable scientific information about the relationship between emotions and heart attacks or other illnesses is a form of malpractice, in the same way that not informing a patient of available drugs that could lower his risk of heart attack would be malpractice. As long as a doctor delivers the information with empathy, acceptance, and an emphasis on the facts and science, and as long as he provides opportunities for the patient to make healthy changes in his life, the data and the doctor can only help the patient, not hurt him.[14]

Beginning to Read the Body

At the beginning of every reading, I get only a person's name and age. Without knowing anything more about him or her, I call and describe over the phone what I'm going to do and not do in the reading. The client and I are not having a physician-patient relationship, and I'm not doing psychotherapy. I don't offer a specific diagnosis and treatment. I tell the clients that I assume that they are working in a healing partnership with some physician or practitioner for specific diagnoses and medical treatments. I'm not practicing medicine when I do a reading.

In the reading, I describe the emotional setting of the person's life as I intuit it. What she does, or did, for a living, any active issues around growing up, any active issues regarding any emotional relationship she is in. Then I describe her physical body from head to toe, each organ system. If I detect any abnormalities, I describe the image I receive of that aberration, but I do not attribute it to a specific disease. I describe any further emotional patterns or images in her life that I see as setting the scene for health or change in the specific organs in her body. I explain that any symptoms she feels in her body are a part of her intuitive guidance system telling her that specific situations in her life need to be changed.

When you begin to tap into your body's emotional patterns and the images that the emotional centers of the body can send you, you are practicing medical intuition. This practice will give you more information about yourself and your health—information that is complementary to that which your doctor gives you. Your own medical intuition will give you information about what's happening to your body in relation to other aspects of your life—the emotional aspects, which can have as much impact as the physical, genetic, environmental, and nutritional aspects of illness and health. You can use this information to make changes for the better in your health and life. Just as a medical intuitive reads your memory patterns and their tagged, or associated, feelings in your brain and body organs, you will become more adept at doing this for yourself, with practice. Throughout this book, I recount numerous readings that I have conducted. I hope in this way to help you learn to do this for yourself. These readings will help you get used to the variety of images and feelings and terms I use to read and describe the changes that I detect in clients' emotional centers and organ systems. I hope you'll begin to associate your own images of health and disease with those that you read and in that way begin to develop your own unique language of intuition.

Here is a sample reading as I expressed it to one client. First, I looked at her emotional life:

> I see you as having a lot of chaos in your family between birth and the age of two. I see gunfire and alcoholism. I see you being handed from one family member to another, from parent to aunt to grandparent. It seems as though your life never appeared permanent. You learned that you had to trust different people all the time, and you had trouble figuring out whom you should trust or mistrust. As a result of this very unstable family situation, you never felt that you were a part of any group of people.
>
> I see you as being extremely independent and not wanting to depend on anyone. Whenever you associated with a group or family, you felt like an outsider. You didn't want to be dependent, for fear that once you became dependent, something would change, and you would lose your family.

All the issues in this woman's life revolved around the first emotional center of safety and security in the world, dependency versus independence, having a strong foundation in the family. Looking at her body, I saw that all those issues were affecting the organs in her first emotional center—her blood, her bones, her joints, and her spine. She had chronic arthritis in many joints due to numerous injuries, a number of them from mountain climbing, since she often went off on long hikes in the hills by herself. She had knee problems and had had several operations. She had also suffered multiple infections and immune problems, including pneumonia, anemia, and hepatitis. I said to her:

Why do you get near so many cliffs in your life? Why do you continuously challenge yourself? You always seem to be alone on some mountain rather than with your family. You seem torn between the two options. You feel afraid in the world, but you're chronically forcing yourself to face your fear by getting near one cliff, one physical challenge, after another. You force yourself to feel safe in situations where no one would feel safe. Yet when you're with your family, where everyone would feel safe, you don't feel that you belong.

Have you noticed that you have chronic colds, pneumonias, viruses? Do you get arthritis in your joints, so that they get swollen? When do these get worse, and when do they get better? This is your intuition telling you when you're having problems with feeling that you can't be dependent on a family. You have to force yourself to feel good about yourself by becoming independent and facing one struggle after another in the world. Your body's trying to tell you this.

Do you remember the woman with hives whom we talked about earlier? If I were reading that woman I'd say, "I see that your mother-in-law can get underneath your skin really easily, because you feel unsafe and vulnerable to her verbal attacks, even though she's in your family, a place that should feel safe and nurturing. And when she gets under your skin, your blood boils, but you can't fully express your feelings, for fear that you'll have to leave your family, and you'll have no support in the world. As a result, you swallow your feelings, and they simmer beneath the surface. I wonder if you have boils beneath your skin."

Sometimes my intuition will give me a picture of a memory stored in a person's body, sometimes in the image of another person. Once, in reading a woman with breast cysts, I saw the image of an adolescent boy projected visually on her lungs. I told her I saw her spending an inordinate amount of time nurturing (fourth emotional center) an adolescent boy with asthma, and I wondered if this was her son. She said, "Oh, no, that would be my brother when I was growing up." Then I was able to see why taking care of her brother was an important issue in her life. I said, "I wonder if a lot of your personality and self-esteem, how strong you feel in the outer world, is based on a pattern of nurturing others rather than being in relationships where people can love you and nurture you back." She agreed that this was so.

By educating you about the link between emotions and disease, medical intuition empowers you. The insight you gain from an intuitive reading, or from paying attention to your own intuitions, can add greatly to your understanding of the emotional factors associated with your physical health or illness. You can gain intuitive understanding by tapping into your own intuition network, by scoping out which emotional center has an imbalance between power and vulnerability, which emotional centers and their associated organs trigger painful memories or call your attention to emotional situations that you need to examine.

That's what happened with the woman in the following story. A colleague who is a gynecologist had a patient who kept coming to her with terrible vaginal infections. No matter what medicine my colleague prescribed, the infections stubbornly refused to clear up. As it happened, the patient was a married woman who was having difficulties with her husband. Ultimately, she found out that her husband was having an affair, but she held on to the relationship for two more years until she finally got up enough courage to let go and get a divorce. Soon after that, the infections stopped. The woman never dealt with the underlying issues in her relationship with her husband, however.

After she had been divorced for a while, she began to date a nice man whom she liked very much. She felt much relieved to be part of a partnership once again, since she'd never really liked being alone. All went swimmingly for a time. Then one day, significantly, she came down once again with one of those vaginal infections from hell. At first she didn't think much of it. But a little voice kept nagging her—the voice of intuition. She didn't want to listen. She didn't want to hear what her vagina was telling her. She didn't want to focus on the fact that the honeymoon was over and that the same kinds of problems that had destroyed her marriage were cropping up again in this new relationship. The infection persisted. And persisted. Then one night she woke with a start from a dream. She didn't remember the dream, but she was aware of a nagging feeling in her heart—and a nagging feeling in her vagina. She felt that perhaps this man, like her ex-husband, was having an affair.

Finally she took the muzzle off her intuition. She learned, as she had suspected, that the man she was seeing was indeed having a simultaneous affair with another woman. She broke off the relationship, and the infection cleared up.

She then went into therapy and dealt with the emotional patterns of her relationships (second emotional center, vagina) and with her problems with autonomy, knowing when to hold on and when to let go, allowing a person to have space in a relationship versus desiring intimacy. She realized that she needed to be alone for a while to focus on healthy patterns in relationships. She also acknowledged and appreciated the fact that the intuition of her vagina would protect her and keep her honest in her endeavor to learn how to stand on her own two feet while maintaining a solid relationship, how not to lose sight of "you versus me versus us" in a relationship.

We are not responsible for our illnesses, but we must be responsive to them.[14] If we unmuzzle our intuition and learn to listen to the language of our bodies, we too can become empowered. We can learn to balance power and vulnerability in all the emotional areas of our lives. We can use the information our intuition sends us to map out a better course for our lives and build a foundation for a healthier, more balanced life in the future.

SIX

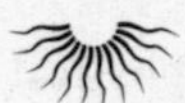

Blood and Bones: Helplessness and Hopelessness

The first emotional center contains memories that are located in the blood and the bones, the immune system, the spine, and the hips. Emotions and memories stored in this center have to do with issues related to your family; your physical safety, security, and support in the world; and to hopelessness and helplessness.

When I was an intern, one of my first patients was Mrs. O'Halloran, an eighty-four-year-old woman on the hematology-oncology rotation. She was bleeding internally throughout her body, and her blood platelet counts were dropping. Her chart indicated that she had recently fallen and broken her hip. Mrs. O'Halloran had lived alone for many years, and had always been proud of her independence. Yet shortly after I entered her room, she confided a new truth to me. "I don't feel safe living alone anymore," she said, but she was at a loss as to what to do next. "I don't want to be a burden on my family," she fretted, "but I don't want to live in a nursing home, either."

Mrs. O'Halloran had a broken hip and an immunological problem with her blood. Her physical ailments were in anatomical areas located in the first emotional center. She was also feeling a lack of safety and security, and she was worried about having to be supported by her family, emotions that are likewise empatterned in the first emotional center. She felt hopeless and helpless in her situation.

Over the course of her stay, Mrs. O'Halloran's blood counts continued to drop. Sitting alone in her room, she received a series of intravenous medicines in an effort to stop her own immune system from producing the antibodies that were destroying her blood cells. But in fact, she developed side effects to the very medicines we were giving her. She became psychotic, paranoid, agitated, and unable to trust anyone.

Despite her emotional and physical pain, Mrs. O'Halloran gradually began to bond with me, to trust me, and to respond positively to my visits. Mostly, I just listened to her talk about her fears, and made her feel safe and secure so that she could express her feelings as the medicines finally began to take hold. By the time she was ready to leave the hospital, she had found peace in the prospect of a new life as she entered a nursing home, which would help provide her with a new family, new social support, and the feeling of safety and security.

Mrs. O'Halloran's feelings of vulnerability, her problems with safety and security in the physical world, and her issues about family support and being a burden on her family were very much related to her blood disorder and her hip fracture. Emotions and memories encoded in the first emotional center—lack of safety, hopelessness, helplessness,[1] trust, family, and social support[2]—affect the health of our blood and immunity, bones and joints (see the following figure).

Family is fundamental. There's no place like home.

These are truths we learn in earliest childhood or perhaps even in the womb. They're reflected throughout our culture. Think of Dorothy, wandering through Oz in a determined search to find the way back to Kansas, repeating "There's no place like home." Think of your mother, reminding you as you went off to college to call home frequently and always to remember that nobody will love you the way your family loves you. Or your father exhorting you that "In the end, all you have is family." The family is our most important source of love and support. It shapes our perception of the world and our attitudes toward others. The life process that makes us who we are begins at home, with our family of origin. Later, we form and find "families" at school, in marriage and relationships, at work, at our places of worship, and in society at large.

Families don't just shape our lives; they also shape our bodies.

First Emotional Center

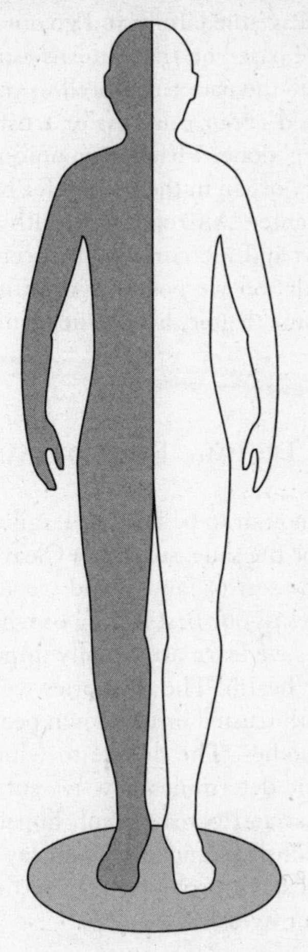

Because family is the foundation of our emotional and physical lives, the first emotional center is the foundation for all the other emotional centers in the body. What we learn from our family of origin is reflected in our adult ties to family substitutes and the way we regard the world in general. How do you look at the world? Do you feel safe and secure in it or fearful of it? Do you trust or mistrust people? Are you independent or dependent? All of these attitudes stem from your family, your framework of support and interactions.

What you learn in your family also affects the organ systems of your first emotional center: your blood and your bones. The memories that are stored in the body organs of that center reverberate throughout your life. When you leave the family and go out into the larger world, you experiment in life based on the patterns established in your family. You try to re-create the patterns, stored in your brain and body, of what you have learned about mistrust or trust, safety and security, belonging yet standing alone. That's why, uniquely, every other emotional center and every organ in the body refer back to this first, foundational emotional center. All roads to health lead back home. We build on the emotions and memories of this center all our lives. The firmness of the foundation we possess will influence everything else we do, and will, to some degree, help to determine our state of illness or health.

WISDOM AND TRAUMA, EMOTIONS AND MEMORIES

We're not all lucky enough to be born to families like those of Ozzie and Harriet Nelson or the sane, suburban Cleavers. Each of us, however, is born into some sort of family, and we all start life with some sort of group that gives us our first feeling of who we are, our sense of identity. The attitudes we learn are equally important to our physical development and our health. The memories we create of our experiences in the world with trusted or unknown people are stored in both our brains and our bodies. The degree to which we perceive these memories as traumatic determines how we suffer or flourish in our lives. Memories of loss and bereavement, hopelessness and helplessness, shape our relationships and goals and lay the groundwork for whether or not we'll have problems in the first emotional center, health or disease in our lives.

The Biology of Belonging

From the first, family gives you a sense of belonging, of being part of a group that supports and sustains you. This sense begins forming in the womb, when you're literally a part of your mother, and continues after birth, in the family that supports your life and fulfills your needs. At the same time, however, family teaches you about boundaries, about where the world ends and you begin. It prepares you to develop a sense of strength in yourself as an individual.

Our whole lives are a process of slowly disengaging from the family and becoming independent individuals, while retaining the sense of belonging to a family or tribe. We begin our lives completely enmeshed with the mother through the placenta and umbilical cord. As soon as the cord is cut, the disengagement, ever so subtly, begins. Eventually, we begin to notice that our parents form a separate unit within the family and that sometimes we and our siblings aren't a part of it. Sometimes Mom and Dad go into their room and shut the door. The gap between enmeshment and disengagement grows. We go to school. Finally we go off to college or a job and now just call home once a month. We're independent, but we still have a metaphorical umbilical cord in the telephone, sustaining the all-important sense of belonging and support we need to function optimally in life.

If we lose or never acquire that sense of belonging, the consequences can be grievous. And they aren't simply emotional. They're physical as well.

Research has shown there to be a biology of belonging, an actual biological nutrient passing between people who live together, eat together, sleep together, a nutrient that has physical and metabolic consequences.[3] When people are together in a communal situation, their biological body rhythms become synchronized and regular. In one study, the individual members of B-52 bomber crews were all found to have similar levels of adrenocorticoid output while they were working together.[4] The other girls in my college dorm and I used to realize we were all having our period at the same time every month when the bathroom would suddenly run out of toilet paper. Similarly, research has shown that women who have close relationships with men actually have more regular periods and fewer problems with infertility.[5] It appears, believe it or not, that something in male armpit sweat helps regulate the menstrual cycle.[6] Apparently, even something potentially offensive, like body odor, has biochemical usefulness in helping us bond to one another.

I was struck by the pervasiveness of our need to bond when I went to a rodeo with some friends one Fourth of July weekend. First, there were the cowboys, all duded up and swaggering around the corral, getting ready to compete for money and prizes. Before the show began, though, all these potential rivals huddled together at the center of the ring for an opening prayer, in which they asked God to help them use their gifts as horsemen and wranglers to the best of their abilities. They had to bond as a family, in the identity of cowboydom, before they became individuals who would go out and compete against one another. I was reminded of the saying, "The family that prays together stays together." Second, there were the sheep. One segment of the show was a sheep-riding competition for children. The sheep bucked wildly to throw their pint-size riders off their backs. As soon as each child fell off, its sheep would take off for the far corner of the corral, frantically looking for the spot where the rest of the flock huddled in the safety of numbers. I watched this happen over and over again, until at last a dozen or more sheep stood crowded together in a single corner of the ring. Alone in the ring with the kids on their backs, they had acted panicked and terrified; once back with the flock, they calmed down. They felt safe and secure. They were home again.

We're just like the sheep. Being together in close and constant fashion the way we are in a family—eating, sleeping, conversing, playing, working, praying—causes us to synchronize our biological watches. All our body rhythms, having to do with sleeping, eating, dreaming, hormones, immunity, cortisol levels, heart rate, and endocrine systems, are governed by metabolic regulators that make them function in healthy fashion.[7] Every single system in your body, in others words, is regulated by the interaction of belonging. But what happens when this closeness is disrupted, when we're separated from the family or group?

Scientists studied the effects of isolation by putting people into rooms alone, without companionship, and observing what happened to their biological rhythms. Since it had long been believed that human body rhythms were synchronized with the light, the lights in the rooms were set to go on and off at regular hours to imitate the cycles of sunlight and darkness. To the scientists' surprise, however, they found that the subjects' body rhythms weren't regulated by the light alone, and they became unstable. The researchers then instituted a system of bells signaling the subjects in their rooms at regular intervals that someone would be coming to collect urine samples. Something remarkable happened. Even though the subjects were all separated from one another, their body rhythms were once again found to be in sync, as each adjusted to the cycle of the urine collector's arrival.[3] It was as though, in their social isolation, they became bonded over the issue of urine. It's amazing; people will find any subject to bond together over, even urine or body odor. They will seek out any port in a storm and fixate on the smallest scrap of human contact to restore the sense of belonging that makes our bodies function in a stable, healthy manner. Without the stable, secure contact of a regular visit from the urine collector, the subjects' sleep, eating, hormone, cortisol, and other cycles became disordered.

Family, a sense of belonging, is fundamentally important for health in our bodies.[2] Social interaction plays a vital role in everyday regulation of our body systems. If you isolate yourself, you remove the metabolic regulators that are present when you interact with a group, and your rhythms—your life, it seems—go kind of kaflooey. When I went away to college and left my family for the first time, my sleep cycle went completely kaput. I started sleeping seventeen hours a day. I was a mess. Changes in your work shift, a change in the group you belong to, can produce the same kind of effect. You can't think straight, your sleep-wakefulness cycle gets messed up, you get weak, you catch more colds, you get fatigued, you become depressed, you lose your appetite.

Most of us ultimately adjust to the change. We find new regulators. Those who don't, though, are in trouble. Studies on sensory deprivation looked at loners, including explorers, mystics, and sailors and at those who were thrust into solitude, like prisoners in solitary confinement and brainwashing victims. They found that such individuals, after extended periods of solitude, had problems with concentration, attention span, restlessness, and anxiety. Their thoughts become disordered, they didn't eat well, they had hallucinations, they lost weight, they lost sleep, and their muscles became weak. Eventually, they moved into despair and ultimately depression.[8]

Despair, loss, bereavement, depression—these are the emotions that can overwhelm us when we lose the nutrient of belonging. All these emotions are stored in the first emotional center. They are the symptoms of grief. They're the same symptoms we get when someone we love leaves us or dies. The feeling of separation or grief, therefore, might actually be due to the fact that your body is missing a real nutrient. I know a woman, Fran, who grew up in a terrible, violent, chaotic family. Eventually she left home, moved away, married, and started her own family. But Fran always says that whenever she has to leave her new family, even for a brief period, she gets a deep-seated feeling of grief in her chest. While she's away from home, she has trouble eating and sleeping. She feels the grief in her bones, down to the very marrow. She's physically starving for the nutrient of belonging to the family she has created. My aunt Rose loves to visit, but the instant the sun begins to set, she's on her feet saying to my uncle, "Joe, get the car. We need to go home." She has to go back to the mother ship, where her biological regulators are. It's almost like a diver who notices on his regulator that he's running out of oxygen and knows he has to go back to the surface. If Aunt Rose, like the diver, doesn't get back to dry land, the cycles in her body go haywire.

In grief or bereavement, you experience not just emotional loss but also physical loss. You lose interaction with a person, and thus your body loses its whole sense of how to regulate its organ functions. Our clocks lose their settings. We lose the proper beat to the dance of life. When you are pining away for someone, your organs may be crying out for contact. Your body temperature turns cold and icy, you long to be touched, you long for the smell of that person, you long for the rhythm of the days and the things you used to do with that person. You're like the person in the Dionne Warwick song, "I Just Don't Know What to Do with Myself." You're like the woman who loses her husband and finds she can't sleep in the bed they shared, because her body is pining for the other body and the organs with which it was in sync. Now her body is on its own. It's lost. And now it's vulnerable.

Here's an example of how the mind-body network sends you intuitive messages:

THE LOST SHEEP
CHRONIC FATIGUE AND FIBROMYALGIA

The Reading. Lucy Graham, age forty-five, called me from India requesting a reading immediately. It was an emergency, she said. I wondered what kind of problem could require such urgency. Looking at her intuitively, I could see two things right away: she was financially comfortable and able to draw on a lot of family money, but she was full of grief and pining away for a lost relationship or relationships. I couldn't see a past for her at all. I saw her floating in space with no connections to anything and no roots. She was like a satellite disconnected from the mother ship, with nowhere to land. She gave me a strong sense of being like an orphan. She felt like a sheep that had strayed from the fold.

In her body, I saw a slow heart rate, some shortness of breath, and stiffness in her joints. I wondered if she had an autoimmune disorder. I also saw lifelong problems with anxiety and depression.

The Facts. I asked her why she was in India, and she told me she had left the United States and her entire family fifteen years before to study transcendental meditation with a guru in New Delhi. She had been living there ever since. Having no financial

> needs, she didn't work, and she didn't even speak the language. In other words, she had very few human contacts and no regular routine of connection with other people.
>
> Lucy confirmed that she had depression, chronic fatigue, and fibromyalgia, a joint ailment associated with immune dysfunction.

Lucy's was a clear-cut case of lost metabolic regulators. She had lost the nutrient of family contact, even contact with her homeland. She was like a diver in the water who had run out of oxygen. Alone in a foreign country where she couldn't even communicate with other people, she was grief-stricken and homesick. She was literally pining for human contacts—contacts who spoke her own language, ate her kind of food, wore her kind of clothing, shared the social mores she had grown up with—who would restore her body's natural rhythms (note the slowed heart rate and shortness of breath). She was separated from her family and had established no other family to support her. The memories of her loss were stored in her bones and joints and immunity. They were part of her intuitive guidance system, telling her in a number of different ways that she didn't belong where she was. After she had ignored these for a while, the intuitive signals got louder, and she developed fibromyalgia. The path she had chosen and pursued for the past fifteen years was no longer right for her. Her body's intuitive guidance system, in the first emotional center and its organs, was telling her she needed to move. On some level, she had heard her own intuition, because her emergency call was a way of reaching out for contact, for connection with the mother country and the mother ship. And that call was as desperate as a baby's cry for its mother's milk.

Lucy was taken aback by my reading and said at the end of the phone call that she would have to sit in a meditation retreat for the next month and meditate on whether or not she should return to her homeland.

Does her experience resonate with a situation in which you find yourself now or one in which you felt as if you had lost your connection to the mother ship? Are you isolated from your family of origin, or have you left another family group that helped you define yourself and your purpose in life? If your body is pining for connection, it may tell you this by giving you fatigue, depression, and problems with immunity. If you are feeling alienated from your old crew, you need to find a new one to sail with, one that will make you feel as if you've reached a safe harbor.

If you've recently lost a loved one, or if major changes have occurred in your social support system at work, at church, or even in your bridge club, you need to take extra good care of your physical health. You need to get the right dietary, nutritional, and exercise regimen, but you also need to create new social bonds and friendships to replenish your nutrients of belonging.

Loss and Health

Depression is a biological change that occurs in us when we're separated from the object of our love and support, from a social connection that helps regulate our bodies. This connection begins in utero and continues when a mother holds her baby in her arms. But what happens when the baby is taken from the mother and loses physical contact? Scientists now know that physical contact is so essential to babies' well-being that if you don't touch them, they actually lose weight and eventually die. That's why hospitals have volunteers who come in and hold abandoned or incubated babies for several hours a day. Close proximity and touching release norepinephrine and dopamine, two chemicals that are presumed to stimulate growth in the brain.[3]

If you're separated too early from your family, literally or figuratively, the loss can have physical and emotional consequences throughout your life. Scientists have theorized that isolation, not belonging to a family, is stored in a person's early childhood memory and disposes him or her to cancer. Feelings of isolation and a lack of meaningful relationships give rise to a sense of hopelessness, helplessness, and despair. This carries over into later life if the person isn't able to negotiate his or her sense of loneliness in the world. And the hopelessness ultimately renders the individual more vulnerable to cancer.[9]

With this theory in mind, researchers studied the effects of premature weaning on rats. The average nursing period for newborn rats is twenty-one days. But in one study, researchers removed selected young rats from their mothers at fifteen days, leaving the rest of the litters to continue nursing as usual. Forty-five days later, when the rats were full-grown, the researchers injected them all with cancer cells. Bingo! The rats that had been prematurely weaned and taken away from their mothers developed cancer more often than the lucky brothers and sisters who had been allowed to spend the appropriate amount of time with Mom. The researchers' conclusion? Premature weaning leads to a greater susceptibility to disease.[10] I call this the Bambi syndrome.

THE BAMBI SYNDROME
A CASE OF LUPUS

The Reading. Vanessa reminded me of Bambi. When I read her, I saw a little orphaned fawn, staring at the world with big eyes fringed with long eyelashes and full of vulnerability and naïveté. She was frozen at an age of innocence and completely lacking a sense of security. She was porous, and the winds of people's pain and anger blew right through her.

I saw that her past was full of death. Person after person, many of them significant, had left her life. Everything in her first emotional center was in turmoil. I saw one remaining person in her family who was difficult and caused her a lot of emotional pain. This person was greedy and self-centered, went after what he or she wanted and didn't care who got hurt in the process. This person was like a bag of pain and anger, which Vanessa tried, not very successfully, to absorb and diffuse.

Vanessa had problems with focus, attention, and memory as well as sadness, melancholia, and depression. I saw her having problems with decreased vision. I also saw a lot of fatigue in her body. I saw her as emotionally vulnerable as well as physically vulnerable to things in the world that were unsafe. She didn't know what to trust or mistrust. And just as she was porous to people's emotions, anger and rage, she was also porous to viruses and contracted repeated infections and colds.

The Facts. Vanessa's parents had died when she was a child, her father when she was four and her mother when she was six. A number of other relatives also died. The only person she had left was a brother, who was alcoholic, depressed, and frequently suicidal. This brother was full of anger and rage and was prone to violent outbursts. Vanessa was deeply affected by his rages and tended to take them personally. Yet she clung to this brother as her only lifeline, the only family she had. She was like someone who had fallen out of a burning boat and grabbed hold of a shark because it was the only thing in the water that could keep her afloat. Any port in a storm, as they say.

Her many losses and the resulting feelings of hopelessness had strongly affected her immunity. Emotional vulnerability became physical vulnerability. She had developed lupus, a blood disorder in which the immune system makes antibodies against all the tissues of the body, especially the joints. She also was very prone to infections because of her blood and immunological problems. The entire world was a pit of danger to her. She couldn't escape her feelings, or the feelings of others. It was hard for her to

> see anger and rage in the people she most wanted to trust. She didn't want to see that someone very close to her, the only remaining member of her family, was not trustworthy at all. Unfortunately, she had lost her eyesight and developed chronic pain and depression.

Vanessa's was a difficult case, because she was so alone in the world and her brother was her only source of any sense of belonging. His effect on her was so corrosive, however, that she would have been better off to let go of him and to try to establish a different framework of support from other people, a new family of support with which to bond. Vanessa had experienced premature weaning from her mother and father when they died during her early childhood. Traumatic memories of these premature weanings had been empatterned as excessive vulnerability in her blood and immune system, the organs of her first emotional center, and as excessive emotional vulnerability to the moods and anger of others. Her repeated colds and immunological problems were part of her intuitive guidance system telling her that something near her could not be trusted and wasn't safe for her. Vanessa, however, didn't want to look at this, because it was too painful to acknowledge that the only family member she had left was no family at all.

Having a toxic relative is indeed a difficult situation for anyone to deal with. If you are in the middle of such a situation, ask yourself this question: What are the good and bad consequences of having this person in my life? Then divide a sheet of paper into two columns and list all of the ramifications of knowing and seeing this person. Put the pluses on the right and the minuses on the left. If the minuses are greater than the pluses, the cost of having the person in your life is too high and the toll on your health will eventually be too heavy. You need to divest yourself of this person. Before you perform this friend-ectomy or relative-ectomy, seek out the emotional support of a minister, a therapist, some other kind of counselor, or a friend or relative to help you through it.

Premature weaning represents loss and bereavement—an untimely separation from the mother, who is the first person to give you a sense of belonging and family support. When your mother nurses you, she literally passes on, through the breast milk, immune molecules that will protect you from bacteria and viruses.[11] She's physiologically transferring safety and security in the world via little molecules that move into your bloodstream saying, "I am safe, you are safe, we are all safe."

She lays the foundation for a strong first emotional center. Even if a mother doesn't breast-feed, she transfers this same sense of well-being through her interaction with her child, through holding and touching, which releases growth hormones, and through cooing and playing. If you don't get enough of this from your mother, you don't get a sense of belonging, and that affects your body. Your internal organ processes aren't regulated.

From your mother, or your family, you learn about life the way you learn to ride a bicycle built for two. The person in the front, your mother, regulates, and the one in the back, you, pedals along. As you ride with your mother, you learn how to pedal. Then eventually, you're on your own bike, and because you have an internalized sense of what pedaling was like from your mother, you can pedal on your own. If you didn't get that sense of how to pedal, though, you're going to be a little loose in that department. You're going to have problems with safety and security in the world, you're going to be afraid to get on the bike, you're going to be afraid you'll fall and hit your head, you're not going to know how fast or slow to pedal, you're going to be dependent on others, you're going to want someone on the bike with you. Or you're going to be hyperindependent: you're going to say I don't need you, I can do this myself. You're going to have problems in the first emotional center. Vanessa had to ride alone too early in life and learn to pedal by herself. She never quite gained confidence on the bike, so she became susceptible to every emotional and physical bump on the road of life, and she became vulnerable and receptive to illness, especially colds and flu.

Unfortunately, many people suffer from figurative premature weaning: for one reason or another they don't receive a sense of safety and belonging. Perhaps they actually lose one parent or the other through death or divorce, or their particular family dynamics re-create the effects of separation or loss. What happens then?

Studies have shown that when you remove a mother prematurely from a child, the child goes through two phases: protest and despair. In the protest phase, where the child doesn't understand or believe that the mother is gone, he goes around and tries to look for her.[12] He looks anywhere he can, searching to reestablish the lost bond. I watched a nature program on TV about this very subject. It was like the little children's book, "Are You My Mother?" where a baby bird falls out of the nest and runs around asking everything from a cow to a bulldozer "Are you my mother?" In the TV show, a baby hedgehog got separated from his mother and the rest of the litter. He spent the rest of the hour wandering around the desert looking for his mother in all the most unlikely places. He went up to an antelope, which looked at him coldly and leaped away. He went up to a zebra, which ignored him. He went up to a porcupine, which curled its back and shot a quill at him. That program really got to me. I've always had problems in my first emotional center, and I don't have a strong sense of belonging. I must have seen something of myself in that little hedgehog, because that night I dreamed that I was trying to have a relationship with a porcupine! In any case, the porcupine did it for the hedgehog, because the poor thing went squealing off and hid in a hole. He moved into the despair phase. That's when the offspring sits and hides from his predators and just gives up.

Notice how closely this pattern parallels depression. You go through the protest: this can't be happening to me; you can't have left my life. Then you go through the despair, and eventually you reach depression, where you want to hide under a rock. Basically, what happens when a child loses his mother is the same as what happens when someone leaves our life. Throughout our lives, whenever we encounter loss and grief, we re-create emotionally, nutritionally, and biologically the loss of the bond we had when we were young.[13]

Many studies have looked at the effects of parents' closeness to a child, and at the age of the father at a child's birth. They found that these two factors were predictors of early death, suicide, mental illness, high blood pressure, heart disease, and tumors.[14] The more distant the parents and the older the father, the greater the risks of physical and mental complications.

This may be bad news for seventy-year-old fathers and would-be postmenopausal mothers, but it's information that can't be ignored. Knowing that one can count on certain things being permanent in life is vital information for an infant's sense of security and safety. It's like playing peekaboo with a baby. When you hide your face behind your hands, the baby becomes alarmed, because when she doesn't see you, she believes that—*poof!*—you've truly disappeared. She delights at your reappearance because you've reassured her that indeed you are still there for her. She has learned an important lesson about her safety and security in the world and about your trustworthiness. As the child grows, she learns this lesson again and again in other ways. There's a scene in the movie *Phenomenon* where the character played by John Travolta, having learned that he has a brain tumor and is going to die, gathers his girlfriend's two young children to talk about the inevitable. The children are angry and scared because he's going to leave them.

The Travolta character is eating an apple. As the kids pummel him with their anger, he holds out the apple to them. Take a bite of this apple, he says. This is my apple, I grew it. When you eat a piece of it, you'll know you'll always have me inside you. After he dies, the kids are comforted by this understanding of his continued symbolic presence inside them, in their tissue, their blood and their bones, the very marrow of their being.

If you don't have the opportunity to talk about the apple, like the rats that were weaned prematurely, if early bonds are severed or weakened, this loss gets stored in memories in your blood and your bones. You learn that the world is not safe, that you cannot trust people, and you don't understand how you can help yourself. You have learned helplessness and hopelessness, and this lesson will affect your health.

The Social Network

All through our lives, long after we have left our first home, we continue to form families in our search for this vital sense of belonging. These families aren't just biological. We develop entire social networks that act as families to support us and to make us feel safe and secure in the world. The knowledge, the intuition, that supportive interaction among people is our lifeblood drives us to do this. If we don't get enough support, our bodies speak up. In fact, the bigger our family in the world, the better off we are. Just as it's not good to stand completely on our own, it's not good to depend on too small a circle of friends and relatives.

Scientists hold that social networks and social support play a role in the ability of our blood cells to resist infections. The blood cells can protect you from a wide variety of health perils, including low birth weight, arthritis, tuberculosis, depression, even death. And social interaction decreases the amount of medication people need and accelerates their recovery from illness.[15] One study looked at surgical patients who were divided into two groups, one that received special care and one that didn't. The anesthesiologists were told to talk to one group while medicating them, extending support, encouragement, and reassurance. They did not extend such support to the other group. The patients who received special care were found to need less pain medication after the surgery and were discharged an average of 2.7 days earlier than the patients who received no special care.[16] I have a little bit of a diminished first emotional center, and I've always had a friend scrub in for my surgery and provide support. I know this support helps to keep post-op infections at bay.

Social support is known to affect immunity.[2] If you don't feel safe and secure and have a sense of belonging, if you feel helpless in the face of what you're dealing with, helplessness gets encoded in your body. Your white cells speak to you through intuition: "I am not safe. I am vulnerable." And the infections will come in and take root.

A very recent study demonstrated this dramatically. Researchers asked 276 volunteers to list their social contacts, meaning the number of people they saw or spoke to over a period of two weeks, and the various categories to which these people belonged—spouse, children, other relatives, neighbors, friends, colleagues, and so forth. Then they were all subjected to cold viruses. The results? Those who had three or fewer different types of relationships got the most colds and were more susceptible to the viruses. Those who had six or more different types of relationships got the least and, when they did develop colds, had the mildest symptoms.

This isn't what you'd expect, is it? You'd think that having more friends, more relationships, would expose you to more germs and therefore cause more colds. But germ theory obviously doesn't offer the full answer to why we get colds and infections. Actually, people who have fewer friends (and come into contact with fewer germs) are more susceptible to colds.[17] This may be so because they probably experience stress from being alone most of the time and not feeling safe and secure in the world. Not having a sense of belonging creates stress. That stress causes the adrenal glands to release norepinephrine and suppress the immune system in the first emotional center.

Can having more friends really make your blood stronger so that it can fight infections more effectively? And can having fewer friends really make you more vulnerable? The answer is yes. Having just one solitary source of support, like some couples who invest everything in each other, is not good for the blood and bones. Staying socially active, with a wide network of friends, is a way of life that's emotionally empatterned in all the organs of your first emotional center. In contrast, isolation leads to feelings of insecurity, and your blood, immunity, and bones will let you know it.

You probably know some women who gave up their jobs as soon as they married and invested themselves completely in their husbands' lives. Not only that, but they gave up all their girlfriends, too. Then their husbands had to be not only their mates but their best friends and employers and everything else as well. I call this the "eggs-in-one-basket syndrome." This situation is bad for a person's health. People with a more diverse social network live longer than people with fewer relationships, and having few friends is a greater health risk than smoking, obesity, and other factors.[18]

THE EGGS-IN-ONE-BASKET SYNDROME IMMUNE SYSTEM WORRIES

The Reading. Mark was a thirty-two-year-old man whom I envisioned immediately as single, thin, extremely meticulous, and good-looking. In fact, I saw him as looking like a Greek god, with chiseled features. He even reminded me of Michelangelo's *David.* I immediately envisioned a gay man, although I wasn't sure of this point. I didn't want to fall into the stereotype that Jerry Seinfeld refers to when he says that people always think he's gay because he's single, thin, good-looking, and tidy. I also saw Mark as involved in an unbalanced relationship with a much older partner, who had more power in the relationship than Mark did. I saw him living and working in a family or group of people where he was the low man on the totem pole. It appeared that all of his relationships, however, were going to end.

I saw that the ending of his relationship and his lack of status within his family were going to affect Mark biologically. In his body, I saw potential changes in his immune system. Otherwise, however, I saw no real physical problems, and no present illnesses.

The Facts. Mark told me that he was very worried about his immune system. He was indeed gay and had been involved in a long-term relationship with a man thirty-five years his senior who was also the powerful head of a large, influential business consulting firm. Mark worked for his lover in the firm, but in a lowly position. He had few alliances with others in the firm, which was also part of a spiritual community. The power balance in the relationship was thus predetermined by both the partner's greater age and his powerful position. He was the general; Mark was the enlisted man. Most significantly, however, the relationship was coming to an end because the older man was dying of cancer.

Mark faced a whole series of issues revolving around "us," around independence versus dependence and sense of self versus sense of belonging. He was overly enmeshed with the older man, who was many things to him: lover, employer, father figure, best friend. With his lover dying, Mark stood to lose all the eggs in his solitary basket. He was about to lose his family—both the family represented by his partnership and the family of his workplace, where he would have even less status than before, and the family of the greater community in which the firm existed.

In fact, Mark had always had problems with family. He had gained no self-confidence from his mother, and his father had been cold and distant. His relationships with older men represented an almost constant effort to earn his father's love. The loss of that lover would be like a loss of his very lifeblood. And Mark intuited that. He knew his situation was precarious even before he got on the phone with me. His life was like a house on stilts by the ocean. One huge storm wave could wipe out his entire social network. This lack of a sense of security and safety was stored in his first emotional center and stood to affect the organs associated with that center—his blood and his immunity. Even though he wasn't ill and his partner didn't have AIDS, he was worried about his immunity. This was his intuition telling him that there could be consequences for his health unless he changed his situation, which was what I had seen in his reading as well.

Mark was right to be worried. He was about to be uprooted and to lose his family. Studies of AIDS have shown that among HIV-positive patients, those who had supportive families and were at peace with their identities tended to live longer than those who didn't have families that supported them.

Mark needed to follow his intuition. He needed to develop a greater sense of security and safety, to build a more stable foundation for his house of life. Stilts would no longer do. They may have sufficed when he was in his teens, but now he was becoming a mature man, and he needed a mature and stable sense of belonging. He needed to build relationships that had a balance of independence and dependence as well as a balance of power. He needed to find another tribe, another family system, one that would support him. Before he was uprooted in spite of himself and wilted like a geranium without a new pot, he needed to start preparing the soil in a new location where he could put down his roots and flourish. Moreover, he needed to find out why his relationships were always so unbalanced, why he was always the younger partner, the one with less power. Examining this question in the light of his memories and past experiences would help him adjust his environment to create a better fit, and it would also help him adapt by making changes in himself that could help him build a healthy future.

When we were talking, Mark realized that he had always wanted to pursue a career in counseling. His overinvolvement with his spiritual community, however, prevented him from finding the time to pursue a career. In order to take the first step toward his goal, he said that he would get catalogs from some local colleges and enroll in night courses toward a degree. In this way he could slowly begin to become a member of another community that would support him in his goal. This was a good resolution, because it would have been just too much of a physical and mental shock for Mark to have left the first community completely, without having prepared to transplant himself in another environment.

Clearly, a feeling of helplessness and a feeling of social support are encoded in our blood and our bones. If your social support is taken away, then you—and your white cells—may "perceive" the world as unsafe. You may be more susceptible to infections. Or your bones may know the same thing, and your joints may swell, or some other ailment may crop up. In fact, studies have shown that when a person with low social support loses his job, the likelihood that he will develop swollen joints increases tenfold.[2] Where you're affected depends upon your genetic makeup and your particular area of vulnerability. If something like rheumatoid arthritis or arthritis runs in your family, your problems are more likely to show up in your bones. If immune problems run in your family, the problems are more likely to go to your blood.

If your family has a genetic disorder, you need to find out which members of the family developed the disease and whether they share certain emotional patterns. Strive to be a black sheep in your family—don't follow the flock. Be different, break the emotional, social, and physical patterns. Stand out from the family context in your actions, relationships, diet, exercise, career—even in the car you drive. If your family drives a Buick, buy a Volkswagen. And get support from a group of people who have changed their lives for the better.

The Power and the Vulnerability

In the first emotional center, and in each of the other six emotional centers, it's essential to have a balance of the emotions that appear powerful in the outer world and also of those that appear vulnerable in the outer world. An excess of either power or vulnerability can set the scene for disease in the organs associated with the emotional center. An imbalance of power in the first emotional center can set the scene for disease in the blood, immune system, bones, and joints.

When I was four years old, I couldn't wait to go to school. As soon as I was old enough for first grade, I was out of the house every day like a shot, rushing a mile to the school, and in my seat by the time the bell rang.

I had an excess of power and not enough vulnerability. I was full of the power of the first emotional center: independence, resourcefulness, a sense of safety and security in the world. I never knew how to hold back, sit still, and let things come to me. I was the original go-getter. Usually patients whom doctors see frequently have an excess of the vulnerability of the first emotional center: dependence, helplessness, a strong sense of belonging, but a mistrust of the world outside the door. They have too much of the "holding back" aspect of this emotional center and not enough development of power in the outer world, not enough "get up and go." Doctors often do not know how to help these people.

Our emotional centers contain contrasting sets of emotions, the powers and the vulnerabilities, which we must balance for the best health. We need some of each for a happy, healthy life. When an imbalance occurs, our intuition knows it, and it speaks to us through our bodies, sending illness our way.

In the first emotional center, the power, or yang, half grounds our feelings of strength as an individual. If we have a healthy sense of self and power in the first emotional center, we are independent, resourceful, fearless, and trusting. We feel safe and secure in the world. If we have an *excess* of power, however, we verge on becoming isolated and we feel all alone in the world. We tend to reject support or help from others, we are fearless to the point of recklessness, and we are overly trusting of the goodwill of others.

The vulnerability side of the first emotional center influences our sense of belonging, even as we understand that there are boundaries between us and the rest of the world. If we have a healthy vulnerability in the first emotional center, we have a strong sense of belonging, we're willing to depend on others when necessary, we're willing to accept help from others, we're able to feel fear, and we don't trust everybody indiscriminately. If we have an *excess* of vulnerability, though, we're overly dependent, hopeless and helpless, fearful and distrustful of everyone and everything.

In the language of the emotional centers, power is not always positive or vulnerability always negative. Independence isn't "better" than dependence, and so on. Sometimes dependence and helplessness are important, because at times it's important to allow ourselves to be helped. Fearfulness, the capacity to feel fear, is vital at times, because fear can save us from danger.

The ideal is a balance between power and vulnerability. Look at the table below and measure your power-versus-vulnerability quotient. Grade yourself on a scale from 1 to 5 on each quality listed. If you're unsure where you fall on the scale, ask yourself if you ever hear yourself making the following statements. These well-worn phrases have become clichés, but they do accurately express our feelings:

- "That's okay, I'll do it myself" (independence).
- "No one's ever there for me. No one cares" (poor sense of belonging).
- "No one's helping me" (helplessness).
- "If you want something done right, do it yourself" (self-sufficiency).
- "The world is a dangerous place" (fearfulness).
- "You can't trust anyone but yourself" (mistrust).

If you consider yourself highly independent, you might give yourself a 4.5 on independence and a 2 on dependence, the ability to accept support from others. After you've graded yourself on each emotion, add up the numbers in each column to find your total power and your total vulnerability.

Power	**Vulnerability**
Sense of self	Sense of belonging
Independence	Dependence
Self-sufficiency	Helplessness
Fearlessness	Fearfulness
Trust	Mistrust

How did you do? I scored 23.5 for power and 2.6 for vulnerability. Not very good if we're looking for balance, is it? The truth is that I find it easy to be out in the world, but I have difficulty forming close relationships with all the inherent feelings of vulnerability and dependence that involves. But you've probably figured out by now that I have a lot of problems with bones and immunity. You probably had me tallied up before I did. Congratulations, you're a medical intuitive!

Whether we're powerful or vulnerable in the first emotional center, and all the other emotional centers, depends on two factors. First is the matter of temperament. Each of us comes into the world with certain "soul qualities," a genetic wisdom in our blood. We all know toddlers who want to be independent from the first. They wean themselves early. "Okay, Mom, I've had enough," and they're out of there. They're always charging into situations and want to do everything for themselves. "I do it, I do it," they cry, eluding Mom's grasp, grabbing the stroller and taking off down the street. They can seemingly slide away from a relationship like they are Teflon. Then there are the babies who seem to be stuck to their mothers with Velcro. They want to nurse forever, they hang back shyly in group situations, and they wrap themselves around Mommy's legs at the approach of every stranger.

Your temperament is set. The second factor that determines power or vulnerability is your memories. Your experience of life in the first emotional center and how they're encoded in your brain and your body will further influence your psychological state and your health in the organs of that area. You may be born with an independent soul, but if you have traumatic experiences in the first emotional center, that quality may be either curbed or exacerbated. You may become too powerful in the first center; someone else may become too vulnerable.

The science shows that an excess of either power or vulnerability sets the stage for illness and disease. One study looked at men who were trying to give up drinking. Some tried to stop on their own; others joined a program like Alcoholics Anonymous. The findings were striking. The men who tried to quit on their own were *twenty times* more likely to contract tuberculosis or other infections.[2] These men evinced an excess of power. They were overly independent—and they got infections. In the germ study discussed earlier, the people who got colds were likewise too much alone and didn't have a wide enough network of associates to give them a strong sense of belonging. The people who didn't contract colds in that study, on the other hand, demonstrated a healthy balance between independence and dependence. They were extroverted enough, had a strong enough sense of self, to collect a wide variety of friends and social contacts; these contacts, in turn, gave them a solid sense of belonging.

Remember when you were in school and there was always at least one kid on the playground who was bundled up in a scarf and hat or earmuffs on the mildest day in September? Who always carried a pack of Kleenex in her lunchbox? She seemed to be hermetically sealed, living life in a Ziploc bag. She was the one whose mother would call her back to the house on a rainy day to put on her boots. You can just hear that child's mother: "Come back in here! You can't go out in the rain like that. You'll catch your death of cold and get an infection. See? Your nose is running already." Mothers like this one have difficulty with their children's individuation and independence. They may also lack a sense of safety and security. The message they're sending their children is that being on their own isn't safe, that the world isn't a safe place, and this message goes right to the children's blood. Their white cells understand that the world is a dangerous place, and if there's one tiny perforation in their Ziploc universe, that'll be it! They'll have an excess of vulnerability in the first center, and it will result, ironically, in decreased immunity against the very germs that their Ziploc bag is meant to protect them from.

THE ZIPLOC SYNDROME
MOTHER-SON AGORAPHOBIA

The Reading. Martha, a forty-eight-year-old woman, called on the scheduled day for her reading with a sudden and unusual request. She no longer wanted a reading of herself, she said. Could I please read her son instead? I explained that I couldn't do that, because she had signed a release form for herself, not for a third party. I was intrigued, though, because her request had signaled me immediately that there was some clear problem at issue.

Martha agreed to proceed with a reading of herself. When I looked at her intuitively I realized at once that her primary sense of identity up to that point had resided in her being a mother. I saw that now her soul was asking her to branch away from that identity and give wing to some other facet of her personality. She, however, was afraid to leave the security of her established identity as a mother and move out into the world and develop some other sense of purpose.

At the same time, I saw someone else in her life who was having a great impact on her heart. This person was a young male, in his teens, who looked thin, wan, and pale. I saw this young person spending a lot of time in front of the computer, surfing the Net. He rarely went out and had few, if any, nonvirtual friends. He was also sick a great deal, with constant and repeated infections. I saw that he had difficulty seeing the world as a safe place and that this belief affected his health.

The Facts. Martha confirmed that the young man I saw was her son. She also confirmed that he had frequent infections, pneumonias, and other illnesses. As a result, he had to stay home a lot. I realized now why Martha had wanted me to read him. In fact, it was impossible to read her without including him. They were truly an enmeshed family, almost one person, as if the umbilical cord had never been either physically or emotionally severed. This was a problem. They had problems in the area of independence versus dependence, the first emotional center.

Martha suffered from agoraphobia, a fear of the outside world and of leaving home. Her son, meanwhile, had "immunological agoraphobia": he was afraid to leave his family even to go to school or have friends. Memories in his first emotional center told him that the world was not safe. This had set the scene for his blood and immune system problems.

I told Martha that she had to kick her son out of the nest, however painful that might be. The more he stayed at home, the worse it was going to be for him, because he would never learn that he could survive in the world. He also wouldn't individuate from her, and that would affect his ability to have healthy relationships with other people.

Martha's response was amazing. She began to get tearful on the phone. "But," she said, "the outer world *isn't* safe for him. He doesn't have the skills to survive there." Martha was teaching her son that the world was a stressful, scary place and that he wouldn't be safe unless he stayed at home. She was teaching him to be helpless and hopeless. *Her* memories, in *her* first emotional center, had been transfused into his, or, even more likely, she and her son shared one emotional center between the two of them. Consequently, every time the son left the house or tried to individuate from his family, he got sick.

I told Martha it was critical for her to move beyond the mother role and find another way of being for herself. Even though it felt good to be needed, to have a stable place, a family, in which she felt she belonged, it was no longer good for her own emotional health or for that of her son for her to continue with this outgrown behavior. If she loved her son, she would have to push him out of the nest and let him fly. As matters stood, he had too much vulnerability in the first emotional center. The fact is that the way you develop your immune system is to individuate from the family and go out into the world, where you meet other types of bacteria and learn to live in harmony with them. The world becomes safe by virtue of your very presence in it. If you don't go out there and stand on your own—with the support of your family—and if you don't create a healthy balance between independence and dependence, you can't build up your emotional strength and your immune defenses. And you could get sick.

Issues around (1) safety and security in the world, (2) trust versus mistrust, (3) independence versus dependence, (4) hopelessness and helplessness, (5) a sense of self versus sense of belonging, and (6) loss of a loved one with its inherent grief and depression are all stored in the first emotional center. People who have difficulties with these emotions have problems with the organs in the first emotional center, the blood and immunity, the bones and the joints.[1,2,19,20,21] They also have higher levels of corticosteroids, which are immunosuppressants, in their bodies. Scientific studies have suggested that these people are more susceptible to diseases in their blood, immune system, bones, and joints. They are more susceptible to chronic fatigue, fibromyalgia, rheumatoid arthritis, lupus, HIV, frequent colds and infections, and osteoporosis.[1,2,19,20,21]

THE POLLYANNA SYNDROME
CHRONIC FATIGUE AND FIBROMYALGIA

The Reading. Deborah was a forty-eight-year-old woman who came across like Pollyanna. She was overly hopeful and always looked on the bright side—but often unrealistically, sometimes to the point of deceiving herself. Consequently she failed to identify and possibly avert potential problems in her life. She had a very childlike approach to life. She trusted too easily. At the same time, she was fiercely independent.

On the one hand, I saw her as having an unusual circle of friends who supported her like a family. On the other hand, I felt that her ability to negotiate relations at work was not well developed. I saw her working in another group where she was low man on the totem pole. She felt safe at home with her friends but unsafe and even subject to victimization at work. In fact, I saw someone near her who was bitter, irritable, and nasty to her. This made her feel unsafe and under siege. She denied the attacks were even taking place, however, and claimed, "Oh, the woman's all right."

I saw issues around trust versus mistrust, safety and security in the world, and a sense of belonging in a family, all of which were affecting her body in the form of joint stiffness and tenderness and some mild neck stiffness. She had decreased range of motion in the joints, coupled with fatigue. I saw her as stuck and unable to move forward out of her situation. This stagnation in the world was affecting her ability to walk.

The Facts. Deborah had a group of friends among whom she felt happy, loved, and supported: her twenty-four pets—cats, dogs, birds, and a snake. Her other friends were her colleagues at the university where she was a professor. Among them, Deborah was under attack. The ringleader of the assault was a senior professor, a woman in her seventies who had organized a signature drive within the department to deny tenure to Deborah. Four months later, Deborah had come down with chronic fatigue and fibromyalgia, a condition causing stiffness and reduced mobility in the joints.

Deborah was a classic example of someone who failed to recognize what the emotions in her first emotional center were telling her: I'm stuck. I trust the wrong people, and they eventually victimize me. Where in the world do I belong? As a result, the emotions were shunted into the organs of her first emotional center. Although she had known her colleague was difficult from the start, she had chosen to trust her completely and without reservation. She had ignored her intuitive guidance system, which was telling her not to trust this woman. She had refused to recognize that this person could cause her problems.

This was a pattern; she had done the same with her ex-husband, an angry man who had placed her under siege during a lengthy and messy divorce. As a result of her illness, she had gone on disability and was working part-time. She told me she suffered from "oppressive" aching and bouts of pain where she had to stop whatever she was doing and lie down.

Deborah had made the intuitive connection between her condition and the problems with her colleague. Withdrawing from the scene, however, was not the best way to cope with the situation. She believed she had won by getting workmen's compensation, but I told her this was the exact opposite of what she needed to do. She needed to go back and reclaim her power within the university family—get her soul back, so to speak. She also needed to adapt by realizing that her child-like approach to life, trusting everyone even though her intuition told her to be careful, her refusal to see the train coming until it had run her over, cast her repeatedly in a victim role and affected her sense of safety and security in the world. In fact, she was afraid to go back to work full-time because of that very lack of a sense of safety. But I told her she couldn't hide behind her illness. She had to go back and resolve the conflict before she could have a better, healthier life.

COPING AND ADAPTING

We can become reconciled to the memories stored in our first emotional center, the emotional patterns and imbalances that can set the scene for disease in our blood, immunity, bones, and joints and keep ourselves healthy. If we listen to our intuition, the emotions and illnesses of the first emotional center can be healed. We can use the skills of coping and adapting to bring about changes that will make us happier and healthier in this area.

When we cope, we change our immediate environment to help us feel whole and healthy. We can cope by broadening our social networks, forming a diverse set of friends, family, and colleagues so as to build a healthier balance of dependence and independence. This gives us a greater sense of belonging as well as a sense of safety and security. We can also create changes by *adapting*—that is, by changing ourselves to fit the world better. We can look inside ourselves and work to change qualities in ourselves so that we're better able to withstand stresses and assaults from the outside world. We can work at learning whom we should trust and whom we should view with caution. We can learn healthy ways to adapt to the world and not allow ourselves to remain hopeless and helpless for long. We must feel our grief, sadness, and sense of loss fully, accept it, and move forward in such a way that our grief doesn't turn into depression.

Studies have looked at the concept of hardiness. What kind of personalities are better able to handle stress and change in life? Researchers looked at two groups of business executives: both were highly stressed, but one group exhibited a high instance of illness whereas the other group had no illnesses. The scientists found that the individuals with high stress and no illness had a strong commitment to themselves, had a vigorous attitude toward the world around them, looked for meaning in the events that took place, and believed that they had some control over every situation. The executives who succumbed to illness, on the other hand, felt powerless, were nihilistic, and believed they had little or no control over what happened to them. They felt that they were the pawns of outside forces.[21]

Healthy people accept change and view it as a challenge and an opportunity to grow. When faced with stress, they may feel hopeless and helpless for a moment, but they will pick themselves up and go into action. In looking at victims of extreme events, such as survivors of concentration camps and disasters, researchers have found that those who did well and had good emotional health were those who had a hardy attitude. They didn't succumb completely to feelings of victimization. They had the ability to snap back. At the same time, they didn't become overly hardy and refuse to acknowledge the grief and pain of their situation.

The key is balance. You can't be overly hardy. You must fully express and resolve the pain and stress of an event. If you don't do this, the organs and cells of your body—the messengers of your intuition network—will present you with symptoms in your blood, immunity, bones, and joints, letting you know that you have unresolved conflicts in your first emotional center. But you must also remember that being overly vulnerable will break down your immunity.

The actual stress of a life event won't have as much effect on you as the way you *perceive* that event. Our personalities are molded from our very beginnings by our families and by our experiences. But personality isn't cast in concrete. We are ever-changing and ever-adapting. Change is always possible and, with it, a better, healthier life.

SEVEN

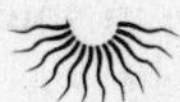

The Sex Organs and Lower Back: Relationships and Drive

Like birds that fly from the nest, most of us reach a point at which we're ready to leave home and go out into the wide world to make our mark. We're driven to pursue and acquire whatever we believe will bring us happiness—a career, money, position, sex, marriage or other partnerships, and children. At the same time, it can be difficult to take the steps toward autonomy that will enable us to fly away from the nest. We worry about individuating from the family, about holding on or letting go, and about gaining control in the outer world. We crave autonomy, but we doubt our ability to be independent. When we enter into an intimate relationship with a partner, we sometimes have difficulty maintaining our own sense of individual identity.

Emotions related to all these issues are stored in the second emotional center. Located in the pelvis and lower back, the second emotional center encompasses the male and female reproductive organs; the kidneys, bladder, and urinary tract; the lower gastrointestinal tract; and the muscles of the lower back. Memories and emotions stored in these organs have a dual aspect: they deal with our drives and how we go after what we want in the world; and they deal with how we manage the relationships we form as we leave the family and establish ourselves as autonomous individuals (see the accompanying figure).

WHAT'S DRIVING ME?

Have you ever wanted something and yet been so afraid to go after it, or felt so bad about wanting it, that you never did anything about it? You secretly liked that cute guy in your high school algebra class and you thought he liked you, but he was going steady with a friend of yours. Your guilt kept you from pursuing a relationship with him, but then you were outraged when another girlfriend, not so doubt-ridden as you, used every trick in the book to steal him away successfully for herself?

The fundamental conflict of the second emotional center is the conflict of autonomy versus shame and doubt, or initiative versus guilt. It has to do with knowing what you want and how you go about getting it. The actions you take and the way you feel about your behavior can affect your health in the organs of this area.

Keith had always wanted to become a lawyer, but he had doubts about whether he could do the course work. For most of his life, he put the thought of law school aside. When he was in his thirties, however, married and with a family, he found himself thinking once again about applying to law school. Keith's present job, like most of his earlier jobs, was unfulfilling and not quite what he wanted. He had gone from one job to another, perpetually in search of the proper fit but never finding it. Yet he had stayed with each job longer than he should have because he always doubted his ability to perform well in the next job. In everything he pursued, his ambition was neutralized by phobia and fear.

Now he felt the itch to go after what he had thought he wanted all his life. Not surprisingly, however, his established pattern held. Worried that his going to law school would be too much of a burden on his family, he hesitated to fill out the applications. His wife, however, was enthralled by the idea of becoming a lawyer's wife. She selected a school in a city she liked, filled out the applications, arranged interviews for her husband, and basically powered him forward, like booster fuel in a disabled rocket.

Keith entered law school, but from the start he had a difficult time. He missed his job and the friends he had made there. He had a hard time forming new relationships and dealing with new challenges and

Second Emotional Center

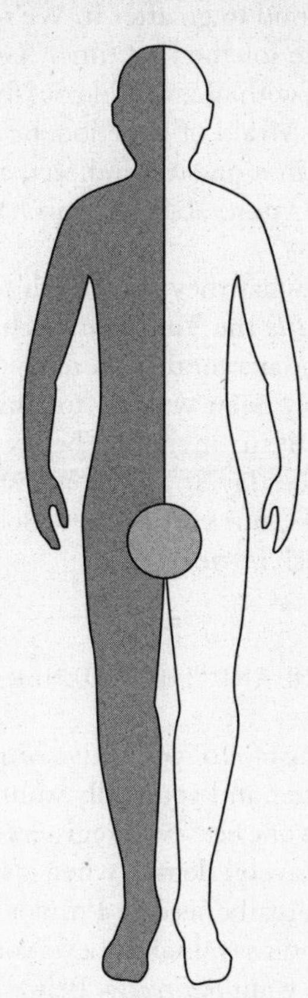

POWER

Drives

- **Active**
- **Uninhibited**
- **Direct**
- **Go-getter**
- **Shameless**

Relationships

- **Independent**
- **Needed by others**
- **Takes more**
- **Has well-defined boundaries**
- **Assertive**
- **Protects**
- **Opposes**

VULNERABILITY

Drives

- **Passive**
- **Inhibited/phobic**
- **Indirect**
- **Waits for things to come**
- **Shameful**

Relationships

- **Dependent**
- **Needs others**
- **Gives more**
- **Has poor boundaries**
- **Submissive**
- **Needs protection**
- **Cooperates**

struggles. In his first year of law school he developed kidney stones. And his was the mother of all kidney stone cases. He got not one or two or three but *eight* kidney stones. For a young man with no history of or predisposition to kidney ailments, this was unheard of. Keith's condition forced him to take a leave of absence from law school, to the great dismay of his disappointed wife.

What was Keith's intuitive guidance system, through his kidneys, trying to tell him about his life? Speaking to him through the second emotional center, it was telling him that he had to find out what or who was driving him. What did he want, and how was he going to get it? Keith wanted to go to law school, but he had doubts about following that dream. This happens to many of us. We want something, but we have doubts about going after it, or we feel ashamed or guilty about going after it, or we're afraid to go after it. We're like the teenage boy asking a girl out on a date for the first time. "Gee, Mary, I don't suppose you'd want to go out with me, would you? No, I guess not. You're probably all booked up." Afraid of rejection, he approaches the object of his desire backwards, in a passive, indirect, and shame-filled way. He's exhibiting too much vulnerability in this half of the second emotional center.

Other people go after what they want with too much intensity. In the movie *Sleepless in Seattle* the Tom Hanks character, a young widower, finally works up the nerve to ask a female colleague for a date. The woman has obviously been waiting for this moment for a long time. He barely stutters out the invitation before she informs him that they'll have dinner on Tuesday at a certain restaurant. Such overeagerness and shamelessness, not surprisingly, doesn't get her very far. She has exhibited too much power.

THE POWER AND THE VULNERABILITY

How do you go after things? Are you active or passive? If there's one drumstick left on the platter and you really want it, do you grab it and start munching before anyone else even registers that it's the last piece? Or do you coyly (and passively) demur when it's offered to you? "No, no, you go ahead. I don't really need it. I'm not that hungry. I'll have another piece of bread," you say, making everyone else feel guilty and thereby getting what you want *indirectly*. Being direct versus indirect, uninhibited versus inhibited, guiltless versus guilt-filled, shameless versus shame-filled are all powers and vulnerabilities in this area. Are you a go-getter, or do you sit back and let things come to you?

Keith, the man who wanted to be a lawyer, had an imbalance on the vulnerability side. Still full of doubt and fear, he went after what he wanted in an essentially passive, indirect way—through his wife. He didn't have the requisite drive on his own, so his wife kindly propelled him forward before he was ready to go. His body, however, promptly told him that this wasn't right for him. It's very meaningful that he developed kidney stones. Stones weigh you down so that you can't move forward.

Keith had an idea of what he thought he wanted in the world, but he wasn't sure about it, and he didn't know how to go about getting it.

He also had doubts about his abilities and guilt about his family and his wife. The worst reason to go after anything—a relationship, money, a career—is out of guilt. If you're not driving yourself out of your true heart, if guilt or shame is driving you, or if your parents or in-laws or husband or wife is pushing you, it won't work. You may go to law school because your mother said, "Of course you're going to law school. Your father was a lawyer and your grandfather and your uncle. What's wrong with you?" But you'll never be a happy lawyer, and you may also be setting the scene for illness in the organs of your second emotional center. You're better off getting that social work degree you wanted.

Many people find it difficult to decide how to deal with their drives. Women, especially, feel bad about being active and powerful. By asserting their drive, women often take people aback and make them uncomfortable, even today. A woman friend of mine who's a well-known lecturer was recently invited to speak at a major conference. The man who handled the arrangements, however, kept trying to persuade her to lecture for free. My friend stood firm. The man offered her a pittance, barely an honorarium. She insisted on receiving her full fee. In exasperation, the man finally snapped at her, "Is that all this means to you—money?" (I'd like to hear him say that to Colin Powell or Lee Iacocca!) To her credit, the woman laughed. "Yes," she replied, "that's about it." She didn't turn vulnerable and collapse into guilt or shame. She was powerful and shameless, going after what she wanted without doubting herself.

If you really want something and you have only one last chance of getting it, then it behooves you to increase your intensity, to assert your power absolutely, and to go after it actively, directly, shamelessly, and in uninhibited fashion. You have to behave like the hero of a 1940s movie who's standing on the station platform desperately scanning the faces in the train windows for the woman he loves. He's never told her how he feels, and she's about to ride out of his life forever. As the train slowly pulls away, he catches sight of her, leaning out the window and mournfully waving to him. He struggles for a moment with the vulnerability of going after her. Then, at the last moment, as the train picks up speed, he leaps aboard, shouting that he adores her and needs her. Shameless and uninhibited in a way he's never been before, he makes a scene, takes the power, and goes after what he wants, without fear or doubt.

Creation and Creativity

Creation and creativity are in the second emotional center. In this area you need a balance of power and vulnerability and a clear understanding of what your drives are. These attributes are essential to your health. In our society, go-getters and people who are driven are generally admired, because they represent so much power. In truth, however, asserting *too* much power in the way we go after our desires can be as unhealthy as being too vulnerable and passive. Going after everything with equal intensity and determination, seizing control and being completely active in the outer world, and being a guiltless, shameless go-getter can be counterproductive and have an impact on certain organs of your second emotional center.

THE ROLLING-STONE-GATHERS-NO-MOSS SYNDROME
A CASE OF INFERTILITY

The Reading. Marcy was a forty-two-year-old woman I saw intuitively as extremely well groomed, neat, and meticulous about her personal appearance and her surroundings. I saw her as highly successful in her work, which involved a great deal of traveling. She never allowed herself to nest in one place. She was very strong in the outer world, had a lot of drive, autonomy, and control. I also saw her as happy in a good relationship but ambivalent about the vulnerability and dependence that a relationship entails.

In her body I saw problems with weight in the past, and I wondered if she had suffered from anorexia or bulimia. In addition, I perceived that she had spent many years maintaining a rigid exercise schedule, to keep her body a perfect size 6. I saw her as having fertility as an issue, coupled with the desire to be fiercely independent and free from limitations, which gave rise to competing goals. She wanted desperately to keep control of her body size at all times, and that ran counter to the reality of having a child and being a mother.

The Facts. Marcy, at 5 feet 4, was a very successful vice president of a large management consulting firm, a job that entailed frequent coast-to-coast travel. She was seldom in one place for very long. She confirmed that she was indeed meticulous about her appearance and her environment; she even prided herself on always having sparkling windows at home and at work. She'd had a weight problem and some bulimia as a young woman, but had worked very hard, through diet and exercise, to control her weight.

Marcy had spent most of her adult life focusing all her drive on her career, climbing the corporate ladder to success. Then, in her thirties, she had married a wonderful, nurturing man. They talked about starting a family, but Marcy was concerned about balancing children and work. She was also concerned about being dependent on her husband. She had finally decided, however, to start a family. For four years she and her husband had tried to conceive a child. Failing with the natural method, they had tried virtually every fertility aid on the market, from in vitro fertilization to Chinese herbs. Nothing worked. Marcy was infertile, and she wanted to know why.

Marcy was a true child of the baby boom generation. Women of this generation aren't interested in vulnerability. We are admired for being powerful, not for being soft and vulnerable like our mothers and the other women of the fifties. We didn't listen to Dionne Warwick sing "I just don't know what to do with myself." We listened to Helen Reddy sing "I am woman, hear me roar." We were told not to wait for men to open doors for us. We were told not to be passive, inhibited, indirect. We were told to leave the home, go out, and make a big splash in the world.

This was what Marcy had done. But now she found herself facing some difficult choices. She loved her job, her perfect figure, and her constant travels, and her energy was concentrated on all the running around she did. This, however, made her a rolling stone, and a rolling stone gathers no moss. By staying constantly on the move, she never allowed anything to take root, including a baby. Her drives were focused on autonomy, not on belonging to a family. Moreover, Marcy disliked the idea of staying home with a child, which she believed would make her financially dependent on her husband and therefore needy. She had told herself from an early age that she would never depend on a husband for her living. And she had one final problem: she didn't want to lose control of her body; having worked so hard to get in shape and stay trim, she dreaded the body changes that pregnancy and childbearing would wreak.

All this made Marcy ambivalent about having a child. She was ambivalent about ceding her power in the outer world, her control over her body, and her position in her relationship with her husband. At the same time, she wanted to please her husband. And her parents and in-laws were pressuring her to produce a grandchild. This obviously caused her some guilt.

Marcy's solution was to go after a baby the same way she had gone after her career. She would produce a baby the way she produced at work. This is the baby boomer way. Women like Marcy, career-oriented, goal-oriented, hung up on control, do this all the time. At forty, having achieved success in their careers, they decide they're ready to have a baby, and they are determined to produce the perfect baby, what Dr. Christiane Northrup calls "the Neiman Marcus baby." But it's not as though you can just order the child of your choice from a catalog. Nor can you go to the drive-through window and pick one up, despite the fact that we're a drive-through culture. There's a drive-through window at a popular place here in Maine where they make great fish sandwiches. But when people have to wait six minutes for a fish sandwich because it's being cooked fresh, they get really annoyed. When they want something, they want it *now,* and, by God, they're going to *get* it now.

That's how Marcy went about trying to get pregnant, without having decided what she really wanted to create in the world. I go around the medical center here saying, "I'm a woman of the nineties. I can have it all," but I say this tongue-in-cheek. Because you can't have it all. You have to choose. I have in fact had my tubes tied, because I knew I wouldn't be able to do a good job of childbearing and raising, and I didn't want to do a halfway job. I don't do very well in the vulnerability column of this emotional center. Most of my drive is in the outer world, and I wouldn't have much left for children. I do have enough for two cats, however...and my friends' kids as well.

It's no accident that baby boomer women are experiencing the highest rate of infertility in history. Studies have found that infertility is higher in career-oriented women who feel conflicts over the biological wish for motherhood and who are worried about changes in their body image.[1] These women, like Marcy, struggle with the responsibilities of being needed by an entire family. They also feel expectations from others to produce children, but these expectations conflict with their personal goals and drives. This is like driving on two roads that go in opposite directions: it gets you nowhere; you make no progress.

We know that all these emotions can be translated into action in your uterine tract. Some studies suggest that some people with infertility have decreased levels of dopamine and norepinephrine, chemicals affecting FSH and LH, the neurotransmitters that help release eggs.[2] Dopamine and norepinephrine are affected by mood. When your mood is low, you release less LH and FSH, and as a result you have more ovulatory failure and infertility. So if you're not in the mood, you're really not. And neither are your eggs.

Fertility is also believed to be related to receptivity.[3] In an emotionally receptive state, a woman's brain releases oxytocin, a neurotransmitter that causes the vagina to contract and literally become a suction apparatus that pulls in sperm. Emotional stress, however, decreases the production of oxytocin and increases levels of norepinephrine and epinephrine, which suppress the sex hormones, turning off the suction mechanism. A woman having sex under emotional stress, like a woman who's desperately trying to use all of her power to get pregnant but is ambivalent about it at the same time, doesn't produce the suction that makes the sperm come flying in. She's not receptive to the sperm. Receptivity is a function of vulnerability, not a function of power.

To help you become fertile, you need a balance of power and vulnerability in the force that's driving you, because your emotions affect your uterus. A large body of literature shows that ambivalence about having children—in other words, ambivalence about what drives you—is associated with infertility.[4]

When a woman is infertile even though she's ovulating normally, artificial insemination is often the first step she takes in an effort to conceive. For some reason, however, the sperm may not come into contact with the eggs—they're hiding in the closet or under the bed. This happens because, as studies have shown, an emotionally reluctant female who is inseminated is likely to remain infertile, since her uterus will fail to signal her ovaries to expel eggs. After several attempts at insemination, a woman who's ambivalent about having a child, even on an unconscious level, may actually stop ovulating.[5,6] It's as though her body says, "Uh-uh, we're not going to do this. Lie low, eggs; you're not going anywhere."

Women who are excessively focused on the goal of having a child have also been found to release eggs prematurely, before they're ripe enough for fertilization.[7] In other words, if you're not ready to have a child, then neither are your eggs. And they'll tell you that you need to reexamine the central drives in your life.

Driving too hard toward getting pregnant can have dire consequences for your ovaries. If you take fertility drugs, you may be setting the scene for ovarian cancer. In fact, studies suggest that infertile women who use fertility drugs have a threefold increased risk of ovarian cancer.[8] What are fertility drugs but booster rockets? So your ovaries aren't powerful enough to push out the eggs? We'll put booster rockets on them. But ovarian cancer has been shown to be related to the number of ovulations a woman has in her lifetime.[9] If you give a woman drugs that cause a lot of ovulations, what do you think is going to happen? It's a case of buy now, pay later. You can't push this process. You can't change your power-vulnerability balance by unnatural means. You have to pay attention to the emotions of the intuition network, the emotions of your second emotional center that may be related to infertility.

Infertility in men is also related to ambivalence. Men with infertility and low sperm counts are more anxious about being criticized at work, have difficulty resisting demands in their work, and have more feelings of guilt than men with no fertility problems.[10] Family stress can also affect sperm count and motility.[11] In addition, the stress of work can make your sperm not work. When men feel guilty, their sperm counts drop. The less they're able to resist demands at work, the less they're able to ejaculate. So they work harder and harder to pay the bills for the infertility treatments. But guess what? Unfortunately, the more they spend, the less value their currency has. Or, as in basketball, the more you shoot under stress, the less you score.

Once again the drive in the outer world is competing with the drive in the inner world to have a child. These men are splitting their drives. They're under pressure from different directions, facing demands at work and at home, and they feel they can't meet them all. Their power is split, and they just don't know which way to shoot.

Infertility is also closely related to problems in relationships. Issues having to do with relationships are the twin aspect of the second emotional center and are discussed in greater detail later in this chapter. Problems in this area of your life can set the scene for illness and difficulties in the organs of this emotional center. Many studies have shown that conflicts in relationships between men and women are related to infertility. Many women with infertility actually have an aversion to sex and experience sexual disharmony in their relationships. Frequently, when they find a more suitable mate, they become fertile.[12] Some couples try to have a baby to cement their shaky relationship. Although neither the man nor the woman is found to be infertile, the woman can't conceive no matter how hard they try. When they try in vitro fertilization, something remarkable happens. The eggs and sperm are placed in a dish, and the eggs are observed visibly rejecting the sperm as they move in for contact. Science suggests that the woman's body is actually making antibodies against the sperm.[13] This is nothing less than rejection of motherhood at the molecular level or, at the very least, rejection of a particular father. It's also a perfect illustration of intuition speaking loud and clear.

You know how some women are never satisfied with any man who comes their way? Scientists have actually identified a gene known as the "dissatisfaction gene."[14] In experiments with flies, researchers have found that females who possess this gene are extremely choosy and find no male to be good enough for them. They're like the person in the Rolling Stones song—they can't get no satisfaction. The female flies with the dissatisfaction gene reject all male suitors during mating rituals and, in the end, never lay a single egg.

Marcy didn't have problems with her relationship, but she may well have had her own sort of dissatisfaction gene. She was at least unconsciously dissatisfied with the idea of staying home to raise a family and giving up her power while her husband brought home all the money. She needed to decide what sacrifices she was ready to make. She needed to find out how having a child would tip her more into the vulnerability category and how she felt about that. Did that make her feel guilty? Would she be unable to ask for things if she didn't have her own money? How would she feel if she went to her high school reunion, where her old classmates would show up as presidents of their own companies, swimming in stock options? Would she be filled with shame having to say, "I've been staying at home taking care of kids for seven years"?

You have to examine your drives very closely. If your have a 100-watt bulb, but you're burning 70 watts during the day at work, do you really want a child to be incubated under only 30 watts of energy? On the flip side, if you have a very important drive to produce in the outer world and be autonomous, then staying home so your children can have a 100-watt experience isn't necessarily going to work out, either. Your bulb is going to dim over time. You're going to look like a cat that doesn't like where it's living. Its fur gets matted and dull, and it stops grooming itself. That's just what happens to a lot of women who stay home with their kids but find it not fulfilling enough for them. They stop grooming themselves, stop bothering with their clothes, their hair starts to look flat, lifeless, and dull. They do what the man who stayed home with his kids did in the movie *Mr. Mom.* He grew a beard, gained weight, and sat around watching TV and eating tapioca pudding with his kids. He gave up because he wasn't fulfilling an important drive in his heart.

You have to know what you truly want; only then can you be successful in going out and getting it. Marcy's intuitive guidance system knew this, and it was trying to tell her so. All she had to do was listen.

Marcy had too much drive in the outer world to have a child in her inner world—her uterus. Not having any at all can be just as self-defeating and risky for the organs of the second emotional center.

> When Candy called me for a reading, I saw her as a completely autonomous young woman without any support whatsoever. Unfortunately, she didn't do autonomy well. She wasn't rooted in the world. I saw her as having just come out of a bad relationship, and I could tell she was living from hand to mouth. She was a very dependent person, but she had never formed a good, solid relationship with a partner. I saw her as having no work skills of any kind. She had attended junior college for one year. She had no career, and no drives in the outer world at all. She was one of those people constantly saying, "I don't know what I want. What do you want?" All she wanted was to stay home and have kids. The guy she had been involved with, however, was ambivalent about getting married and had left her.
>
> Most of her body was normal, but in her pelvis I saw two objects, one with the number 12 on it and the other with the number 8. They looked almost like billiard balls.

Candy had recently had two miscarriages in a row, one at eight weeks and the other at twelve. She wanted to know what she could do to change this history so she could carry a child to term. I told her I was very concerned, because she was in an overly vulnerable state. She hadn't developed power in the world at all. Her nearly complete passivity and dependence had actually driven her last partner away, leaving her alone and without support.

In fact, premature births are known to be related to emotional factors in the mother. These include ambivalence about having a child, being fearful about the ramifications of having a child, and having trouble accepting responsibility. Emotional factors and stress can precipitate changes in your body's hormones, especially epinephrine, which can trigger premature labor contractions.[15] Women who have frequent miscarriages have been found to be excessively conforming, adaptable, submissive, compromising, and compliant. All of these are vulnerabilities, and Candy had them all.[16] These women are less able to be direct and have poor problem-solving skills. They're more dependent and more likely to feel guilty than other women. They have difficulty openly and directly expressing anger or hostility in a way that relieves their frustrations. And their primary way of feeling good about themselves is by filling others' needs. Most of these women's strengths were in the vulnerability column, not the power column.

A pregnant woman's view of pregnancy and childbirth is also closely related to her attitude and relationship to her own mother.[17,4] If a woman has a good relationship with her mother and pleasant memories of it, she's likely to have a warm longing to be a mother herself. If she has a bad mother-daughter relationship and painful memories of fighting, tension, and struggle, and if she's ambivalent about having to meet the needs of a dependent child, then she might on some level resent the fetus as something that will drain her energy. She may fear losing her freedom and being tied down and burdened with the responsibility of motherhood.[18] Candy's mother had been very much like her, married at sixteen and soon struggling with the burdens of a family.

Candy's problem was that what was driving her to create in her inner world wasn't balanced with success in the outer world. She had no real support, so she already had a diminished first emotional center. In the second emotional center, she had all the traits of vulnerability and none of power. In other words, her eggs were all in one basket. She confirmed that she was very inhibited, fearful, and phobic about doing anything in the outer world. She had a math phobia and had dropped out of junior college because she didn't like computers. As a result, her search for some means of power in the world could be accomplished only through a husband. She had become so needy, dependent, and passive, however, that she couldn't sustain a relationship. Her partner felt swallowed up and overwhelmed by her neediness. She expected him to take care of the entire left-hand column of the power-vulnerability chart. Until she took some of the power for herself she would probably continue having problems with her efforts at creation.

Holding On and Letting Go

In our struggle for autonomy, learning when to hold on and when to let go in any relationship is a delicate task. It takes a long time for many of us to master it. People tend to be either Velcro or Teflon in temperament, either hanging on for dear life or never bonding to anything. How many people do you know who stay too long in jobs they hate or in marriages that aren't working? What about people who never really leave their childhood home at all? People who have problems with this issue set the stage for illness in the organs and tissues of the second emotional center.

HOLDING ON FOR DEAR LIFE
A CASE OF COLON CANCER

The Reading. I could see that Harriet, at age fifty-three, needed to break away. She wanted to achieve something in her life, but she was attached to a group of people among whom she had very little power. Part of her realized this, and she had a sense of loss and disillusionment over it. I saw that she would make the necessary changes to try to break away from this group but that the process would be very painful because of her long attachment. I saw her beginning a new project but having difficulties, especially in raising the money she would need to make a go of it.

Harriet's body seemed normal until I got to her bowels. There I saw lesions, inflammation, and irritation of the colon in the rectal area. I also saw some kind of degeneration in her right hip.

The Facts. Harriet, a longtime partner in a successful weight-loss organization, had always enjoyed her work. However, she now felt her future there was stymied. She had come up with her own weight-loss and dietary program, which the president of the organization, with whom she had once had a close relationship, refused to implement. Harriet wanted to go out on her own and establish her own clinics. Most of her funds, however, were tied up in the weight-loss company. She was having difficulty persuading the president to buy her out, and she didn't want to force the issue. She had moved to another state to distance herself from her former business partner, but she continued to work for the company's clinic in her new place of residence. She couldn't move forward with her own project until she got her money.

In the meantime, she had developed a severe degeneration in her right hip. And she had colon cancer.

Harriet believed she had made the break and let go of her previous attachment, but in fact she was still joined at the hip to her old organization. Ironically, her degenerating hip was the right hip, which is where many men keep their wallets in their pockets and where she carries her purse. Beneath the hip, her colon was affected, too.

Harriet was being too passive in her efforts to establish herself as an individual and set up her own business. She couldn't assert herself to demand her money back and go after what she wanted. She was fearful of leaving the nest and full of doubts about her ability to fly on her own. All this had affected the organs of her second emotional center, which were speaking to her about the need to develop the assets of the power column, let go of what no longer worked for her, and act on her drives.

THE GOLDEN HANDCUFF SYNDROME, OR "TAKE THIS JOB AND—" A CASE OF LOWER BACK PAIN

The Reading. I saw Donna in a work relationship with a group of people where she had very little power. She couldn't express her identity and be fully who she was, but she couldn't get up the initiative to leave, either. Her response to her dilemma was to throw herself into more projects than she could handle, which just dissipated her energies and caused her anxiety and tension.

I saw that Donna, at age fifty-one, was slightly overweight due to her stagnation. I also saw fatigue and a constant low level of depression. And I saw chronic lower back pain.

The Facts. Donna was a nurse on a surgical ward. She had liked her job—until managed care came to her hospital. Previously the staff had worked together smoothly toward the common goal of caring for patients and making them well. It was like the crew of a skiff, everyone rowing in rhythm and the boat gliding along purposefully. But then managed care became the new coxswain, shouting, "Hurry up! Produce! Produce!" and everyone lost the rhythm. All the oars were going in different directions. Donna tried to produce more and more, but she was being paid less and had an ever-decreasing feeling of fulfillment. She knew she should get out of the boat, but she was afraid of jumping out and swimming alone. She hated her home, but she still wanted to be in it.

She had begun having chronic lower back pain, which she believed was due to stress from her job. She had consulted numerous doctors and medical practitioners, including an osteopath, an acupuncturist, and a homeopathic physician. This was another reason for her unwillingness to let go of her job: she needed the medical insurance. So she was caught in a vicious circle: she stayed with a job that made her ill because it paid for the treatment of the illness it induced.

Lower back pain is the number one cause of workmen's disability in the United States, not just for furniture movers or dockworkers but for white-collar workers as well. Lower back pain among office workers has created a boom in the ergonomics industry, leading to elaborately designed office furniture and equipment to promote proper posture and reduce muscle strain in workers. Guess what, though? Most of these efforts don't make a bit of difference. A recent study found that educating office workers in ergonomics did not significantly reduce cases of lower back pain and disability.

This doesn't surprise me, because lower back pain is part of our intuitive guidance system, which is telling us that something is out of kilter with a drive we have in the world, in this case a drive related to work. You're in a job, and you're ambivalent about staying or leaving, holding on or letting go, and going after something else in the world that's more in keeping with what you really want to do. This was Donna's problem.

There are many psychological reasons for poor, pain-producing posture. We create memories, laying down emotions in the tissues of our bodies, without even knowing that we're feeling them. We might not consciously know we're fearful or angry, but we feel stiffness or tightness in certain muscles. People who are depressed or unhappy with where they are in life most frequently create more tension and tightness in certain muscles.[19] Backache and increased muscular tension occur when people can't go after something they want or can't take steps to resolve a conflict because they're afraid of retaliation. So they stay where they are, they hold on like Velcro instead of letting go. They suffer the golden handcuff syndrome and assume and maintain a rigid posture, which sets the scene for lower back pain.

Donna's drives in her job—her desire for work she loved as well as for money and power—were being inhibited, and she felt unfulfilled. But she was holding on, afraid to let go. In fact, she was right not to leap too quickly. If she suddenly and completely changed her identity she could cause herself even more illness. Her first emotional center, her sense of support, could be jarred and her back could get worse. She needed to take the ficus approach. You can't move a ficus tree abruptly from one end of the house to the other. It doesn't like that and will drop nearly all its leaves if you move it too far. You have to move it a little at a time, a foot or two, to get it accustomed to a new spot. That's what Donna needed to do. She needed to let go a little at a time, and establish a new identity in increments. Rather than giving up nursing all at once, I suggested perhaps she should try working with patients individually, doing a little counseling, and then gradually increase the counseling while cutting back on the nursing, until finally one took over the other. In that way she could gradually accomplish the difficult task of letting go and moving on to a new drive.

Work is a vital human drive in the outer world. But drives in the outer world must be balanced with strength in the inner world of relationships.

"YOU AND I" VERSUS "WE"

Partnership and Healing

The second emotional center concerns relationships, one-on-one intimacies, and the inherent paradox they contain. After all, we've just spent all this time talking about the drive toward autonomy that's housed in this center. At the same time, however, we also have a drive to be in a relationship with another person. In fact, seeking out a satisfying relationship is one of our most important drives. But why do we want that? Why would we want to leave our family to establish our autonomy, only to turn around and immediately go after something so much like the family we just left? People need people, to quote Barbra Streisand. Partnership is healing. That's why we seek it, the way plants seek the light.

Being in a relationship can affect your immunity and protect you from disease. Men actually have a physiological and immunological need for a woman's presence. Studies on mice have shown that when male mice with tumors are housed with two or three females, their tumors progress less rapidly than when they're housed alone or with other males.[20] As for men, it's been found that single men die earlier on average than married men do. Women, on the other hand, live longer if they have close female friends, as do female mice, whose tumors grow more slowly when they're housed with other females. Relationships, in other words, aren't just partnerships with members of the opposite sex. For women, it seems that close friendships with other women are as important as partnership with a man.

In any case, relationships are critical. The end of a relationship, whether through separation, divorce, or death, is known to be one of the most stressful events in life, and to have significant health consequences.[21] The health of a relationship can affect your physical health. Improvement in a person's marriage, for instance, can help to alleviate chronic pain, especially in the lower back.[22] When someone with lower back pain and marital problems undertakes marriage counseling with his or her partner, the lower back pain often improves significantly, without benefit of surgery or medication, as the relationship improves.[22] It's easy to see, in this instance, how the back pain may be the intuitive guidance system telling the individual that there was an emotional pain in his or her second emotional center and that that area of his life required an adjustment.

Relationships and Boundaries

Achieving a balance between relationships and drives looks tricky. At first glance, it seems that the drive for autonomy and the drive for relationships are in conflict: we want to stand alone, but we want to be with someone. How, you ask, can you be alone and live with someone at the same time?

It's really quite simple. Here's what happens when people get married or form a relationship or partnership: You and I, two individual entities, are linked together by a new entity, "we." Being united, however, doesn't mean that we cease to exist as individuals. When we come together as "we," a collective entity, we still acknowledge that you will continue to exist and I will continue to exist as whole, individual human beings. Now, however, we've added a third identity, which brings us together as one united being. We still keep our separate, individual boundaries and perimeters intact, however. People complain about prenuptial agreements, saying they're indicators of mistrust and anticipation that a marriage will end, but I see them as documents that symbolically acknowledge and enforce the boundaries. They say that even if "we" cease to exist, you and I will still remain with our perimeters intact. And this is good.

Setting up and maintaining boundaries in relationships is extremely important. It's important to know what's to be shared and what's to be yours and what's to be mine. A lot of people aren't able to do this. They lose their boundaries as soon as they enter a relationship. How many women give up everything—job, career, even friends—as soon as they marry, and merge into their husbands, like the bride in the movie *My Best Friend's Wedding*? In the rapture of love, they talk to their girlfriends about "we" this and "we" that to such an extent that the friends get nauseated. These women lose themselves in the "we" word. They become surgically attached at the hip to the new lover.

You can lose boundaries in other relationships, too. Friends tell me I have no boundaries in my close friendships. My friends can come to my house at any time and take whatever they want, because I'm overly trusting (trust and mistrust from the first emotional center) and therefore overly giving.

A relationship has to have boundaries, and it has to have a balance of power and vulnerability. It's not good for one partner to have all the power and the other all the vulnerability. When Freud was teaching, he developed a mentor-protégé relationship with most of his students. When they graduated, he gave them rings, almost like wedding rings. But if in the course of their careers they ever disagreed with him, he would take the rings back, as he did, famously, with his most celebrated renegade disciple, Carl Jung. Giving the rings and then taking them back was an extremely controlling power play on Freud's part. It would have been devastating to a student to lose the great Freud's ring. But Freud was making the point that he was always the lofty teacher and the protégé was always the lowly student. His followers had to be passive and obey all his rules, or else. They could not individuate from him. He had all the power, and they had all the vulnerability. It made for a very unclean relationship.

The power in this part of the second emotional center is in being independent, being needed by others rather than needing others, taking more rather than giving more, having well-defined as opposed to poorly defined boundaries, being assertive rather than submissive, protecting instead of being protected, opposing versus yielding. If you have a balance, you know that you will sometimes be dependent in a relationship—you'll have to ask your partner to hold the ladder while you paint the bedroom wall. But there will be other times when you're down painting the baseboard and you don't need any help or support at all. There will be times when you need others and times when others need you. There will be times when you're assertive, and times when you're submissive.

In our society, of course, men tend to be acculturated to be powerful in relationships, while women are acculturated to be vulnerable. I once watched a television show about abusive relationships. A husband explained his view of why he wielded all the power in the relationship. "I was just trying to protect you," he said to his wife. Letting herself be protected, always being submissive, the wife had yielded all her power and control; she had let her husband become all-powerful in the marriage, while she had all the vulnerability. And the result in this instance was abuse.

Women know all about getting together with a girlfriend who's in an unbalanced relationship and listening to her moan, "He doesn't write, he doesn't call"—that tired old line. Ever used it yourself?

Women in a relationship like that tend to suffer from poor boundaries; they are overly dependent and needy, and they give more than they get. But it can just as easily be the man who's needy. In the movie *Moonstruck,* the Cher character was initially in a relationship where she was clearly dominant. She pressed her fiancé for a wedding date, then prepared to make all the arrangements for the ceremony. All he had to do, she said, was show up. In restaurants, he'd order a dish he liked, and she'd cancel it saying it wasn't good for him and order him something else. She was the assertive and powerful one. It was clear the relationship was off-kilter and really going nowhere. Then she met the baker. This guy was more her match, and their relationship had a better balance. They traded the power. She would be assertive sometimes, submissive others. She learned to yield to him on some occasions, and to oppose him at other times.

The person who handles the money in the family (money being another issue of the second emotional center) usually has the most power. A friend of mine, a teacher, married a banker. My friend was intelligent, but she had a little bit of a phobia about balancing her checkbook. Every week, therefore, on payday, she'd hand her check over to her husband, and he would give her $25 spending money (yes, this was in the nineties). Talk about keeping someone on a short leash. If she ran out of cash and asked him for more, he'd demand to know what she'd spent it all on. His rationale was that he was "protecting" her from spending more. He was protective; she was protected. My friend was so submissive, in fact, that when you asked her about this patronizing arrangement, she would defend it. "Oh, it's much better this way," she'd say. "He's much better at taking care of the finances than I am." Plenty of women, though, control the purse strings in the family. In many families, the mother is the dominant figure and carries the money. In a restaurant, after dinner, the mother silently hands the money to the father under the table so that he can pay the check.

It's not healthy for your relationship, your emotions, or your body when one partner has all the power and the other has all the vulnerability. In fact, either position can be painful. You have to learn to understand the joys and benefits of the opposite position, of being vulnerable when the occasion calls for it and of seizing power when necessary. Failure to do that can set the stage for illness in the organs of the second emotional center.

RELATIONSHIP ON ICE
FIBROID CYST

The Reading. I had some difficulty with the intuitive reading I performed on Ruth. I could see her clearly as an attractive, well-groomed woman in good overall physical condition. But in the area of her relationships, I encountered some confusion. I saw her involved in a decades-long dead-end relationship. Yet I had trouble envisioning her partner. I would get images of a conventional-looking, slightly overweight, balding, 5-foot 10-inch man; then they would suddenly change into pictures of a tall woman with shoulder-length hair, dressed in flashy, colorful clothing and wearing bright jewelry and bold makeup. I didn't know what to make of this. Was my client's partner a man or a woman? I asked Ruth directly, and she replied that he was a man. Still the images of a woman would flash before me. I wondered if Ruth could be caught up in an *M. Butterfly* sort of situation. In that play, based on a true story, a man has an affair for two decades with someone he thinks is a woman, but who turns out to be a man.

Physically, I felt a heaviness in Ruth's pelvic region and wondered if she had a frozen-solid cyst in her uterus.

The Facts. Unlike me, Ruth wasn't confused about the sex of her partner. For twenty-one years, she had been involved with a man who was a cross-dresser. She was confused, however—if not in near-despair—about the future of their relationship. For two decades, she had hung on, dependently and submissively waiting for her lover to decide whether or not he could marry her. She was frozen in the relationship, unable to move forward. In her uterus, she had developed a large calcified, or frozen, fibroid tumor.

Ruth's fibroid cyst was the physically embodied memory of her frozen relationship with a man who held much more power in the relationship than she. She had spent two decades giving and giving to this man while receiving little in the way of commitment in return. She was afraid to ask him directly for a commitment because she didn't want to appear needy, desperate, and dependent. She preferred to hint at what she wanted, being indirect and passive.

More research needs to be done in this important area, but there is evidence that stress in a relationship can affect the uterus. Stressful events in a woman's life can cause the adrenal glands to produce more steroids, which trigger uterine bleeding.[23]

It was important for Ruth to take more power in her relationship and make a decision about whether to stay with her partner or leave him. Only by achieving a balance of power and vulnerability in her approach to relationships could she release herself from her frozen state and move forward in the world.

Relationships and Sex

An important part of a healthy, balanced relationship is the ability to talk to your partner. You have to be able to communicate in order to negotiate issues having to do with power and vulnerability, needing versus being needed, taking versus giving, and so on, and so that you can agree on establishing boundaries. Successful relationships based solely on sex are extremely rare. Generally, even if two people agree in principle that all they want from each other is sex, at least one of them secretly wants much more than that. Or eventually one person or the other person will feel the need to explore the possibility of relating on a level beyond the purely physical. A relationship in which physical intimacy occurs without emotional intimacy can serve as a prime staging area for disease and disorders in the organs of the second emotional center, specifically the sexual and reproductive organs.

Women who blindly engage in relationships that never go beyond the sexual suffer from what I call praying mantis syndrome. When praying mantises mate, the female rips off the male's head and continues the act. This frequently happens when women choose a partner. They fall in love with a guy from the neck down. They have a sexual relationship that disregards the man's brain and basic personality. These women have what I call head-pelvis disconnection syndrome. The following may seem an obvious, commonsense statement, but since so many women and men don't seem to practice it, I'll say it anyway: you have to ground your attraction to someone's body with an even stronger attraction to his or her brain.

I worked with a machine called an aggreganometer in the medical lab when I was doing blood research. Occasionally the machine would blow a fuse, and I'd have to take it apart, replace the fuse, and put it back together. Being a bit of a mechanical klutz, I'd usually have a couple of screws left over when I was finished, and I wouldn't be able to figure out where they went. But the machine would seem to be working fine, so I'd just leave them on my desk. One time my supervisor came in and noticed the screws on my desk in a paper cup. "Where did those come from?" he asked. "They're just some leftover screws from the aggreganometer," I replied casually. He grabbed his head with both hands. "Those are grounding screws!" he cried. "You've got to put them back in or you'll electrocute yourself."

Relationships need to be grounded, too, or you can get burned emotionally and physically. You have to know what each of you is feeling and what your boundaries are. If you don't, your intuitive guidance system, through the organs of your second emotional center, will signal you that there's a problem in this area of your life. I know a woman who has sex with men indiscriminately. She meets men in airports, on planes, in hotels, and at conferences and invariably ends up in bed with them. But that's as far as it goes. No relationship ever develops. She waits for weeks after the encounters for the men to call her, but they never do. This woman has problems with boundaries. Either she has no boundaries whatsoever or she takes cover behind the Berlin Wall. In her work she watches her back and her turf intently so that no one can ever take advantage of her, but meanwhile, she repeatedly lets men take advantage of her. She's either a wide-open window, letting in all the vermin of the world, or an Anderson double-glazed thermal pane, sealing everything out.

It didn't surprise me when this woman developed cervical cancer. Distinct emotional patterns have been found to predominate in women with cervical dysplasia and cervical cancer. They're likely to have had sexual relationships at an early age, to have a relatively high number of premarital sexual experiences and extramarital affairs as well as several marriages and divorces.[24] More than half of these women grew up in homes where the father had died or deserted the family. Essentially these women never had adequate love from a man as children. Their later sexual behavior is like a cry for love, an effort to find what they couldn't get at home. Without an internal representation of love, they constantly try to fill the empty hole inside them with an abundance of unbalanced relationships.[25]

In women with cervical disorders, love and desire for a loving relationship is often a major reason for their willingness to have sexual intercourse. Very frequently they don't even enjoy sex.[26] Yet they tend to be selfless and willing to do whatever pleases the man, physically and emotionally. They usually give more than they take. In fact, a study of fifty-one women with cervical cancer found that those whose cancers progressed most rapidly were the ones who put more into the world than they took from it.[27] Like Sandra in the story below, these women usually have endured lifelong loneliness and a sense of hopelessness about changing the quality of their lives and relationships. In their relationships, they tend to be overly cooperative, passive, and unassertive. They make themselves too vulnerable, and they don't maintain firm boundaries.

THE PRAYING MANTIS SYNDROME
CERVICAL CANCER

The Reading. At thirty, Sandra was experiencing emotional and physical distress and wanted to create new patterns of health in her life. I saw her as a diminutive woman with a very slight build. I saw that she had had many short-term, unstable, sexually intimate relationships since her late teens. This history of unstable sexual relationships was associated with her relationship with her father. I could see painful feelings and memories around the fact that her father frequently left the family for weeks at a time during Sandra's childhood. His absences made her feel empty, unloved, and abandoned.

In Sandra's body I saw severe chronic cervical irritation and a recent bloody discharge from her uterus.

The Facts. Sandra had cervical herpes and a history of venereal warts. A few days before her reading, she had aborted a pregnancy that had resulted from a three-week relationship with a man she hoped would marry her.

Sandra had only recently, however, separated from her husband, John, after a two-year marriage. She could only speak a little bit about her father, but she admitted that during her childhood he had served in the merchant marine and had frequently left home for months at a time. She wished they could have been closer.

In addition to her health, Sandra was worried about money. She and her estranged husband together owned a lucrative business, and Sandra was having difficulty imagining what she could do for a long-term career apart from her husband. She was unsure of her drives in the outer world. Her financial assets and employment were usually controlled by the men with whom she was sexually involved.

Sandra felt hopeless about her life. She was frightened about her physical condition, and she felt powerless around the men she attracted and with whom she had relationships. Her emotional pain about her sexual relationships, money, and power or control issues was stored in her second emotional center. As a result, the organs located in this region were speaking to her through pain and disease via her cervical dysplasia, herpes, and vaginal warts.

Sandra was driven by the desire for a loving relationship with a man to fill the void that had been left by her father in her childhood. Cervical cancer has also been associated with a certain coping style. Susceptible people tend to be passive, pessimistic, submissive, and indirect in forming a relationship. Those who are more resistant to this cancer have a more active coping strategy.[28] Immunologically, if we don't cope well with stressful environments or relationships, our adrenal glands produce more sex steroids, making us more susceptible to an illness like cervical cancer. Researchers can almost predict which women with abnormal Pap smears will develop an invasive cancer. It will be the one whose boyfriend or husband runs around a lot, is unfaithful, and drinks too much. She'll say, "I should have left him, but I couldn't because of the kids." Her intuition told her what to do, and she even heard the warning but didn't act on it. She chose to be passive, submissive. Such women take the blame for problems and shoulder most of the responsibility out of a sense that others need them. The women who don't develop cervical cancer, by contrast, usually know the limits of their responsibility to others and to themselves, and they're able to adapt, to change as their lives change.[27]

Another classic example of how emotions and memories having to do with sex and relationships are stored in the body concerns chronic pelvic pain.[29] Survivors of childhood sexual abuse and women with painful sexual relationships are prone to chronic pelvic pain.[30] Yet often they don't recognize what their intuition is telling them through the organs of their second emotional center.

TRAUMATIC MEMORIES
CHRONIC PELVIC PAIN

The Reading. When forty-two-year-old Katrina called me, I saw her sitting at a desk, being inundated with material by two different bosses and passively doing whatever they asked of her. I also saw her as having had a very painful past with at least two men, who were not her bosses. I saw this pain encoded in her pelvis in the form of a great deal of scarring, setting the scene for chronic pelvic pain. I also saw that she had problems with depression and substance abuse.

The Facts. At first, Katrina denied having had any painful relationships with men. In fact, she was adamant. There had been none, she said. She didn't currently have a boyfriend. She was focusing on her career, she said. She confirmed, however, that she did have chronic pelvic pain. It was so bad that it had required four operations, none of which had helped. She wanted desperately to know what she could do to free herself from this pain.

When we hung up, I was confounded by Katrina's reading. Had I misread her emotional past? Fifteen minutes later she called me back. Oh, yes, she said, she'd forgotten. At the age of fifteen she had been abducted while walking home from school, driven to a remote location, and raped by two men.

Katrina hadn't mentioned the rape because she hadn't viewed it as a relationship. Yet clearly it was the source of her physical troubles. A huge literature chronicles the connection between chronic pelvic pain and previous sexual abuse. Sexual trauma, especially in childhood, is known to help set the scene for pain in the genital and urinary tract as well as for eating disorders and obesity. Women who experienced sexual abuse in childhood are also more likely to exhibit self-destructive behavior to escape their memories of trauma.[30]

Katrina's was a clear case of emotional dissociation and conscious forgetting of a traumatic memory. But the memory was stored in her pelvis, the symbolic area where her trauma had occurred. Katrina had never faced and resolved that memory. She had never learned the skills to deal with the ways in which her past trauma disturbed her current relationships. As a result, she was repeating the pattern of powerlessness that had marked the incident in her teens. She was passive and submissive toward her employers, anxious to please, and giving more than taking. At the same time, she was avoiding intimate relationships with men. She was throwing herself into her career, a drive in the outer world, but failing to balance it with a healthy relationship in her private life. Her intuitive guidance system, through her pelvis, was speaking up with the message that her life was out of kilter and giving her an opportunity to do something about it.

BALANCING RELATIONSHIPS AND DRIVES

In the second emotional center, relationships and drives are intertwined. And they're both necessary to our health in this area. You can't have one and not the other.

Relationships, indeed, are a vital drive in their own right and represent an essential counterpoint to our drives in the outer world, for money, power, careers. Men who lose their jobs do better at carrying on with their lives and avoiding illness if they have a strong sense of family support and a high degree of satisfaction with the relationships in their lives.[19] This makes a lot of sense. If you lose your job, you lose one major drive in your second emotional center. If you have problems in your relationships, too, then you'll be vulnerable to symptoms in this emotional center.

The following story illustrates the intricate interplay between relationships and drives and their potential impact upon a person's health.

ROOSTER WITHOUT A HENHOUSE
POWERLESSNESS AND PROSTATE CANCER

George, age fifty-four, had always been the proud patriarch of his family. The son of immigrants, he had worked his way up the corporate ladder to a highly paid, high-ranking position in a major investment company. He had a beautiful wife and two wonderful children. The family enjoyed all the trappings of George's success—a magnificent home with a pool, several cars including a Volvo and a Jaguar, a membership in the local country club, and a golden retriever named Muldoon. George was a pillar of the community, an officer of the Lions Club and the Rotary, and an informal adviser to the mayor of his town.

At home, George was the supreme master. He not only brought home the bacon, he also controlled all the money, and paid the mortgage and the bills. He was very protective of his daughter, Sally, when she started to date. His wife, Karna, stayed home to raise the kids and did some volunteer work. She never held a job, even after the children went to school. She and the children submitted to George on all major family decisions. Karna, in fact, suffered from depression, but she never made a move to oppose her husband, assert herself in the marriage, or find a drive outside the home.

The family was riding high when George was suddenly

indicted in an insider trading scandal. The fallout was devastating. He was convicted and sentenced to two years in prison. All at once, this powerful man, who had wielded so much control in the world and at home, was stripped of everything. He no longer had any power or any control, anywhere. His family visited him in prison and communicated daily at first, but soon the cards, letters, telephone calls, and visits became less frequent. George railed against the enforced passivity of prison. He was consumed with guilt and filled with shame over what had happened.

Meanwhile, Karna was gradually becoming a new woman. At first she was grief-stricken and fearful when George went off to prison. But then she brushed up on her typing skills, got a secretarial job, and started earning her own money. She took some trips. She started to get used to being alone, independent, and answerable to no one. Her children still needed her, but for the first time, she found out what it was like not to need others to give her a sense of strength. She learned to be assertive and to set limits. Her depression lifted. She felt empowered, and she began to make decisions for the family, which she had never done before.

When the two years had passed, George prepared to come home. He requested that the whole family be there to meet him. The kids came home from school, and they tied a yellow ribbon outside the house to greet the returning patriarch. They arranged themselves in their old positions in an effort to re-create the family they had once been.

But things were different now. George had trouble finding work. He began to gain weight, grew a beard, and wandered aimlessly around the house. The children had gone off to college, had started to individuate, and no longer looked to their father as the unchallenged head of the household. Karna, meanwhile, was enjoying her power in the outside world. She had received a promotion and was now taking paralegal courses at the local university. She felt somewhat estranged from George. He wasn't the man she had married.

The power balance in the relationship had completely shifted. Karna was making most of the family decisions now. With their children gone, she told George she wanted to sell their large house and move into a smaller one. When he got into several accidents with his Jaguar, Karna insisted that he sell that, too. George had lost his power in the family. Now he was also losing his possessions, the symbols of his status and wealth. Soon thereafter, he began to have pain while urinating. He went to the doctor and learned he had prostate cancer.

George's condition was related to the loss of his great power in the outer world as well as to the loss of power in his relationships. He had experienced a complete reversal of his position in both areas of the second emotional center, and this set the scene for changes in his prostate, an organ of the second emotional center.

How do we know that feelings of power in the outer world—sex, money, jobs—and issues of power and vulnerability in a relationship can affect the health and potency of a man's sex organs? Studies on rhesus monkeys support this conclusion. They found that when a male monkey asserted himself to become dominant in his group, to seize the power, his testosterone levels would increase. In contrast, the testosterone levels of submissive, or defeated, males, who enjoyed little or no power or status within the group, would decline.[31,32]

Social status, after a brief stop in the brain, apparently shoots directly to the pelvis. Scientists studied a fish known as *haplochromis Bertoni*. They found that in aggressive males of this species who commanded large territories and kept contending males at bay, the brain cells in the hypothalamus, which controls testosterone, would swell, correspondingly enlarging the sex organs—in other words, the fishes' balls; when people talk about a man having "a lot of balls" it seems this can be literally true.[32] These fish were then able to mate six to eight times longer than other fish. And they would develop extraordinarily bright coloring that contrasted with the drab beige coloring of the ordinary fish. So not only were these fish getting all the chicks, they were also wearing the power suits (and probably driving the flashy cars).

In his heyday, George had been like the macho fish or the rooster in the henhouse. Powerful, socially prominent, dressed in power suits, he had swaggered through life. But then he suffered a reversal. The fact is, it's great to be king of the hill, but one negative aspect of it is that when you're on top, everyone wants to pull you down. It's a dog-eat-dog world even if you're a fish, it seems. The brilliantly colored fish in the study didn't live happily ever after with all the girls and the real estate and the power jobs. Their beautiful colors were like a red flag to predators and competitors, the next fish looking to make it to the top. If they were defeated in the power struggle, the previously macho fish suffered a reversal of the process they had earlier undergone. Now the cells in the hypothalamus shrank, and their testosterone went down. Their balls, if you will, got smaller. At the same time, their beautiful colors began to fade, and soon they were reduced to wearing the beige leisure suit of the middle manager.

The fish teach us a neat little lesson about the need for a balance between power and vulnerability in what drives us. Obviously, you can't just marinate in machismo, be nothing but a go-getter, and hang out in the power column of the second emotional center. Excessive power can actually make you vulnerable to something else in the end. The predators may come and get you. And then you'll shrivel and shrink.

When George lost his power and status in the community and in his relationships, he was like the fish whose brain shrank and whose balls shriveled. The balance in his life shifted entirely from the power column to the vulnerability column. At the same time, his wife got the balls in the family and donned the power suit. She moved into the outer world and into the power category while he moved into the vulnerable category. The accompanying stress affected his health. Stress is believed to be a contributor to cases of enlarged prostate. Stress goes to the hypothalamus, which affects the pituitary gland, causing an imbalance between androgen and estrogen and leading to prostate enlargement.[33]

But George's case had to do with more than stress. His intuitive guidance system was telling him that affairs in his second emotional center were out of whack. In fact, his second emotional center was on the verge of devastation unless he acted to right it quickly. He had to restore a balance not only between his power and vulnerability in both drives and relationships but also between the two halves of his second emotional center. For if your whole life is your job and you have poor relationships, then you're missing one side of your second emotional center. You have no balance, and you're vulnerable to illness here. Conversely, if you have great relationships but no balancing drive in the outer world, you can be equally vulnerable.

In the second emotional center you can't have all your eggs in one basket or the other. You have to distribute them between the two.

EIGHT

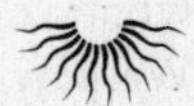

The Gastrointestinal Tract: Responsibility and Self-Esteem

In the heart of the hit musical *A Chorus Line*, one of the characters, wondering if she'll ever make it as a dancer, sings a song of self-doubt and questioning. "Who am I anyway?" she ponders. "Am I just my résumé?"

This question reverberates in every person's consciousness. As we strive to make our mark on the world, our sense of identity and self-esteem is intimately bound up with our work or our task in life, with how well we do it, and how others perceive, assess, and acknowledge our performance.

This concern is at the heart of the third emotional center. This emotional center has to do with the "me against the world" element of our lives. In our quest to establish ourselves as powerful in the outer world, we struggle with our feelings of adequacy or inadequacy, with competitiveness and aggression versus noncompetitiveness and defensiveness. We struggle to develop a sense of responsibility, to set up boundaries, and to understand our limitations. Memories related to these emotions are stored in the organs of this center, the organs of the gastrointestinal tract, including the mouth, the esophagus, the stomach, the small intestines and upper colon, the liver, and the gallbladder (see the accompanying figure).

THE POWER AND THE VULNERABILITY

Some of us are driven to succeed. We strive for a sense of competence and adequacy. We're highly competitive, ambitious, and aggressive in the execution of our labors, whatever they may be. We take our responsibilities very seriously. We play to win, at everything. Society rewards us for our accomplishment, through money, recognition, and continuous encouragement, and this keeps us going. Having become powerful and successful, we perceive ourselves, as others perceive us, to be riding high.

At the same time, however, we're riding for a fall. Wanting always to win, never accepting the possibility that you might lose at something, displays an excess of power in the third emotional center. Unbalanced by a realistic ability to tolerate inadequacy and incompetence in ourselves at some levels, this overabundance of power can help set the stage for disease in the organs of the third emotional center.

THE CORPORATE TAKEOVER
A CASE OF ULCERS

The Reading. When Peter called me for a reading, I intuitively saw a forty-five-year-old man who worked in an intensely competitive setting, where a corporate-takeover mentality prevailed and where there was a lot of vying for power and control. I saw that Peter was very good at what he did, extremely competent and highly skilled. He had reached a point, however, where his work was no longer fulfilling to him. He was beginning to question his purpose and whether he could meet his growing spiritual needs in some other way. Moreover, although he had successfully acquired more and more corporate territory, I saw that he had lost his job after attempting to acquire some sort of account that belonged to somebody else.

In Peter's body, I saw that he had the capacity to form blockages in the coronary artery. This was not bothering him at present, however. When I got to his esophagus, I began to see inflammation, and then, in his stomach and duodenum, I saw large bleeding holes.

Third Emotional Center

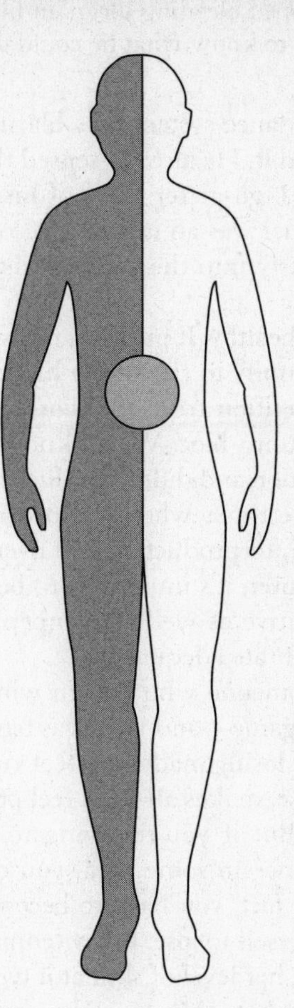

POWER

Adequacy
- Skills
- Competence
- Making it work

Responsibility
- Being caught in the middle

Aggressiveness
- Threat
- Intimidation
- Territoriality

Boundaries

Competitiveness
- Winning
- Gain

VULNERABILITY

Inadequacy
- Inferiority
- Incompetence
- Giving up

Irresponsibility
- Addiction

Defensiveness
- Restraint
- Entrapment
- Avoidance and escape

Limitations

Noncompetitiveness
- Losing and conceding
- Loss

The Facts. Peter had for many years been a highly placed executive with a Fortune 500 company. He had competed intensely and with great success against others for power and control over various accounts and territory. He stumbled, however, when he tried to take over a very special account: he had had an affair with his boss's wife. When the liaison was discovered, he was transferred to a less desirable job within the company. Ultimately, he was forced to seek work elsewhere, and he landed a job with another Fortune 500 company, a competitor to his previous employer.

Peter had developed bleeding ulcers in his stomach and duodenum and wanted to know what he could do about them.

Peter's intuitive guidance system was blaring like a siren, and on some level he had heard it. He already sensed that he needed a change from the high-powered, go-getter ways of his past. His yearning for something more spiritual was an intuitive recognition that he needed to move more vigorously into the vulnerability column of the third emotional center.

Competition can be healthy. It puts you in a situation where you and others have the opportunity to rise to the highest level of your ability. If you eliminate competition from the world, you get the old Soviet Union and the Communist bloc. We all know they didn't last. Their citizens had no motivation and didn't produce to their maximum level of ability. But there are times when competition, the mere desire to win or lose, can be counterproductive and overbearing. For health in the third emotional center, it's important to be able to lose as well as win, to be noncompetitive as well as competitive, to tolerate inadequacy as well as to celebrate adequacy.

We've all known someone who had to win at everything—every argument, every chess game—and who was basically a boor. He never wanted to lose, because losing made him feel vulnerable and incompetent. Winning, of course, makes all of us feel powerful and wonderful and very competent. But if you're trying to acquire new skills or increase your competence in some area, you can't expect to win the first time up at bat. In fact, you have to become noncompetitive and perhaps even allow yourself to lose. I play tennis regularly with a good friend, but I don't have her level of skill at it (yet). I almost always lose to her, which I admit I hate. My game has been improving, though, and one evening not too long ago I was actually ahead of her in a match, four games to two. At that point, though, I told her that I wasn't going to try to win the next few games; I was going to work on my racquet skills and shot placement instead. This wasn't easy for me; like most people, I hate to lose (which I did), but it was necessary if I hoped to acquire the skills and achieve the level of competency that would enable me to give my friend a real run for her money on the court.

In the same way, while we all want to be competent and adequate, we have to accept that we're going to be inadequate in certain areas of our lives. No one can be good at everything. We have to tolerate inadequacy in ourselves and in others as well. I don't always do really well at this. Some people, however, are so afraid of failing that they never complete their tasks. They wait and procrastinate.

The figure illustrates the power and the vulnerability of the third emotional center. What's your power-vulnerability quotient in this area? Do you see yourself as competitive, as someone who always has to win? Is being competent at everything you do important to your self-esteem? Or do you feel so inadequate that you never finish anything you start? Do you consider yourself responsible and committed, or do you avoid responsibility, because it makes you feel trapped, and do you seek escape in addiction? Are you aggressive in the face of challenges and threats, responding by being intimidating, or do you tend to run and hide, avoid and escape? Lastly, are you territorial? How do you manage your boundaries and territories? Do you establish boundaries around you in your life and work? Do you have to have things just so? Are all the magnets on your refrigerator lined up? All the socks arranged perfectly in your dresser drawer? Are the dollar bills in your wallet lined up according to denomination? Do you go after the boundaries of others, seeking to expand your territory and avidly guarding your own turf but not understanding your own limitations? Or are you hobbled and frustrated by limitations, feeling trapped and restrained?

Do you hear yourself saying things like "I always have to do everything myself" or "If you want something done right, do it yourself"? That may mean you're excessively responsible. If your mantra is "I need to be number one" or "If I'm not the best at something, I'm not going to do it all" (that's mine), and if you hate mediocrity, you're probably intensely competitive. On the other hand, if you believe you'll never be good enough, you may be mired in feelings of inadequacy.

For years, Peter strove to be number one. He had stayed almost exclusively in the power column of the third emotional center. Always a winner, he had barely acknowledged the possibility of loss in his competitive pursuits. He had never considered taking a noncompetitive approach to anything. Competition was his reason for being. Highly skilled and competent, he had pursued his goals aggressively and with a strong sense of territoriality. Conquering new territories was his specialty and his primary drive. Moreover, Peter viewed his competitiveness, aggressiveness, and territoriality as the means of meeting his responsibilities in life. By being competitive, he felt that he was being responsible. In fact, though, he was increasing his own boundaries by invading the boundaries of others. Yet winning and succeeding gave him, at least for some time, a strong sense of self-esteem.

At last, however, his intuition and the organs of his third emotional center spoke up with the news that it was time for a change. The competition and territorial aggression in which Peter had engaged for so long were affecting the health of his stomach and digestive tract.

A striking parallel to Peter's case is found in a study of Australian marsupials.[1] Observing the animals during mating season, researchers saw that the males vied aggressively among themselves for both territory and mates. They'd run around fighting and arguing, violating each other's boundaries and grabbing space. The females, meanwhile, sat back and watched. Once the dust died down, they took a look at who had the biggest territory, and then the largest and most desirable female would get up and sashay over to his space, and so on down the line. The males would inseminate the females, and soon after that, they would drop dead. They never even got to see their kids.

Examining the marsupials to determine the cause of death, researchers found they were riddled with stomach and duodenal ulcers. They had been heavily infested by parasites, which had eaten through the walls of their stomach and intestines, right through the boundaries of their guts, and they had bled to death. As the marsupials had threatened and competed with each other, they had increased their levels of corticosteroids, thereby suppressing their immune systems and making the parasite invasion possible. The irony is exquisite. The very thing that they were trying to do, break through others' boundaries and invade others' territory, had been done unto them internally. And it had wiped them out. Some would call this a case of karma cookies, or proof of the Golden Rule, "Do unto others as you would have them do unto you."

The territorial battlefield of the marsupials could be the corporate battlefield of New York City. Like the marsupials, Peter had spent the mating season of his life, his adolescence and young adulthood, carrying out the rituals of enhanced intraspecies aggression and territoriality. This had given him a sense of power, responsibility, and self-esteem. It had also given him ulcers.

The ulcers, however, were the voice of his intuition telling him that he could change his life. Science tells us the same thing. A large body of literature supports the fact that people who are very ambitious, very striving, highly competitive, have a higher incidence of ulcers.[2] But let's revisit the case of the Australian marsupials. Researchers gave each of the male animals a piece of land—his own little house with a picket fence, as it were—and prevented them from competing and invading each other's territory. What happened? The males no longer dropped dead after impregnating their mates. They lived to see their children be born and to watch them grow up; they were able to grow old with their mates, and they lived twice as long as they had before. Changing their ways had changed the state of their health and the quality of their lives. It could do the same for Peter.

Is this an argument against any kind of competition, anytime? Am I saying we should all be like the marsupials, let the government issue each of us a plot of land and a Ford Escort and then settle for mediocrity? No. As I've said before, competition can be healthy at times, but unbridled competition can be bad. It's necessary to find a balance between the two extremes. We need to learn how to be the best at some things while allowing ourselves to be mediocre at other things. It's possible living twice as long did not make all of those male marsupials happy. Some of them may have experienced long life simply as double the time in which to be miserable. Longevity doesn't necessarily equal happiness. The point is that in Peter's case, his own intuitive guidance system was telling him that all-out, intense competition and striving ambition were no longer fulfilling to him. He needed to find a better balance in his life, as do most of us.

WISDOM, TRAUMA, AND GUT FEELINGS

The organs of the third emotional center are more closely aligned with our emotions than the organs of almost any other area of the body. This intimate connection may be due to the fact that the first way we interact with the world is through the digestive tract. From the moment we put our mouths to our mothers' breast, through all our other relationships, food and eating, and therefore the GI tract, are central and essential to our lives. It makes sense, therefore, that we can feel our emotional connections at the gut level.

As far back as the 1800s, physicians talked about patients being "gut responders," and they spoke of the guts as communicators of our feelings. Just think of the emotional language we've built up around the stomach and the gut. We get "butterflies in the stomach" when we're anxious; we can't "stomach" someone we dislike. When something we hear disgusts us, we say it makes us "want to throw up." When we get an intuitive insight, we describe it as a "gut feeling." Other organs of the GI tract are included. When we're depressed, we feel "down in the mouth." When someone's wrong, we make him "eat his words." The organs of the third emotional center are thus related, generally speaking, to anger, disgust, fear, depression, vengefulness, and intuition.

In the early nineteenth century a man named Alexis St. Martin accidentally shot himself in the abdomen.[3] The wound was large, and it never healed. Through a small hole in St. Martin's abdominal wall, you could clearly see his stomach lining. The famous surgeon William Beaumont undertook a study of St. Martin, to determine what effect the man's moods would have on his stomach. He observed the lining changing color as a given emotion caused the release of more or less acid in the stomach. Whenever anger caused St. Martin's face to go red, the stomach lining would also turn red. This was the essence of mind-body (or in this case mind-stomach) medicine. Every emotion St. Martin felt—anxiety, resentment, frustration, anger, happiness—was literally revealed on the video screen of his stomach wall.

How does the brain translate emotion and memories of an event into a physiological change in the stomach or any other part of the GI tract? Rich nerve fiber connections exist between the brain and the gut.[4] A large network of fibers of the autonomic nervous system—which fires the brain without our being consciously aware of it—runs from the brain down to the gut, where the nerves actually wrap around the tubelike intestines like a radial belt on a tire and cause them to contract. When you describe something as "gut-wrenching," that's exactly what you mean: when you feel an emotion, the fire from the nerves branches down, wraps around your gut, and clenches it.

Rich connections also exist between the amygdala in the temporal lobe of the brain and the stomach.[4] These connections allow our intense emotions—fear, anxiety, anger and rage, threat, intimidation—to be felt in the stomach and abdomen. Since the amygdala plays an important role in memory, it can also moderate the degree to which adverse or traumatic experiences can produce changes in the GI system. In animals the amygdala controls whether the animals feel resilient (powerful) or vulnerable in stress situations. The more helpless the feeling in the face of threat, restraint, and aggression, the greater the individual's likelihood of developing ulcers.[4]

People have known for ages that many different emotions are related to ulcers. Feeling threatened, for example, causes the brain to signal the stomach to secrete more acid while reducing blood flow to the lining, thus setting the stage for ulcers.[4] Some scientists have theorized that ulcers are caused by an overgrowth of a bacterium known as *Heliobactera pylori* in the stomach.[5] Since, however, all of us have

Heliobactera pylori in our stomachs—just as we all have E. coli in our intestines, and all women have yeast in their vaginas—there must be something about the environment in some people's stomachs that makes them more susceptible to the bacteria's overgrowing. Scientists believe that stressful life changes, feelings of threat, and being trapped or restrained can alter some people's immunity and cause the bacteria to overgrow, setting the stage for ulcers.[6] It's as if *H. pylori* is the bearer of bad tidings, but not necessarily the bad news itself.

In fact, the sensation of being trapped, of having no escape from something, has been shown to contribute to ulcers.[6] The incidence of ulcers shot upward during the blitz in London in the 1940s, when people were trapped in their homes and unable to go outside, unable to defend themselves against the threat of annihilation from Hitler's bombs.[7] People who can't escape from a situation have been found to have higher levels of free fatty acids in their blood, indicating stress, which can set the scene for ulcers to develop.[8] Hospitals today commonly put long-term and intensive care patients—patients who are confined to very restricted quarters for long periods—on antacids after a given period of time because such patients are known to have a higher than normal rate of ulcers, arising from the stress of entrapment and restraint.

Chronic anxiety, worry, and rumination are also closely associated with ulcers,[9] as is perfectionism.[10] In addition, decreased self-confidence can cause a drop in blood levels of the hormone somatostatin, which prohibits the stomach and intestine from functioning properly, thus setting the scene for ulcers and other GI problems.[11]

YOU'RE ON MY TURF
A CASE OF CROHN'S DISEASE

The Reading. I could see that sixty-year-old Marshall was a man with a lot of creative vision. He would get an idea of how something should be done and express it openly with a strong sense of focus. However, he had little tolerance for disagreement and for failure. At the same time, I could see that he worked with someone who sat in judgment on him and had the power to block his vision. I saw him as having problems with authority repeatedly over the course of his life, engaging over and over again in struggles over territory and boundaries. This caused Marshall a lot of anguish, which would churn inside him.

In his body I saw redness and inflammation in the lining of his stomach and duodenum and all along his colon. I also saw scarring of the liver due to past drinking and scarring of the lungs from past smoking.

The Facts. Marshall was a foreman in a newspaper printing plant. He was in charge of the loading dock. And he had problems with his boss, with whom he engaged in repeated power struggles over what he viewed as his turf. He had ideas about how things should be done, including where boxes should be placed, which his boss would frequently override. This agitated Marshall considerably. "On my loading dock," he said, "I want things done my way." He had a strong sense of territoriality and turf-consciousness.

In his youth, Marshall had had similar problems with his father, a strongly authoritarian figure who always wanted everything to be done his way. Marshall had always sought but seldom won his approval.

Marshall confirmed that he had Crohn's disease, a condition in which ulcers spread from one end of the GI tract to the other. In the past, he had also smoked and suffered from alcoholism.

Marshall had problems with boundaries and limitations, and he allowed his self-esteem to be too dependent on the approval of others. Here was a man whose sense of who he was, and how powerful he was in the world, was based completely on how competent he was at his task in life and how that competence was acknowledged by others, especially his superior. His task was organizing boxes on the loading dock, and he took it seriously. It was his responsibility, his turf, and he drew carefully delineated boundaries around it. You have probably known someone like this, someone whose desk always has to be a certain way, who labels his rulers and pens and arranges objects on the desktop with nearly straight-edge precision. Then Marshall's boss would come along and suggest that perhaps *this* box should be moved over *there,* and Marshall's whole world would crumble. His self-esteem, his ability to feel good about himself, would suffer, because the mere suggestion that a box should be moved appeared to him as a challenge or threat to his responsibility, his territory, his boundaries. Feelings that his territory was threatened would churn inside him, he would ruminate over them ceaselessly, and they would affect the organs of his third emotional center.

In addition, by challenging Marshall's decisions, his boss, in Marshall's eyes, was failing to acknowledge Marshall's skill and competence at his job. This was a replay of Marshall's difficulties with his father, who had never recognized his son's competence or adequacy. In fact, Marshall was typical of people with ulcerative colitis, who have been shown to retain a deep psychological attachment to a key figure in their lives, which they transfer to other key figures as they get older. These people are also known to have an almost life-or-death need for another person's approval in order to be able to feel good about themselves.[12]

When Marshall's boundaries and self-esteem were threatened—if his boxes were moved, for example—he plunged out of the power category of the third emotional center and right into the vulnerability category. He felt inadequate, incompetent, defensive. With someone else calling the shots and limiting his authority over his boxes, he felt trapped and restrained. He felt, in short, horrendous. For years he had tried to seek escape from these feelings in addictions such as smoking and drinking, which medicated his feelings of anger and inadequacy. He had, in fact, tried to quiet his intuition, but it was still speaking to him through his disease, telling him that he needed to stop depending on external approval for his self-esteem and learn to manage his anger over the invasion of his boundaries by others.

RESPONSIBILITY, COMMITMENT, AND ADDICTION

One of the largest issues associated with ulcers and other ailments of the third emotional center is the issue of responsibility and its related trait, commitment. As we perform our work in the world and gain skills and confidence, we're faced with the need to develop a sense of commitment and responsibility. We learn, to greater or lesser degree, how to promise to dedicate ourselves to a job or a group or a person for a certain period of time and to fulfill our responsibilities as required. How well we fulfill those responsibilities, based on the emotions and memories stored in the third emotional center, can set the stage for illness or health in this area.

We know that certain emotions, including the feeling of responsibility, can affect the gut. When a child first goes out into the world, off to school, and takes on his first responsibilities in life, he often gets *stomachaches*. The anxiety, the worry, of his responsibility, perhaps his desire to become adequate to it, all affect him in the gut.

As we gain more responsibility, we can be more strongly affected. Scientists took a pair of monkeys and put them together in a cage. One was designated the "executive monkey,"[12] while the other was his underling. The underling was wired to receive electrical shocks. The executive monkey, for his part, was given the ability to control the shocks his employee received by means of a button in the cage. So one monkey got the pain, while the other got the responsibility. Which monkey do you think developed ulcers? Wouldn't you think that the monkey getting the shocks would get the ulcers? It wasn't so. The monkey with all the responsibility, like the corporate executive in charge, got the ulcers.

Lots of people, of course, have a great deal of responsibility but never develop ulcers. In some cases it's possible to predict, in a given situation, who will get an ulcer and who will not. One study looked at a group of military trainees with a tendency to secrete excess pepsinogen, a chemical that influences the development of ulcers. Within this group, those that developed duodenal ulcers were the ones who had difficulty dealing with issues of control, responsibility, and helplessness.[12]

There is some suggestion that family environment, and the emotional memories thereof, can help set the scene for GI problems in children, including eating disorders, anorexia, and ulcers.[13] I knew a young man whose parents divorced when he was eighteen. Afterward he felt forever torn between his responsibilities to the two of them. His father would plead with the boy to spend Friday and Saturday nights with him, the very times the son most wanted to be with his friends. His mother would complain that he didn't spend enough time with her, and she begrudged the father any time with the son at all. The son complained that he felt literally torn between the two of them as he tried to fulfill his responsibility to both parents. Eventually he came down, fittingly, with Crohn's disease, in which the lining of his GI tract sloughed off in large tears.

The emotions and memories you carry stored in the organs of your third emotional center, plus your ability to balance power and vulnerability in this area, can set the stage for health or disease here.

CAUGHT IN THE MIDDLE: THE WEIGHT OF RESPONSIBILITY ULCERS AND OBESITY

Felicia was the oldest of eight children in a strict Fundamentalist family. As the eldest, she was always responsible for her brothers and sisters. Whenever her parents went out, leaving the children at home, they would tell her that she was in charge and that they were counting on her to keep the other children in line. Felicia's brothers were little hell-raisers, however, and hard for anyone to control, let alone a young girl who wasn't much older than they. They routinely got into terrible mischief, once even setting fire to a barn near their home. Whenever something like this happened, Felicia was blamed. She soon realized that the only way she was going to earn love was to be responsible.

As she grew older, this conviction began to rule her life. Moving into the working world, she gravitated toward administrative jobs where she was in charge of running things. Because she was highly competent, she soon became the top administrator in her firm. She handled all the details, put out all the "fires," and managed everyone as though the firm were a family of kids who were out of control. When squabbles arose among her colleagues, she would act as mediator and attempt to smooth matters over, but she always felt caught in the middle.

Over the years, Felicia gradually became obese. All her weight was in her torso, especially around the stomach; her arms and legs remained surprisingly slim. In addition, feeling caught in the middle, Felicia began to suffer from abdominal pain that she couldn't understand. One day, she had a severe attack of nausea, vomiting, fever, and chills. Finally going to the doctor, she learned she had ulcers.

Felicia is a poster child of illness in the third emotional center. Do you frequently feel caught in the middle? Do you carry the weight of responsibility for others? Are you always putting out other people's fires? Felicia's difficulties with the issue of responsibility clearly stemmed from emotions and memories stored in her brain and in her body from childhood. To prove that she was indeed responsible, she was determined to become competent and adequate at whatever she undertook, which happened to be jobs that tested her responsibility. She developed, indeed, a hyper-responsibility that was guaranteed always to keep her in the power column of the third emotional center. This meant, however, that she lacked the ability to stand back, watch others make errors, and let them assume responsibility for their own problems. She believed that it was her responsibility to prevent errors from occurring. Otherwise Mommy and Daddy would come home and blame her for whatever had gone wrong.

Her overdeveloped "responsibility gland" had helped set the scene for Felicia's ulcers. Ironically, they were exacerbated by another aspect of Felicia's nature. Despite her responsible image, Felicia had difficulty making commitments. In actuality, she avoided making new commitments in her work or her personal life because she dreaded taking on the additional responsibility they would entail. At the same time, she believed it was her duty and obligation to take on the responsibility. Being asked to make a commitment would lead to feelings of entrapment that echoed a childhood experience. When Felicia was a young girl, her parents had disciplined her by shutting her in the dark basement for several hours and ignoring her weeping and pleas to be let out. Feelings of entrapment, as we have seen, help set the scene for ulcers.

Meanwhile the weight of all the responsibility she had carried for so many years came to appear on her physically in the form of the excess weight around her midsection. The location of the weight is significant. As a child, Felicia had felt caught in the middle between her parents and siblings; as an adult, she was caught in the middle of all the people she worked with and was responsible for. Her heavy torso and abdomen were the physicalized memory of Felicia's childhood trauma.

Can stress over responsibility and commitments lead to weight problems? Can it set the scene for problems in how our bodies handle carbohydrates, fat, and calories? Scientific studies suggest that certain stress and emotions can affect a person's metabolism, or ability to break down food. Stress has been shown to change the way the body metabolizes fat.[14] Emotions also affect the way we metabolize sugar.[15] Emotional upheaval, adverse life situations, and severe frustration can contribute to the onset of diabetes, a metabolic problem related to carbohydrates (or sugar) and fat, and can aggravate the course of the illness.[16] One study suggests that diabetes in some children intensifies when the children experience stress related to issues of responsibility and parental control.[17] Emotional stress increases the level of cortisol in the bloodstream, in turn increasing insulin levels, while at the same time causing greater insulin resistance. The body wants to store more of what you eat into fat.

Felicia always wanted to be in the power column of the third emotional center. She felt it her duty to be responsible for everyone else and, simultaneously, never to let anyone else be responsible for her, because that made her feel vulnerable and dependent. If she was invited to a party or a movie with friends, she would always insist on driving her own car so that no one would need to be responsible for her—and so that she would never feel trapped. In fact, there is literature that suggests that people with ulcers and GI tract problems have issues related to dependence.[18] Although people with this issue have an intense desire to be loved and cared for, which was in fact a driving motivation for Felicia, they feel ashamed of this or afraid that the need won't be met, so they overcompensate by becoming ambitious, displaying excessive strengths, and appearing to need no one. But Felicia's intuitive guidance system knew that her soul was crying out for this to change.

While Felicia had an overly responsible approach to life, others find responsibility overwhelming and seek escape from it, either by avoiding it entirely, or by finding refuge in addiction.

DROWNING HER SORROWS
A CASE OF ALCOHOLISM

The Reading. When Maureen, at age forty-eight, called for an intuitive reading, I saw at once that she had unresolved grief over someone close to her who had recently left her life and with whom she'd had a difficult relationship. I also saw that she was carrying a heavy burden of emotional stress at work, where she was responsible for the care and nurture of a large group of people who were in great need.

Physically, Maureen appeared to me as a slightly overweight woman prone to excess alcohol use. I saw that this was damaging the organs in her third emotional center, primarily her liver and pancreas. I even noted that her damaged liver could be diagnosed with blood tests that would show elevated liver enzyme levels in her blood.

The Facts. Maureen was a psychotherapist with a large practice of patients who suffered from extreme physical and emotional abuse. At present she was finding the emotional burden of their care overwhelming. These feelings had been exacerbated by the recent death of Maureen's father, an event Maureen was finding especially difficult to process because she had never resolved her feelings about her father's inability to nurture her while she was growing up. Maureen was contemplating cutting back the number of patients in her psychotherapy practice so she could sort out her feelings of grief over her father's death.

Maureen's physician had recently notified her that her blood tests showed liver damage due to excess alcohol consumption.

When I later met Maureen, she was drinking wine while adding cooking sherry to a stir-fry she was preparing for lunch. She was trying to numb her grief over her father's death as well as soothe the emotional difficulty she was having dealing with her patients by filling her stomach with alcohol. In fact, Maureen was torn by issues of responsibility. She was still living in her father's house. She wanted to sell it, but she felt a responsibility to keep the house in the family, as her father had wished. Maureen's addiction, drinking, covered up her feelings of inadequacy about the responsibilities she had trouble handling. The alcohol soothed her. That's the purpose of most of our addictions, many of which, interestingly, involve putting things in our mouths. That's because eating is a primal act that makes us feel warm and safe and puts a good, fuzzy feeling in our bodies.[19]

An addiction, however, doesn't have to involve a substance. You can be addicted to work. We all know the kind of person who never wants to go out for a drink on Friday nights with the rest of the office because he has so much work to do. Work is the only god he worships. Or we have a friend who can't miss her daily run; she'll never commit to any engagement because she has to be sure she'll be able to go for her run. Other people are addicted to soap operas. Addiction in its essence is a means of escaping from responsibilities and commitments in the outside world. Alcoholics are always missing their commitments, showing up late for work or appointments. But they're deeply committed to their addiction, which is the only commitment they can handle, especially since it lets them off the hook for everything else. At bottom, this kind of addiction often covers up deep-seated feelings of inadequacy, aggression, and low self-esteem.

FOOD IS LOVE
A CASE OF ANOREXIA-BULIMIA

The Reading. In my intuitive reading of Andrea, age forty, I saw in her past an emotional situation in which she had been involved with someone who was trying to balance two different things. I couldn't tell what exactly this person was balancing, but I saw that he wasn't doing a very good job. Eventually the person had had to choose between the two things he was balancing, and his choice had had a very deep effect on Andrea.

I saw that this choice had also had an effect on Andrea's body and that it was related to her physical condition, which I had some trouble discerning. Andrea's organs all seemed normal, but I saw that her arms and legs looked emaciated, while her abdomen was huge and balloonlike. This was very confusing to me.

The Facts. When she was twenty years old, Andrea had had an affair with a married man. Eventually his wife had found out about the affair, and the man had been forced to make a choice between his marriage and Andrea. He had decided to drop Andrea and go back to his wife. This decision had a profound impact on Andrea, who never again had a close relationship with a man. Instead, she had thrown herself into her work, becoming a professional chef and a photographer. At the time of the reading, she was also writing a book.

Despite my image of her as having a huge abdomen, Andrea, it turned out, was actually anorexic and extremely thin; she also suffered from bulimia, in which a person binges on food and then purges it by inducing vomiting. What I had read in her was not the true appearance of her abdomen but her own *perception* of its appearance.

After the breakup with the married man, Andrea clearly suffered from feelings of inadequacy and loss of self-esteem. These she tried to regain by throwing herself into her work. However, she undermined these efforts by turning work into an addiction. One addiction, to her lover, had thus been replaced by another. Her total absorption in her addiction allowed Andrea to avoid other commitments and responsibilities, including other relationships. It allowed her to pull herself out of the competitive arena and to escape or avoid threatening situations that might arise as other relationships offered themselves up to her. Andrea was thus dwelling completely in the vulnerability column of the third emotional center.

Meanwhile, she began to use food to fill in the hole her lover had left behind. Her approach to food was addictive as well. By taking in food, she imported a sense of love and fulfillment, a good, fuzzy, protective feeling that made her feel warm and safe. Like the true addict, she either abstained completely (anorexia) or binged uncontrollably (bulimia). She used food as a metaphor for love, which could bring her the self-esteem she lacked. Andrea said herself that she often used food to fill up the "black hole of emptiness" she felt inside her, the area where self-esteem is stored in the third emotional center.

Food is intimately associated in human culture with love. We all tend to use it as a substitute or a metaphor for love. Just think of those Italian families, where the matriarch runs around the table urging everyone to "Eat! Eat!" because food is an expression of love. Food is especially important to women in filling out a sense of themselves and making them feel whole inside. We all know the woman who's dateless on a Saturday night and drowns her sorrows in a package of Oreos and a pint of Ben and Jerry's ice cream. We all know women who would kill for chocolate when they're depressed, but we rarely hear about men doing things like this. That's because of the way men's and women's brains are structured. In a woman's brain, the areas having to do with food and sex are extremely close together, almost superimposed on each other in the hypothalamus.[20] In men, they're separate and farther apart. For a man, there's food, and then there's sex. For a woman, there's food-sex. This means that as the neurons fire while you're eating chocolates, you have sensations similar to those you experience when you're in love and having sex. Women's receptivity to sex and their receptivity to food wax and wane together, in rhythm with the hormones in their bodies and their menstrual cycles. (Some of my friends have been known to kill for chocolate just before their periods.) So it's no mystery that food and love are a problem for many women and fat is a feminist issue.

Depression can make women eat more or eat less, as can anxiety.[14,15] Emotions can cause the thyroid, adrenal glands, and brain to secrete more or fewer hormones, revving up the metabolism or slowing it down. When I'm having lunch or dinner with a person who makes me feel stressed, I can have a carrot stick dipped in water, cross my eyes, and gain two pounds. On the other hand, when I feel total comfort and unconditional love, I could probably eat everything on the menu, including deep-fried foods with extra butter and double chocolate sauce on my dessert and not gain an ounce. It all depends on how you feel, your sense of self-esteem and acceptance.

Andrea had a severe lack of self-esteem and acceptance after her rejection by her lover. But her body, through her intuitive guidance system, was telling her that she could make changes to enable her to find a new path to self-esteem, adequacy in both relationships and work, and, ultimately, health.

A Question of Temperament

Given the close association between the organs of the third emotional center and our feelings, why is it that all of us don't get ulcers and become obese or develop addictions? The answer lies both in our individual temperaments and in the place in each person's body, the hole, where intuition comes through. Felicia, the obese woman with ulcers, had strong emotional memories from her childhood of self-esteem built on a sense of responsibility, as well as recollections of being trapped by commitment. She also apparently had a temperament that caused her to perceive those memories as traumatizing in such a way that they had a continued effect on her throughout her life.

Other people might experience the same trauma but have different perceptions of it and therefore not experience the same physical problems. I know another woman, though, who had repeated experiences of being restrained in her youth. A hyperactive child, she would frequently escape from the baby-sitter and run wildly out into the town, sometimes with no clothes on. She was so hard to handle and so wild that, for her own safety, her family often tied her down to keep her from escaping. Once she was even tied to her bed with the tow rope from a ski lift; but she still managed to escape. You might think this woman today would have posttraumatic stress disorder, fear of closed spaces, and problems with commitment or being "tied down" in any way. But she doesn't. Her temperament is completely different from Felicia's. She remembers thinking, while she was being tied down with the ski line, "This is no problem. I can get out of this in a flash."

This woman has no problems in her third emotional center because she doesn't perceive her memories of being tied down or restrained as traumatic. Felicia, on the other hand, does perceive her memories that way, even if unconsciously. By learning the language of the third emotional center, part of her intuition network, she began to learn what the ulcers in her GI tract were communicating to her. She learned that her problems with responsibility, commitment, and self-esteem were rooted in trauma in her past and in the memories that had been laid down in her stomach, an organ of the third emotional center. Knowing this, she was able to gain an understanding of her problems and to see that when she had stomach trouble, something was activating her memories, and she needed to attend to some issue in the present that was related to responsibility and commitment. Felicia's intuition had found the hole in her body—her stomach—through which it could speak to her. This is what intuition does in each of us.

NINE

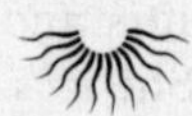

The Heart, Lungs, and Breasts: Emotions, Intimacy, and Nurturance

One of my favorite stories is "How the Grinch Stole Christmas" by Dr. Seuss. I love the part at the end, when the Grinch's pinched heart, previously "two sizes too small," suddenly begins to grow, bursting outward to normal heart size. Why does this miracle happen? Because little Cindy Lou Who and the Whos down in Whoville have showered the mean old Grinch with love.

This seemingly corny Hallmark card–like ending actually mirrors real life. Dr. Seuss may have thought his story about love feeding the heart was just a little fable, but love truly does exactly that. Along with all other emotions, it affects the health and, almost literally, the size of the heart. This was demonstrated by a famous study, in which researchers at Ohio State University set out to raise rabbits genetically to develop hardening of the arteries to the heart.[1] After weaning, the animals were regularly fed a high-cholesterol diet. Once the rabbits were full-grown, however, the researchers were amazed to discover that 15 percent of them had almost completely clear coronary arteries, no signs of serious blockage at all. This seemed impossible, and no one could understand it. It also seemed odd that all the healthy rabbits were in the most accessible cages, the ones that stood at waist level.

Well, guess what? It turned out that someone had showered these rabbits with love. The graduate student in charge of feeding the animals had been in the habit of taking these particular rabbits out of their cages and petting, stroking, and playing with them. The researchers' conclusion: being held, stroked, talked to, and entertained can help to keep the heart's blood vessels clear and even help the heart itself to heal. In other words, receiving and feeling the emotion of love is good for the heart.

Knowing, feeling, and expressing all your emotions—whether of love and joy or fear and anger—is good for your health. It keeps you moving steadily through life. In fact, the word "emotion" derives from a Latin verb meaning "to move" or "move out." This is what our emotions do. They move us in the direction in which we need to go in life. They direct us toward health and fulfillment, like love and joy, or they move us away from the wrong track, like fear and anger.[2]

Emotions are part of the intuition network. They're like a current of intuition that runs through us. When you're able to identify, feel, and say, "I feel sad" or "I feel angry" or "I feel grief" or "I feel fear," you can make the appropriate moves, changes, and decisions that will enable you to experience and enjoy your life to the fullest.

Emotional expression, how we deal with and communicate what we feel, is the focus of the fourth emotional center. Linked with it is the emotional life of our partnerships, the intimate relationships we form with other individuals, since these are the other actors in the play of our lives, the people to whom we express ourselves and our emotions and to whom we speak our lines. In every situation in our lives, we need to understand the function of the emotion we're experiencing, to feel it fully, and to respond to it appropriately. If we're unable to do this, we set the stage for illness in the organs of the fourth emotional center—the heart, lungs, breasts, and the esophagus. If emotions are an intuitive current inside us, then these organs are the speakers that broadcast and communicate it. They'll recognize, respond to, and express our emotions for us in the form of physical symptoms when we fail to recognize and express them ourselves. Understanding how wisdom and pain about emotional expression are empatterned in the heart, breasts, and lungs will help you understand the language of your body's intuition (see the following figure).

Fourth Emotional Center

POWER

Emotional expression
- **Passion**
- **Anger and rage, hate and hostility**
- **Joy and exuberance**
- **Stoicism**
- **Courage**
- **Bereavement**
- **Loss**

Partnership
- **Isolation**
- **Giving help (putting out)**
- **Giving**
- **Fathering**
- **Martyrdom**

VULNERABILITY

Emotional expression
- **Love**
- **Resentment and bitterness**
- **Serenity and peace**
- **Emotional effusiveness**
- **Anxiety**
- **Depression**
- **Abandonment**

Partnership
- **Intimacy**
- **Accepting help (taking in)**
- **Accepting**
- **Mothering**
- **Nurturance**
- **Forgiveness**

EMOTIONS, THE HEART, AND THE INTUITION NETWORK

The heart's relation to emotions, its unique image as the seat of our feelings, is almost mythical. We talk about emotions being heartfelt and about following our hearts. We describe nurturing and loving people as being kindhearted, bighearted, warmhearted; we wear our hearts on our sleeves; we wish for our heart's desires; we hold something or someone in our hearts. The Cowardly Lion in *The Wizard of Oz* wanted a heart for courage, and those who are brave and intrepid are said to be stouthearted or to have a lot of heart. When someone is cold and unfeeling, we say he has no heart. When we want to shut off emotion, we say we must harden our hearts, which, in fact, is literally what happens when we suppress what we feel.

Louise Hay urges us to think of the heart as the center of joy and the seat of emotions in our lives.[3] How well your life's blood flows through your heart, arteries, and veins is linked to the degree to which joy flows through your life. Cholesterol-blocked arteries symbolize a blocking of the flow of joy, or a suppression of emotion. Heart attacks, Hay says, happen when all the joy has been squeezed out of your heart in favor of the pursuit of money, position, or materialistic gain. In fact, it's well documented that a vast number of heart attack victims are so-called type A personalities, often driven men whose passion derives almost exclusively from money, power, and position and who aren't really much of a joy to have around.

Moreover, we know that unresolved and unexpressed anger, sadness, and fear actually cause vasoconstriction, a tightening of the blood vessels connected to the heart. When you feel anger or fear, these blood vessels constrict in response to an outpouring of chemicals from the sympathetic nervous system. In contrast, joy and love open up the blood vessels to your heart, as they did for the rabbits in the Ohio study. Joy and love stimulate the parasympathetic nervous system, which opens the blood vessels and creates more blood flow to your heart.[4] This is not to say, though, that you should never feel fear or anger. Feeling and expressing *all* emotions, in a balanced way, is essential to health in the fourth emotional center.

There are six basic emotions: love, joy, anger, sadness, fear, and shame. All other emotions are shades or flavors of these basic emotions, the way Coke and Pepsi and Diet-Rite are various brands and flavors of colas. Grief, despair, and melancholy are flavors of sadness; rage, resentment, and hatred are shades of anger; anxiety, panic, and horror are shades of fear. Throughout our lives and at various stages, depending on what is happening with us, we all feel these emotions. Emotions, and the memories that embody them, speak to us as elements of the intuition network, intuitive guidance signals that tell us whether we're heading in the right direction or the wrong direction for our happiness and health.

When an emotion feels good, we know we're on the right course. Feelings like joy and love are your internal cheering section. They tell you you're succeeding at something, you're on the happy track, and you should keep going the way you're going. They're like the bell that rings on a game show when you get the right answer. You don't just hear that bell. It literally resounds inside you, in the organs of the fourth emotional center, in the heart, lungs, and breasts. Think of it this way: when you hear a band go by in a parade, or you listen to the mournful music of a funeral procession, where do you feel the emotions the music stirs in you? You don't feel them in your toenails or your hair; you feel them in your chest.

Emotions that feel bad are telling us we're off course. Anger, for instance, is frequently a way of communicating to ourselves that things haven't turned out the way we expected. We feel anger when we lose power, status, or respect. It tells us that we're not getting something we want or need, or it signals us that an important or pleasurable activity or aspect of our lives has been interrupted or stopped. Anger can sometimes be protective; it tells us when we're feeling physical or emotional pain, or it tells us when we're being threatened by someone or something. It's like a warning signal in the brain telling you you're off, stop ringing in so quickly, slow down, consider, try another tack. The same is true of fear, which is a strong intuitive guiding signal telling you you're in a new and potentially treacherous situation, to watch yourself, be careful. Similarly, sadness usually tells us we're going somewhere we don't want to go, we're not getting what we wanted, or something important has been removed from our lives.

All too often, however, we don't recognize our feelings. We walk around feeling sad without really even knowing that sadness is the name of what we feel and without knowing *why* we feel the way we do. Our culture and society, in fact, often encourage a detachment from certain feelings. Say you're a child and you're walking down the street with your mother when you run into an uncle on your father's side of the family whom you don't like because once, when you were alone with him, he touched you in a way you knew wasn't good. "Oh, honey, here's Uncle Ned," your mother says. "Shake hands with Uncle Ned." Instead of shaking his hand, of course, you shake your head, pull back, and try to hide behind your mother. You're full of fear of this person who you know instinctively violated you in some way, and you're also angry at being forced to greet him now as though nothing had ever happened. But you can't put a name to your feelings, because the language of your emotions isn't yet fully developed. "I hate him!" you cry. Your mother, embarrassed, scolds you. "Of course you don't hate Ned! He's a wonderful man," she says. "Now, you be good and shake his hand right now!" The emotions you're feeling are being invalidated on the spot. So you begin at that moment to comprehend the language of emotions. All you know is that every time you see this man, your flesh crawls, your heart skips a beat, and you go cold all over. And then you begin to unplug from your emotional intuition network. Your emotions are there to protect you, but you're being taught not to hear or heed them.

This happens repeatedly in our lives. You have no right to be angry, we're told as children, because look at what you have—you have food, you have clothing, think of all the starving children in Africa. You shouldn't be angry, you should be grateful. So you quickly learn to bottle up your anger or to turn it aside. Instead, you hang out with some other emotion, such as shame. Or you get depressed, and you don't know why. People with chronic and severe depression can in fact eventually become disconnected from the language of emotions; they have to be taught to understand it once again. In 1993, Marcia Linehan wrote a wonderful book that helps teach such people how to recognize their emotions and respond to them in an appropriate way.[5] I had a patient once who told me about a trip to the doctor's where a blood sample had to be drawn. "I got very angry" when the nurse approached with the needle, she reported. This sounded puzzling at first, but a quick peek at Linehan's book and the description of the sensations and physical signs that accompany certain emotions soon told me that she meant she was *afraid*.

Most of us don't need a textbook to come to an understanding of our emotions. But it *is* essential that we learn to understand the language of every emotion we feel, its function, and how it's empatterned; to express that emotion fully; and to respond to it appropriately. We have to move with the emotion.

If you don't move with your emotion, the emotion will go into your body and move the cells of your organs instead, possibly in the pattern of illness. In the fourth emotional center, emotions can cause problems ranging from heart disease to stroke to breast cancer.

THE GREAT IMPOSTOR, OR PUTTING ON AN ACT
A CASE OF HEART ATTACK

The Reading. Mike was sixty-two years old when he called me for a reading. I saw a shortish man, about 5 feet 8, overweight and bald. (His baldness is significant because a famous study showed that bald men have an increased risk of heart attacks, due to excess testosterone.) I saw this man as a member of a group that was a family of sorts. He believed that in this family congeniality reigned and everyone worked together. Underneath the surface, however, I saw that he knew this really wasn't true. I saw him as being very angry, resentful, and bitter about not being where he wanted to be in his life. He was getting on in age, and he had considerable grief about not having gotten something, not having won some account he believed was due him. He was in a very competitive field, but he didn't acknowledge the pain, grief, and fear associated with that competition. He kept his emotions sealed behind a brave face and insisted his group was a wonderful, supportive set of people.

In this man's body I saw one distressing area of concern: the blood vessels surrounding his heart were thick and hardened with blockages.

The Facts. Mike was an actor who had had a fairly successful career in movies and on television, although I hadn't recognized his name when he gave it to me. Never the leading man, he had done well mostly in supporting roles. As he grew older, however, even those roles were becoming more difficult to land. My reading indicated to me that he had grief and disappointment over the fact that his career had never been bigger. I saw that he experienced heartache over this and over the fact that his career was now receding as younger people came up to take his place. To my surprise, however, Mike denied that any of this was true. He insisted that the actors with whom he worked were a wonderful, caring, and supportive group. Yes, he was getting fewer film roles, but he was doing a lot of summer stock now, which he said was fun and easygoing, with no rivalry among the actors. He was cleaning up the whole situation and stoically hiding his true emotions, which he refused even to recognize. He also insisted he had no physical symptoms of any kind, and certainly nothing like heart problems.

This reading was very upsetting to me, because I thought that perhaps I had misread this client entirely. Six months later, however, I happened to be reading *People* magazine. And there in the obituaries was a report on the death of this very actor. He had died suddenly of a massive heart attack.

Here was a case of someone who had failed to recognize and respond to his emotions. Suppressed emotions have been shown to play a role in hypertension, which is due to hardening of the blood vessels.[6] In other words, roadblocks to your emotions can cause roadblocks to the flow of blood to your heart. Even if Mike had acknowledged what was truly going on in his heart, he might have been unable to avert the ultimate catastrophe that overtook him.

Studies have also shown that difficulty adjusting to significant life changes often helps to set the scene for heart attacks.[7] It's also been shown that people who suffer a major loss are more likely to die of heart attacks and heart disease in the first year of their bereavement.[8] Widowers over the age of fifty-five have an increased risk of heart attacks in the first six months after they lose their wives. It's quite clear, therefore, that people can literally die of heartache or bereavement. Loss of a loved one isn't the only event that can lead to a heart attack. As a person reaches the end of his career and moves into retirement, grief and bereavement can move in to live with him. The very word "retire" means to withdraw; after a lifetime at center stage, we're forced to withdraw into the wings, and this act can cause profound heartache.

Mike had refused even to admit that his life was undergoing a change. Everything, he insisted, was hunky-dory. He didn't even know that he was depressed and anxious or hostile and angry. Yet those emotions, ironically, are the ones most closely related to heart disease. A survey in a health newsletter for women actually found that 46 percent of the women responding believed their most severe problems were depression and anxiety.[9] And what is the number one killer of both men and women? Heart disease. A study on hopelessness and helplessness, meanwhile, found that middle-aged men who think of themselves as failures may develop narrowed arteries faster and have more heart attacks than their optimistic counterparts.[10] In fact, experiencing hopelessness and a sense of failure has been observed to carry the same risk for heart disease as smoking a pack of cigarettes a day. Not one or two cigarettes. *An entire pack*. Doctors always ask heart patients if they smoke or used to, but they don't ask people if they feel hopeless or hostile or if they believe they're failures, even though these emotions obviously have a great impact on their health.

Notably, if steps are taken to try to change the situation so that a man regains hope and optimism, his physical condition can improve. As Mike headed into a new phase of his life, it was imperative for him to take a good look at his life and at the emotions he was feeling, listen to the body intuition stored in his fourth emotional center, try to understand what it was communicating to him, and try to make the appropriate changes in his life. If he had talked about his separation from his colleagues, his grief about how his life was changing, and dealt with these feelings, expressed them fully, and then started to make plans for the next stage of his life, he might have lowered his risk for heart disease. Instead, ever the actor, I suppose, he played the great impostor and put on an act, hiding behind a facade of stoicism, cheer, and optimism, claiming his life was rosy and all was well with the world. But life and health aren't a movie script, and our intuition network knows when we're pretending. Mike wouldn't allow his emotions to move him forward in the best direction; they moved instead into the organs of his fourth emotional center.

Studies of type A personalities who have had one heart attack show that patients can lower their chances of a second heart attack by learning to express emotions in a non–type A way. Patients can learn to do this through meditation, cognitive therapy, and behavioral modification therapy, but it's important that they seek guidance in doing it.

I did a reading of a stock analyst from Chicago who had had a heart attack. George had been driven by the desire to make a big killing for his clients. Quite literally, making money was like lifeblood to him. He could sniff out a good stock a year or two before it began to rise dramatically. The thrill of the hunt propelled him through his professional life, and like many men in his line of work he gave short shrift to his emotional and personal life and his family.

Of course, because he was human, George did make errors in his stock assessments and recommendations, and sometimes his clients did suffer huge losses, sometimes in the many thousands of dollars. To survive as an analyst in that competitive world, and to nerve himself to take the same kind of big risks, George learned to block out his feelings of sadness, grief, and shame when his deals did not work. He hardened his heart against disappointment and spoke remorselessly about "blowing clients up." Then one day his heart snapped.

George's wife made him call me for a reading after he returned home from his angioplasty, an operation in which the blood vessels are reamed out so that circulation improves. I saw George's coronary arteries surrounding his heart as having been recently festooned with spiky, hard stalactites that prevented the blood from flowing smoothly. At the time George called me, he was in the middle of what doctors commonly call a post–myocardial infarction depression. The way I saw it, however, George was sitting in a hospital bed in his room at home, and was finally feeling the sadness of the realization that his old way of life was over for good and he needed to find a new profession. His depression seemed to me a biochemical manifestation of the fact that, with those spiky stalactites gone, he could finally feel the full impact of the emotions—the sadness, grief, and shame—that he had kept at bay for so many years.

THE POWER AND THE VULNERABILITY

In the fourth emotional center we're concerned with two vital aspects of life: power and vulnerability. We're asking the question: "What feeds my heart?" (and thus keeps all the organs in my chest healthy). The response to this lies in the degree of emotional expression we allow into and experience in our lives. At the same time, a central concern of this emotional center is that of partnerships. This term is different from the "relationships" of the second emotional center. In the fourth emotional center, the paradigm of partnership is "You and I are one." We're concerned with the intimacy and emotional quality and nature of the one-on-one relationships in our lives. In the second emotional center, we view a relationship like a three-legged race. You have two legs tied together, but each of you keeps one leg free, untethered to the other person. You're bound together, but you're still individuals. The partnership of the fourth emotional center is like a potato sack race where you both get inside the bag and move together toward the finish line. You're truly one, a single entity in the world. You have to be able to manage both of these feats at the same time.

The power column of emotional expression in this center includes passion, anger and hostility, joy, courage, and stoicism, being able to contain your emotions when necessary. The vulnerabilities it encompasses include love, resentment, serenity, anxiety, and emotional effusiveness or lability, a kind of emotional incontinence, the capacity to "lose it" when necessary. In the partnership equation, the power column lists isolation, giving help, fathering, and martyrdom, while the vulnerabilities include intimacy, taking help, mothering, and nurturance.

You can see where you fit on this scale. Are you given to wild swings of passion rather than steady, quiet love? Do you express anger by boiling over constantly, or do you simmer and seethe with resentment and bitterness? Are you always joyful and exuberant, or do you tend to be serene and peaceful? Do you approach life boldly, with courage, or are you filled with anxiety? Do you feel, express, and resolve your bereavement and sense of loss, or do you let it linger and darken into depression? Do you understand and accept loss, or do you let it swallow you up in a sense of abandonment? Most of all, do you hide all your emotions behind a brave face, or do you let it all hang out all the time? Or are you, in all or some of these areas, somewhere in the middle, where all of us would like to be?

In your partnerships are you isolated or intimate? Do you prefer to give help or take it? Are you more fatherly, giving instruction and direction, or are you motherly, concerned with warmth, nurturance, and love? Do you tend toward martyrdom, sacrificing yourself and doing everything for others to win recognition, or do you prefer to be nurturing, to help and guide others in achieving self-sufficiency?

As in every other emotional center, a balance between power and vulnerability is the key to health in the fourth emotional center. To have healthy organs here you have to allow yourself to feel both the power emotions and the vulnerability emotions.

Stoicism, for instance, is admired in our culture. In the fourth emotional center, stoicism is a power quality. It's considered a sign of fortitude, and the strength it conveys is often needed and appreciated. When John F. Kennedy died, the world watched in wonderment and admiration as his widow, Jackie, stoically led a bereaved nation in mourning. Her black-veiled figure symbolized courage of the highest order, and no one would have dreamed of reproaching her for shedding not a single tear in public. But excess stoicism, the inability ever to express any emotions under any circumstances, is decidedly not good for you. We know it leads to depression and a variety of other ills. The actor, Mike, was stoic; he had a lifelong history of hiding his emotions behind a cheerful facade. The effect was to push his emotions into his heart and its blood vessels instead, forming blockages there.

Emotional effusiveness is the opposite of stoicism. In our culture, emotional effusiveness is still looked at somewhat askance for the most part. We teach our children not to be excessively effusive when they play sports, not to leap and cry "Yippee!" when they cross home plate after hitting a home run. A high five with a teammate and then a low-key jog to the dugout will do. But we've just talked about how expressing emotion is good for you. Even the British, long famous for their stiff upper lip, appeared to realize this after the tragic death of Diana, Princess of Wales. Pouring out their grief proved a catharsis after a long history of emotional repression. When emotional expression degenerates, however, into a constant weepiness, it can become an excess vulnerability that lays you open to problems and symptoms as well.

Anger is another power emotion. Science tells us that it's healthy to express your anger, and this is true, but if you express your anger to an extreme, if anger is the only emotion you feel all the time, you're headed down a deadly path.[11] Not expressing your anger, though, can be equally poisonous, as we saw with the actor. Keeping your anger close to your chest in a show of stoicism can also affect other organs of the fourth emotional center, especially in women.

CARRYING A GRUDGE
A CASE OF BREAST CANCER

The Reading. Frances Payne, age fifty-two, felt very much like a martyr to me; I saw her as a Joan of Arc type. I could see she was a very bright and gifted woman. But I saw her paired with a partner who was running all the time and who seemed to me exhausted. As a result of his exhaustion, Frances had a hard time feeling a deep connection with him, a hard time feeling loved and nurtured. I told her I thought she had some disappointment in the relationship.

I also saw that Frances had suffered a significant loss, a death of something or someone. I felt that whenever her partner left home, his departure brought up the same feelings she'd had over this loss. I saw a lot of repressed anger and rage. I generally felt that something very big was going on in Frances's life, and that it was difficult to handle.

When I looked at her body, I had an image of a red fuzz ball in the area of her right breast, below the nipple. Scanning further, I noticed another red fuzz ball in her left hip. I also thought I detected some red areas in her liver. And I saw her having problems with memory and changes in the white matter of her brain.

The Facts. Frances was married to a man whose job took him away from home two to three times a week, often for more than one day at a time. Essentially, he was hardly ever home. Frances, however, insisted that she had no disappointment with the relationship. "I'm with a loving husband and he's wonderful, and there's no problem," she said. When I pressed her on this point, she finally admitted, "Well, I suppose sometimes he's not there for me, especially when I get bad medical news."

Frances also insisted she'd had no significant loss of any kind. The only thing that might count, she said, was the death of her father. "But that was four years ago, and I'm glad he died," she said. Her father had apparently verbally abused her all her life. She said her relationship with him consisted of nothing but one endless screaming session, during which her mother would fade into the woodwork. When I suggested she might have unresolved and unexpressed grief, as well as anger, over his

> death, she denied it heatedly. "I'm glad he died," she repeated. Finally, however, she conceded that she might have some unresolved grief over what she would have *liked* the relationship to be, and anger over the fact that he had died before the relationship could change. Frances also had trouble receiving nurturance from anyone. "I wouldn't take an aspirin from anybody," she said.
>
> Frances's comments about her physical health were the most amazing part of our discussion. She told me that she had been diagnosed with breast cancer by a medical specialist. She, however, didn't accept this diagnosis. She said she had guides—internal spiritual advisers—who told her that all she had was an infection in her breast. She was having pain in her left hip, but she believed that was only an infection, too.

Frances's unexpressed grief and anger, with both her father and her husband, and her inability to accept help or nurturance from anyone, fit the emotional profile of a breast cancer patient to a tee. Research has shown a relation between breast cancer and an apparent lifelong tendency to suppress anger.[12] Failing to express your distress can affect your immunity. We all have "natural killer" cells that run around keeping check on our bodies, and if a cancer cell comes on board, they chew it up and spit it out. A person's natural killer cell activity has been found to be an important predictor of whether or not the cancer is likely to spread. If you have fewer working natural killer cells, you have a higher chance of getting cancer. Researchers found that if a woman had unresolved emotional loss in her life, she was more likely to have wiped out as many as 51 percent of her natural killer cells.[13] Clearly, if you're upset, you're better off knowing you're upset, expressing your distress, and resolving it.

Frances was an extreme example of someone who couldn't do this. She was so disconnected from her emotions that she couldn't admit she was still angry with her father and her husband. She had also refused all nurturance and was in denial about her cancer. Frances wasn't allowing her emotions to move through her, nor was she letting them move her to change toward forgiveness. Instead, they were moving matter inside her body, making way for tumors and masses and illness. Because she wasn't changing her emotions, they were changing her, literally, through the structure of her body.

It's perfectly normal to hold emotions in from time to time or to nurse a given emotion for a period. But the key is in the length of time that you do this. The emotion itself isn't a poison that will hurt us. It's dangerous only if it's suppressed for too long. Compare it with sitting in a chair for too long. The act of sitting in a chair isn't itself unhealthy. But if you sit in a chair for seventeen hours and never get up, you're going to be frozen in one position. Sitting in the chair isn't your problem; being *immobilized* in the chair is your problem. In the same way, being immobilized in any emotion is unhealthy, because it's the opposite of what emotion means, which is to move on or out. If you're stuck in an emotion, it's not an emotion anymore. It's a problem.

For instance, take the following client story: Meg was a college professor who had worked in the state college system in Michigan for fifteen years, nurturing her graduate students through their Ph.D. studies. She was up for tenure and had spent many nights and weekends researching and writing papers for academic publication, sacrificing any home life or leisure activities in pursuit of tenure. In her most recent published paper she had alienated some of the bigwigs at the college by expressing a controversial opinion of feminist studies. As a result, she was passed up for tenure.

Meg was furious and grief-stricken. She left the college and started writing a book based on her last paper, figuring she would publish her findings in even greater depth and really get even with the college. Of course, she was not letting go of her desire for vengeance with this emotion as her motivation. Fourteen months after she had left the college, Meg noticed a mass in her right breast, but ignored it for six months before getting a biopsy. It was cancerous.

Meg was scared by the diagnosis and was willing to change her life to heal herself, although part of her still wanted just to focus on her book. When I did a reading for her, I saw an image of a betrayed family member sitting in her chest. This, of course, was the college, which had been a family to her. To her credit, Meg realized that she was filled with grief and rage, and that she needed to let go of the connection to her betrayal—the book—which she had been using to medicate and intensify her feelings of betrayal, anger, and hurt. She took a sabbatical from writing and underwent a course of chemotherapy.

Meg also realized that she desperately missed her friendships and ties to the college and needed to construct another social and emotional support system. She also needed to find another intellectual outlet—although not the book—to use her mental skills and creativity. Meg landed a part-time teaching position at a community college and reconnected with her passion for teaching, which she had missed while she was writing in solitude. The book just was not a sufficient substitute for a professional association with other teachers and students, nor was it a full expression of her skills. Eventually, however, Meg did finish her book. She has been cancer-free for three and a half years.

WHO ARE YOU AT HEART?

Most people, when they're worried about heart disease, think that if they just switch to low-fat cookies, they'll reduce their cholesterol level and be all right. They sit at the table counting pats of butter, eating artificial eggs, and assuming this is doing good things for their hearts. No one has told them about their emotions and the role they're playing in their heart health.

But emotions are critical here. Take the type A personality. A host of studies indicates that type A behavior is associated with hypertension, increased cholesterol, and sudden death from heart attacks.[14] And what are the defining characteristics of this personality? People with type A personality (as of now, we're speaking mostly of men, since few studies have been done on women who might have type A personalities) have an excess of power and a deficiency of vulnerability in both emotional expression and the way they behave in partnerships. Type A's express themselves emotionally with an excess of anger and hostility. They tend to be aggressive, hard-driving, competitive, and impatient. They have a rigid personality structure that makes it difficult for them to experience peace or serenity. In partnerships, they frequently have problems with intimacy, accepting help, and nurturing others. They're always waiting for the next fight, and they aren't inclined to be submissive. This fight mode, or alarm reaction, has been related to high blood pressure and coronary artery disease.[15] To many players on the tennis court, the game is all about competition, not about partnership.

Type A's are like drivers stuck in the power zone, pressing the pedal to the metal. They go 80 mph in a 25 mph zone, cutting people off and saying, "Don't you understand? I have places to go, people to see. I'm on my way to solving the problems of the world." If you know anyone who's a type A, I'm sure you don't think of him as a vulnerable individual. Still, some type A's hide their hostility and direct it inward. When these guys cut you off, they do it with a smile.[11] These people often suffer from high blood pressure. They want to appear compliant and agreeable, but they resent people and have to internalize their thoughts of rage.[11] This type A will keep his smile on in the boardroom until he cuts the deal. Then he leaves the meeting and slams his fist down on his secretary's desk because he's so enraged by all the demanding and demeaning comments he had to listen to from those other guys in the meeting.

In an earlier chapter I described Peter, a hard-charging, competitive corporate executive. His primary physical problem was severe ulcers, which is why I used his story in the third emotional center. But I could see that he had existing problems and potential problems in the fourth emotional center as well. He's a good example of how the emotional centers echo back to each other and even overlap. I noted that he had the capacity to form blockages in the coronary artery. There weren't any yet, but they could develop down the road. His intuition wasn't speaking to him yet through the fourth emotional center, but if he didn't change the way he was heading in life, I knew that eventually it could speak up through symptoms in his heart.

Even though they have trouble with partnerships, type A's are often seen as good providers.[16] Their hard-driving, competitive, workaholic qualities ensure that they'll go out into the world and do whatever it takes to bring home the best bacon available and the largest amount of it. Unfortunately, they frequently don't allow themselves to enjoy the meal with their partners when they do get home. They can't leave their type A qualities at the door. After they have cut off everybody else in traffic and on the job, they return home, to the world of their most intimate partnerships, and keep doing the same thing. They're on automatic pilot, and the car keeps going in the same direction, cutting off everyone in its way, even a spouse.

One study looked at the way type A people communicate in relationships, measuring their heart rate and blood pressure at the same time. Investigators wanted to see whether type A individuals cooperated, competed, punished, rewarded, or withdrew from their partners in relationships. The type A's were found to be excessively aggressive and overly competitive in partnerships.[16] They competed twice as often as non–type A's, punished their partners three times more often, and did not cooperate or reward each other significantly. This excess of power and deficiency of vulnerability influenced the organs of the fourth emotional center. Fluctuations in heart rate were greater in the type A's, and their blood pressure was more likely to go up.

Type A's were more likely to distress their partners when talking to them. Even if the partner was trying to validate the type A's point of view and trying to be conciliatory, the type A's were confrontational and threatening. They were more likely to ignore what their partners were trying to tell them—fifteen times more likely, in fact. That means that if your husband is a type A and you send him a message saying, "Are you listening to me?" he'll probably ignore it. If you plead, "Can you please not put the towel on the bedroom floor?" he'll turn a deaf ear. The study showed that the type A's, in short, were uninterested in true partnership and mutuality. The communication in their ears was unidirectional: they recognized only outgoing calls, not incoming messages. Type A's were non-nurturing and less able to satisfy their partners' requests.

In their relationships, type A's remind me of the monkeys in a dominance study that found that the dominant monkey asserted his authority over the others in his group by never making eye contact with any monkey that approached him.[17] He would always look up and slightly away from the other monkey with apparent indifference. He appeared utterly powerful. Clearly, type A's want always to be in the power column of their partnerships. And they're more comfortable when their partners are in a vulnerable position. They want to dominate, but that can set the scene for their physical breakdown.

A Rock Feels No Pain
A Case of Heart Disease

The Reading. Fred, a sixty-eight-year-old man, didn't want to talk to me. His wife, who had placed the call, pleaded with him to speak with me. Finally he picked up the phone. Now all I heard on the other end was a stony silence. In fact, that's what Fred felt like, a rock or a stone. I thought of the John Donne poem that says that no man is an island, and the Simon and Garfunkel song, "A rock can feel no pain, and an island never cries." I saw him as very good-looking, with cool, icy blue eyes, about 6 feet 1, trim with just a slight paunch, and as someone who prided himself on being a good tennis and bridge player. I saw that he was very stoic, never let his grief or anger show, and expected those around him to behave the same way. He didn't tolerate emotional effusiveness. In fact, he looked at others with extreme disdain, feeling that most people didn't quite measure up to his standards. He was extremely successful and expected his children to succeed. He exercised a great deal of control over his family, but from a distance. I saw him as being very isolated from his wife and children. In fact, I actually saw that he had a mistress, a flashy woman who was the opposite of his conservative preppy wife. I also saw that he had nursed a lot of anger and hostility his entire life. He was like a boiling pot. At present, he had a lot of anger and grief beneath his controlled exterior over some setback in his work.

I could tell at once that Fred had an unusually rapid, although regular, heart rate. His lungs looked boggy and somewhat filled with water. Something in his abdomen looked large, as though there were a balloon inside it. He looked pale and sallow. He looked very weak on the inside, in spite of all the strength he displayed on the outside.

The Facts. Fred was a World War II veteran who had earned a Purple Heart. He'd had a long and successful business career. All his life, his self-esteem had been based on his ability to manage finances. His children were all very successful professionals—doctors and lawyers. Fred was proud that they were able to fulfill their responsibilities in life. He didn't believe in mollycoddling. At one time, his younger son had wanted to pursue a career in fine art, but Fred had refused to pay for the schooling, because he didn't believe in anything so "emotional" and right hemisphere. Although he had a circle of acquaintances at the country club with whom he and his wife socialized, Fred had no real friends or close intimates.

Fred's firm had been sued for financial improprieties, and was about to lose the case. This prospect was devastating, but Fred refused to show any distress. In fact, although he had spent years fighting the lawsuit, everyone said he had faced it like a real trouper and never let on how much it bothered him. He was stoic throughout.

Then, out of the blue, Fred began to suffer from weakness and lassitude. When he consulted a doctor, it was discovered that he was suffering from heart failure with a life-threatening arrhythmia. In addition, he had a virtually irreparable aortic aneurysm, or tear, in his abdomen near the kidneys.

Fred fit all the criteria for type A personality at risk of coronary disease and hardening of the arteries. He felt and acted like a rock, because he thought that to be powerful was to be stoic. Yet he felt hostility beneath the surface. He would release it in nasty and offensive and aggressive ways. He was the kind of man who would turn to a woman having dinner with him and say snidely, "You can really pack it in, can't you?" or "I don't know how you can eat something so rich."

No one really knew him, and no one could ever get close to him emotionally. He was isolated, cool, and distant. It was as if he never allowed himself to be petted, stroked, and entertained. He knew neither how to receive nurturance nor how to nurture. He was immersed in his identity as a father, but not in a nurturing sense, only as a distant, guiding force. His idea of giving help was providing funds and clothing and support. He was never emotionally available, he condescended to waiters and waitresses, and he tended not to look directly at other people but to gaze slightly past them with an air of disdain and superiority, like the dominant monkeys in the study I spoke of.

His keeping a mistress was the outward manifestation of a split heart, which was physically symbolized by his split aorta. Moreover, he had a kind of heart-brain split. He divorced his feelings from his head and didn't believe in anything that was illogical or emotional or limbic or rooted in the right hemisphere. He thought everything should be rational and intellectual. Well, studies have shown that when you have more frontal lobe (rational) activity during an emotional experience, you generate sympathetic nervous system input to your heart and increase the risk of arrhythmia. In plain English this means that if you can't allow yourself simply to feel something fully, if you have to go into your frontal lobe and intellectualize it, you have a higher risk of developing an arrhythmia.[18] That's exactly what Fred did.

All of Fred's emotions were in the power category. But while he looked powerful on the outside, he was actually very weak inside. No joy or love flowed through him, and all the highways to his heart were either completely clogged with coronary artery disease or were ripping apart from an aneurysm. He had no vulnerability to balance the powerful emotions he couldn't express, and they consequently wreaked havoc inside his body.

So if you're a type A, does this mean it's all over for you? Since this is your personality, are you destined to die of a heart attack or heart failure? No. It doesn't have to be that way. One study followed a group of men for two years after they'd suffered a heart attack. Some of these men were counseled and taught how to change their type A behavior, how to talk about their anger and resolve it. Amazingly, they were found to have a lower recurrence of heart problems than the men who received no counseling, even though their blood pressure and cholesterol levels did not change. In other words, when they were counseled to move out of their exclusive habitat in the power column of the fourth emotional center and to balance their lives with a little vulnerability, their health unquestionably improved. When they listened to their intuitive guidance system and made changes in their lives and their emotional reactions, they improved their prospects for health.

We have to understand, therefore, that health in the heart, in the fourth emotional center, isn't just a matter of blood pressure or cholesterol. Nor, of course, is it just a matter of hostility. There are many contributors to heart disease, including diet, fitness, heredity, and behavior patterns, like smoking. But hostility, which is a shading of anger, definitely occupies a unique place as both a component of type A behavior and a component of personality that has been associated with heart disease.[11] Thus, *emotions* or, more accurately, fully expressed and resolved emotions, are critical to heart disease or health.

BOILING POTS, SIMMERING KETTLES: WOMEN AND HEART DISEASE

It seems that "anger" and "man" are two words that just naturally go together in people's minds. And they sometimes go together in a positive way: an angry man is seen as a pillar of righteousness and power. At worst, he may be regarded as a tough bastard who's hard to deal with and gives you a run for your money. But even that description carries a certain amount of grudging admiration. At the hospitals where I've worked, the male doctors who show any forcefulness of temper or are hard-driving and aggressive are universally looked upon with approval as go-getters and movers and shakers.

What happens, though, if a *woman* shows anger? I can't think of the last time I heard anyone speak admiringly of "angry young women." At work, any outbursts on my part get me instantly tagged as an aggressive or angry bitch. Now, this *b*-word carries a much different connotation from the male *b*-word above. It's flat-out derogatory. Nobody would snap to if I spill my anger out the way my male colleagues do; people would just give me the hairy eyeball. I've always thought this was unfair, but there you are.

In our culture, women aren't supposed to exhibit fiery and violent emotions. Because of their fear that they'll be seen as bad people, women generally are afraid to express their anger directly in all its potency. This doesn't mean they don't *feel* the anger, though. It just stays inside them, stewing and turning into resentment and bitterness. And this bitterness can attack the heart just as readily as a man's open hostility. Too many people make the mistake of thinking that when we talk about heart disease, we're talking mainly about men. It's true that previously, almost all cardiovascular studies have been performed on men, but that's rapidly changing as we realize that heart disease is the number one killer of women, too. Shockingly, though, a recent survey found that only *8 percent* of American women know that heart disease is their most significant health risk.

High levels of expressed anger and hostility are related to heart disease in men,[14,11] whereas *low* levels of expressed anger have been related to heart disease in women.[15] Although some men are unusual and some women vary from this generalization, generally speaking men and women are like two sets of pots on a stove. Most men are pots left on high with no lid, so that they boil fast and loud, until they finally and rapidly boil over. Most women, on the other hand, are like a kettle left to simmer for a long period of time, with the top on to hold in the feelings. This kettle makes less noise and is less obvious than the boiling pot, but next thing you know, the water has evaporated and the pot has cracked. There was no noise and little steam, however, so that no one was even aware there was a problem. But there was.[9]

THE SMOTHERED SPARROW
A CASE OF HEART ARRHYTHMIA

The Reading. As soon as I began reading Violet, age thirty-eight, I saw a life full of joy and exuberance. She seemed to me like a little sparrow sitting on a fence, warbling away. She didn't like to complain, and masked everything with her cheerfulness. But underneath her heart, I saw a difficulty, a person who was getting in the way of something Violet wanted. I saw disappointment in her relationship with this person, which was making Violet's healing a challenge. I saw something Violet wanted to do, some life's path she needed to follow, but I saw that she was being held back by this person who had authority over her. This person appeared to be extremely goal-oriented and focused on his own needs to the detriment of the feelings of those around him. In fact, he reminded me of a cat who's just killed a bird. He's sitting on the porch, surrounded by feathers. And the feathers are the petals of Violet's heart.

I saw that Violet was feeling less and less joy and was slowly becoming angry and resentful. Her partnership was not one of equality; her partner was the authority, and she was submissive.

In her body, I saw a little scarring in her lungs from past smoking, and occasional bladder infections in the distant past. But in her head, I saw a kind of fury, what I call a tornado in the scalp. This whirlwind of anger and hostility was buffeting her heart and causing it to race and skip a beat.

The Facts. Violet was a musician who had an intense desire to become an orchestral conductor. She had the opportunity to work and train toward this end with a leading male conductor. Her husband, however, was opposed to this idea. A nonmusician himself, he was threatened by the prospect of his wife's working closely with another man at something in which he could have no part, and he refused to allow her to pursue her plan. Violet was inwardly furious at this, but out of deference to her husband's feelings and jealousy, she had put off her training. However, she hadn't given up on her determination to become a conductor. She continued privately to plan to do it at a later date, thinking she could present the idea to her husband in another way so that he would eventually approve it. For the time being, Violet had put a lid on her own feelings to keep her husband happy, but her resentment simmered.

Meanwhile, she confirmed that she had developed an arrhythmia in her heart.

It didn't occur to Violet simply to defy her husband's wishes. Their unequal partnership made this impossible. Violet had given over authority in the partnership to her husband, but the results of this were causing her great resentment, and this resentment was sitting on her chest. And this in turn was setting the stage for serious heart problems. Sudden death from a heart attack is believed to be due to arrhythmia, a change in the rhythm of your heart. Stress often causes an increase in the production of brain chemicals called catecholamines, which can speed up the heart rate, overstress the heart muscle, wear down its reserves, and enhance a person's chances of developing heart disease.[11] By not expressing her emotions, holding them in and hiding them behind a brave face, Violet was maintaining momentary peace in her partnership, but in the meantime she was potentially doing damage to the organs of her fourth emotional center. Violet was a simmering kettle, in danger of cracking.

Generally speaking, women's and men's hearts react differently to similar emotions in part because men's brain connections to their hearts are different from women's. Men's brains are more lateralized, or compartmentalized.[19] Men have what you could call the Rubbermaid kitchen drawer brain. The male brain, in other words, is like the kitchen drawer with the plastic organizer in it, where you separate all the knives, forks, and spoons neatly into their own compartments. The different functional areas of a man's brain are all neatly divided. When a man talks, one or two areas in his brain light up, while the emotional areas remain separate.[19] Women, on the other hand, have a messier drawer, a less obviously organized brain. The female brain is like the drawer you toss everything into without any order so that everything gets jumbled together—the ice-cream scoop and the lobster cracker, five rubber bands, sixteen twist ties, several shish kebab skewers, and some plastic forks with broken tines. It's obvious that both drawers have their function and utility. Neither one is better than the others. The organization is just different.

This means that most men use one hemisphere of their brains at a time, usually the left. They therefore think more linearly and logically; but when they go into the right hemisphere and feel, their emotions are very intense, because they're concentrated on that one activity.[19] Their feelings boil more rapidly, until they boil over. Most women, however, use both hemispheres simultaneously. That means they have greater and more continuous access to the right hemisphere. And the right hemisphere has richer connections to the heart. This means that most women have greater neurological and emotional connections to the heart than most men. At any time, therefore, whatever a woman is feeling or experiencing can be felt and experienced in her chest. All that simmering, therefore, takes its toll over a longer period of time.[19]

My friend Norma describes herself as a lifelong chronic slow simmerer. She has a lid on her anger, especially when she's resentful or angry toward someone from whom she fears rejection. She learned this behavior in her family; the memories of how her family acted are encoded in the organs of her fourth emotional center. Everyone in her family is a so-called good egg. Growing up, Norma never saw anyone in her family get openly angry at anyone else. (To me, who grew up in a hot-blooded Mediterranean family, this is almost inconceivable!) She was never struck as a child. The members of her family defer their own needs to keep everyone else happy. Everything looked harmonious and placid on the surface, but there was a lot of simmering going on underneath. And indeed, all four of Norma's grandparents, as well as her father, died of some form of heart disease. Normal knows she'll have to break the deadly pattern of keeping a lid on her anger if she wants to achieve real health in her fourth emotional center.

Because women have traditionally kept a lid on their power emotions of anger and hostility, for a long time we didn't worry about women and heart disease. This lack of concern was reinforced by the way women present with heart disease. When we think of heart attacks, we think of the way men have heart attacks: sudden chest pain, spreading to the jaw and down the left arm. A woman having a heart attack, however, may not exhibit these symptoms. She may have abdominal pain and indigestion. She may have no chest pain at all. The first sign of a heart attack in a woman may be congestive failure, with no symptoms of heart attack preceding it.

The idea that women didn't have heart attacks used to be so common that when a woman, especially one in her late thirties or early forties, *did* arrive at the hospital emergency room complaining of chest pains, she was routinely told she was merely anxious, perhaps having an anxiety attack. This isn't the case anymore. At the hospital where I used to work, it became routine within the last several years to give an EKG automatically to any woman who came in complaining of pain anywhere between her abdomen and her neck.

Violet is a prime example of someone who was keeping the lid on her emotions and ignoring a lot of intuitive guiding signals, not listening to that warning buzzer in the body. But she would be in danger if she continued to simmer for too long, if she didn't move with her emotions. Her emotions were telling her to go out and get the job she wanted. In fact, a woman's heart health and her job are related. Women who are employed, especially those who have complex, challenging jobs and autonomy, usually have the best health. On the other hand, clerical women with demanding supervisors who find themselves in job situations where they can't express their anger are more at risk for developing heart disease. You could say that's 98 percent of the women in the United States. Even if they work at home, a lot of them have demanding supervisors in their husbands. You could also say that Violet fits this profile. Her husband exercised supervisory authority over her and put her in a position where she felt she couldn't express her anger. Moreover, he was forcing her to continue in a situation where her heart wasn't in her work. It's not difficult to see that if a woman's heart isn't in her work, it will give out. Taken one step further, if your heart's not in your life, it will not work as well and may help you check out of living.

As our society changes, we're beginning to see a certain masculinization of women's health patterns. Whether this is good or bad, I can't say. All I can say is that if you're doing something that doesn't feel right, your body organs are going to speak for you. The most important thing to remember about anger and hostility and heart disease is that it doesn't matter how you express your anger, whether by boiling over or simmering slowly, in the end, the effect is the same; either route can lead to heart disease. There isn't perhaps any clearer illustration of the fact that either extreme in how you express emotions—through power or through vulnerability—is unhealthy. A constant venting of anger isn't good, but a constant suppression of it into resentment and bitterness is just as bad. Finding a balance and a middle ground can set you on the path to health.

NURTURANCE AND MARTYRDOM

One of the most disturbing health developments of our time is the startling rise in breast cancer among women of the baby boom generation. Where just recently one woman in nine was expected to develop breast cancer, the odds have now increased to one in eight. For the most part, the efforts to reverse these statistics have been concentrated on finding a magic bullet against cancer, a form of chemotherapy or a purely medical cure that takes into account nothing more than the physical and biological contributors to breast cancer.

But we can't discount the significance of emotions and mental attitude both in the spread of cancer and the battle against it. The women of the baby boom generation are subject to a whole raft of emotions that arise out of the cultural changes our society has undergone in the years since they reached young adulthood. Most of these emotions center around the great conflict of the generation—the conflict between motherhood and self-fulfillment through work. Questions of nurturance, women's ability and desire to provide it, as well as their willingness to accept it from others, confront these women in ways that previous generations of women seldom had to deal with. Some embrace the role of nurturer naturally, but others struggle with it. Unsure of their capacity for it, they turn it into a form of martyrdom in which they sacrifice their own needs to take on all the responsibility for others in a conscious act of supreme self-sacrifice that isn't always related to true nurturing. This affects all their partnerships, with spouses as well as with children.

It's logical that the effects of such conflicting emotions should be felt in a woman's chest, the part of the body to which we hold those whom we love, and, most specifically, in the physical symbols of a woman's love and nurturing, her breasts. To maintain healthy breasts and other organs in the fourth emotional center, women need to be able to find a balance between power and vulnerability in both emotional expression and partnership. They need to be able to love others but also to follow their passion. They need to be able to express love, hate, and other emotions fully and not hide them behind a brave face. They need to be able to feel grief and bereavement fully and then release them. They need to feel intimacy in relationships, but also to make time for themselves and isolate themselves from the hubbub of the family when necessary. They need to balance giving to others with taking for themselves.

THE AMBIVALENT MOTHER
A CASE OF BREAST CANCER

The Reading. Samantha, age forty-three, struck me as a highly responsible woman, almost hyperresponsible, and very comfortable with power in the outer world, in a boardroom, and in complicated political situations. I could see, however, that she wasn't dealing well with complicated emotional situations in the inner world of her partnerships. I saw that she was trying to hold something together, but finding the effort burdensome. I saw someone in her life who was depressed or grief-stricken about having lost something and who needed her emotionally. She resented his neediness but didn't express her resentment. I also saw that she had a lot of disappointment and regret with a second relationship of some kind. She seemed to be trying always to balance two things, either taking care of other people's needs and resenting it or doing something for herself but feeling guilty. She felt somewhat stiff and dried up to me, certainly not someone who was emotionally effusive.

Looking intuitively at her body, I noticed a slight extra heartbeat and markings in her lungs. I felt she couldn't take a deep breath. I also saw cysts in her breasts.

The Facts. Samantha had been a major marketing executive, better known and more successful than her husband, who had recently lost his job as a museum curator. This caused him great distress and made him emotionally needy in their partnership. The crux of Samantha's situation, however, was in her rocky emotional relationship with her twenty-one-year-old daughter. The young woman had told Samantha that she was dissatisfied with her as a mother. This filled Samantha with guilt, since she had been ambivalent about having a child in the first place. Having gone ahead and had one, she had then struggled to balance work and family. Her daughter's comment was, to Samantha, a stinging indictment of those efforts and proof that she hadn't succeeded at motherhood and nurturing the way she had always succeeded in the world of work, where her heart truly lay.

A number of years earlier Samantha had been diagnosed with breast cancer. It had recently spread to her lungs. Every time she took a deep breath, the pain was excruciating. Samantha had quit her job and was devoting herself to taking care of her health and her family.

Samantha had an incredible amount of insecurity about being a mother. She hadn't really been interested in being a mother, but she had sacrificed herself to become one because it was the accepted thing to do. After having a child she wasn't sure she wanted, she had tried to perform a balancing act that didn't work. She had guilt feelings about her unsatisfactory relationship with her daughter, as well as feelings of self-criticism about her abilities as a mother, which were reinforced by her daughter, who had apparently sensed her mother's ambivalence and used it as a weapon against her. She also had an unequal relationship with her husband and found herself giving while he was taking. Samantha had given up her job and given herself to the family in self-sacrifice. This very act, however, could be one of several factors that were contributing to her breast cancer. One research study found that thirty-five out of forty-six women with breast cancer had strong self-sacrificing qualities. Moreover, prior to developing cancer, they felt guilty, acutely depressed, vaguely anxious, and strongly self-critical.[20]

Although they don't admit it openly, a lot of women in our society wonder whether or not they should have children. And some quite clearly don't want to have any. The prevailing pressure from society, however, as well as from family, husbands, and friends, leads many of these women to launch themselves into motherhood all the same.

Most people don't realize that you can be a woman in this world and use your creative and reproductive organs for other purposes. Being a whole woman doesn't necessarily mean you have to have children. In fact, having a baby when your intuition tells you not to may be a mistake. For instance, studies have shown that the easiest way to give a rat cancer is to force it to breed and have young when it isn't ready to do so.[21] Scientists prematurely removed litters from female rats and forced the rats to mate and breed again immediately, although they weren't ready to. Most of them quickly developed mammary tumors.[21]

To combat her feelings of guilt and unworthiness as a mother, Samantha had also moved into the realm of martyrdom. A responsible person by nature, she now became hyper-responsible in her partnerships with her husband and her daughter, assuming all the responsibility for making the family work and for supplying the emotional needs of those closest to her. Martyrs, however, are so given to self-sacrifice that they tend to repress their own emotions and to shoulder the burden for everyone they care for. They do this in the belief that they're being nurturing, but in reality martyrdom is very different from nurturing. There's an old saying: "If you give a man a fish, you feed him for a day; if you teach a man to fish, you feed him for life." The second way is nurturing; the first is a form of martyrdom. A lot of women in our society learn to do everything for others. Eventually they develop an overactive responsibility gland, while the other person gets an atrophied one.

This is what was happening with Samantha and her daughter. Her daughter had reproached her for not being satisfactory as a mother, which was tantamount to telling her mother that she expected Samantha to satisfy all her needs all the time. Samantha therefore began to bend over backwards to please her daughter. She quit her job, she decided to take her husband into therapy to see how they could improve the situation for their daughter at home. But what she was practicing wasn't really motherhood. Motherhood is teaching the other person to become a skilled, independent, and strong human being.

What is the essence of nurturance? We might find it in a certain South African fish. The male fish is the social organizer; he plays the role in the outer world. When a predator appears, he calls the alarm. The female fish then opens her mouth and all the baby fish swim in to be sheltered where it's safe and warm. When the danger has passed, the male gives the all-clear, the mother opens her mouth, and all the babies swim back out into the open water, to continue to grow in independence and autonomy. This is the kind of warm, rosy image of motherhood most of us cherish, the mother protecting her babies against the dangers of the world, yet letting them frolic and develop on their own when safety permits. Curiously, though, every once in a while, one of these fish apparently has a problem with the motherhood role. When the father calls the alarm, she won't open her mouth to let the babies in. They either escape on their own or get eaten by predators. Conversely, there is on occasion a mother who'll take the babies in when the alarm sounds, but when she gets the all-clear, she won't open her mouth to let the babies out, and they smother inside her.

Human mothers are sometimes like these two fish moms. There are cold, withholding, and distant mothers who are ambivalent about nurturing. And there are overly protective, smothering mothers who nurture in an excessive, emotionally effusive way. Neither the excessively powerful approach nor the excessively vulnerable approach is good for either the mother or the child. And in fact, both cold and distant mothers and overly protective mothers have been shown to have a high incidence of breast cancer.[22] Women who depend on child rearing as a source of self-esteem and their feminine identity, for instance, are likely to develop more symptoms of menopause and also to be at a greater risk for breast cancer.[23] On the other hand, cold and distant mothers are found to be a recurring element in the backgrounds of many women with breast cancer.[24] In addition, women with breast cancer often had more childhood responsibilities than other women. Frequently they shouldered all the responsibility for the families, and soon found their self-esteem derived from it. They had conflicts with their mothers, had difficulty dealing with and expressing anger, hiding it always behind a pleasant face. They tended to sacrifice themselves and had difficulty asking for nurturance or help from others.[25] Samantha strongly exhibited all of these were characteristics.

There is, however, such a thing as a "good enough mother." Samantha didn't need to sink into the martyrdom role of taking complete responsibility for her daughter. She needed to teach the child how to be responsible for herself, provide her with appropriate support, and then hope for the best. And she needed to balance her power with vulnerabilities, release some of her stoicism, and learn to emote for the sake of a closer connection and more intimacy with her daughter as well as her husband.

For a better chance at health, she needed to let down her brave face and the pleasant facade she maintained in the face of her cancer and learn how to take help as well as give it. We know that the way women respond to their cancer makes a difference in their prognosis. Numerous studies have shown that many women with breast cancer tend to be stoic, to bottle up their feelings, especially their negative feelings, to maintain a cheerful, pleasant facade, to act respectful and cooperative, and to suppress their anger.[12] They keep their grievances to themselves, as though they were holding them close to the chest and nursing them inwardly. And then those emotions may go directly into their breasts.

THE SINGING NUN
A CASE OF BREAST CYST

The Reading. Teresa, at forty-one, was one of the most unusual clients I've ever had. When she called me for her reading, I immediately had a picture of someone almost encased in a voluminous and formal black robe of some kind. I saw a stiff white yoke that surrounded and nearly covered her face and masked her facial expressions. I had no idea what this garment was, but I knew that it was rigid and uncomfortable and made it very difficult to perform normal bodily functions. In fact, I wondered out loud how Teresa managed to go to the bathroom. This costume seemed to be very important, so I went on and on about it in the reading.

As I tried to imagine Teresa's family, I could see no husband or children. There was no ranch house with a golden retriever. Instead, I saw her spending a lot of time with a large group of people who were a quasi-family for her. "I don't understand your living arrangements," I said, "but you're certainly not part of a nuclear family." Where she lived, everyone had the same daily schedule, and Teresa's emotions—passion, anger, hostility—were cloaked by the group's uniform expression of serenity and peace. Emotions and their expression were to be kept secret, as were all physical needs. Among Teresa's clan, however, I sensed many secret relationships as well as an overall lack of nurture and support for Teresa.

Physically, I saw an area of redness in Teresa's left breast.

The Facts. Teresa, as you may already have surmised, was a Roman Catholic nun. She lived in a community of contemplatives, whose rules put strict restrictions on contacts and relationships between members of the order. Apart from praying and eating together, the nuns were forbidden to fraternize and were expected to maintain silence throughout the day. The nuns all wore the traditional habit of the religious, a heavy and uncomfortable black robe with a starched white wimple and veil.

In contrast to others in her order, Teresa had been initially ambivalent about entering the convent after a failed secret relationship with another woman in high school. She wasn't a true candidate for the order. She had entered as a means of protecting herself and finding refuge from relationships in life that made her uncomfortable. Like the character of Maria in *The Sound of Music,* she hid behind the walls of the convent, cutting herself off from emotional and physical needs.

Teresa told me she had a cyst in her left breast that was causing her concern.

There's hardly any stronger personification of sacrifice and stoicism in our society than a nun. Nuns actually *practice* suppressing their emotions. They must never be angry. Researchers have actually been able to predict which women may get breast cancer by looking at their ability to express anger. Those women who are more likely to adhere to social norms and to bend under social pressure were more likely to get breast cancer.[12] Teresa was certainly required to adhere to the social norms of her convent. In addition, women who accept their breast cancer with stoicism have been shown to die sooner than women who express some emotion, any emotion—anger, fear—upon diagnosis, or women who react with some denial but demonstrate a fighting spirit.[12,26] Women who took the fighting spirit too far, however, and began to confront situations they couldn't hope to change, like the death of a loved one, reversed their odds by moving out of the realm of normal fighting to assuming a crusade and becoming martyrs.[27] They moved far too deep into the power category of the fourth emotional center. There was a lot of wisdom in Chief Joseph's vow: "I will fight no more forever." You have to know when to hold and when to fold, when to be powerful, when to be vulnerable.

In Teresa's order, the sisters were supposed to be pious and without bodily needs. Teresa was also never really allowed to seek nurturance from others. Yet taking help and accepting nurturance can be significant to a woman's health if she has breast cancer. Women who *perceive* a lack of support in their immediate environment are more likely to have a recurrence of breast cancer sooner than women who feel they have support.[28] The women who felt they had strong support from a spouse or other intimates had a higher proportion of natural killer cells, the cells that ward off cancer.[13] Martyrs and stoics, as it happens, tend not to have very extensive support systems. If you never ask people to help you, they eventually stop coming by. Then, when you fall, you don't have a net to fall into. If Joan of Arc had been a trapeze artist, I would bet you any money she would have performed without a net.

Teresa wasn't allowed to have a support system in the convent. Yet women with breast diseases need support. When women with breast cancer meet together in an intervention group, they live demonstrably longer than women who don't receive such support. In one study, they virtually doubled their survival time.[29]

Even though being a nun may be a healthy choice for some women with a unique calling, Teresa's intuition may well have been telling her that she was in a place that wasn't right for her, a place that forced her to suppress her emotions and always maintain a joyful outlook. Joy, as we know, is the lifeblood of the heart. But if Teresa's joy was counterfeit, if what she presented was merely the *semblance* of joy, her intuition and her body's guidance system knew this. I knew that Teresa had strong emotions and passion for someone, but it was a passion she couldn't express. This was why I still saw Teresa in the traditional, swathing habit of the order, even though she told me that the nuns hadn't worn the old habit in years. The secrets and secret relationships I saw in her reading reflected the real emotions she was hiding behind her mask of a brave and cheerful face. Those real emotions were going into her system and affecting the organs of her fourth emotional center.

THE WEIGHT OF SORROW

Grief is another emotion we feel in our chests. When we are grieving, we often say we have a heavy heart or we feel a weight on our chests. When we lose something—a parent, a child, a spouse, a job, even a sense of identity—we have to be able to grieve over the loss. If you don't feel your grief, express it fully, and then resolve it, it can affect the organs of the fourth emotional center. For women, this often means the breasts, especially when the loss has to do with an object of love, such as a husband, parent, or child.[30]

The connection between grief and breast cancer has been noted for centuries. As far back as the 1700s, physicians observed that most breast cancers occurred after a disastrous event of life. Listen to this nineteenth-century case of a twenty-seven-year-old woman with cancer in her right breast. When questioned about her emotional life, she denied any problems. It soon came to light, however, that her father had died several years earlier and her mother had gone bankrupt. The young woman had gone to work as a governess. When she discovered a lump in her breast, she waited a year before getting help. Here's a 150-year-old example of a stoic to the *n*th degree, denying and repressing her emotions and then continuing to hide behind a brave face even after she developed illness.[30]

Remember the rats who got tumors when they were forced to breed before they were ready? Those rats had had a first litter of babies removed from them prematurely. There's reason to believe that not having time to resolve their grief over the loss of those first babies before being forced to have a new litter could have played a role in why they developed cancer. In humans, bereavement due to death, job loss, or divorce has been shown to increase the risk of breast cancer twelve times in women who suffered stress over a period of five years.[30] In other words, the five years after someone leaves your life, or you lose a job or get a divorce, are a time when you really want to get in touch with your anger, your pain, even perhaps your joy, if you're glad that something is coming to an end. You should embrace all the different emotions that come with bereavement and loss and with anxiety about what's next in your life, and make sure they're fully expressed and healed, because if you don't, you run the risk that those emotions might be expressed through your intuitive guidance system in your breasts or somewhere else in your body.

We all know that the incidence of breast cancer skyrockets as women reach the time of life when children are leaving home, their husbands are retiring, they may be leaving their own jobs. This is the time of life when the very structure of a woman's identity as a mother, a partner, or a working woman is subjected to losses that a woman might hold on her chest. Dr. Christiane Northrup tells a story about a woman in her early fifties who came to her office. The woman was grief-stricken because her dog had just died, one child had gone off to private school, and another had left for college. The woman had dreamed recurringly that she was nursing her children. She also had a cyst growing in her left breast. When it was aspirated, it was found to be filled with breast milk.

So we see that grief does go right into the organs of the fourth emotional center. Unexpressed and unresolved, it can cause grave illness there.

NO WAY OUT
A CASE OF BREAST CYST AND LUNG CANCER

The Reading. Fifty-two-year-old Helen gave me the sense of being a forced martyr. I had the feeling that she had spent her whole life taking care of someone. This gave her no fulfillment, however. I could see that she actually had difficulty nurturing. She felt trapped, and she was very angry about this. She felt that God had put her into a situation over which she had no control. A huge responsibility had been forced upon her, and she couldn't move.

In Helen's left breast I saw a brownish reddish area, like a hole. Although her lungs looked clear to me, I saw something different about her upper vertebrae, although I wasn't sure what the problem was. It looked humped or degenerating.

The Facts. Helen had a thirty-year-old daughter who had been born with cerebral palsy and mental retardation and required total care. Helen had worked hard to care for the daughter herself, vowing to keep her out of an institution. Her daughter was her chief project in life, since her husband had abandoned both of them when the child was two years old. Helen wasn't a natural martyr, however. She didn't feel fulfilled by taking care of her child. She found it difficult and painful, and suffered guilt over these feelings, which she tried to repress. Yet she felt trapped in motherhood.

Helen had a great deal of grief over the fact that her duties to her daughter had prevented her from fulfilling herself in the outer world, where her heart really lay. She was an RN, and had worked toward a Ph.D. in nursing, but she hadn't been able to finish it because she had essentially alienated her advisory committee with her angry, resentful approach. She found it difficult to be in partnerships or to work with anyone because her anger always got in the way. This only increased her ire. She felt she had sacrificed her entire life to someone else; as a result, she had never had the chance to live her own life.

Helen had had a tumor removed from her left breast ten years earlier, at the time her Ph.D. fell apart. Recently, after protracted efforts, the state had succeeded in finding her husband, only to learn that he was unemployed and unable to pay her more than $50 a week in support. Finally, Helen was forced to put her daughter into a state-run facility, since she could no longer afford to care for her. A week later she had a chronic cough evaluated and was found to have lung cancer, right beneath the spot where her breast tumor had been.

Helen clearly carried a lot of grief in her chest—grief over her lost home, grief over her unfinished Ph.D., grief over never receiving support or nurturance from anyone, and grief over her daughter and her emotions about having to care for her. She had borne it all stoically. But the result was that all this grief, and the anger that stemmed from her sense of forced martyrdom, had bored a hole into the organs of her fourth emotional center and were moving the cells around in the patterns of disease. Instead of stoically bearing her cross, Helen would have done better to listen to the signals coming from her intuition network. Instead of taking on all the responsibility for her daughter for her whole life, she might have done better, difficult as it may have been, to place her in an institution and visit her there or to find some other solution in the middle, one where the act of giving wouldn't literally drain all the blood from her body. She needed to free herself to pursue the path her heart truly desired. Some women's souls are fed by selfless acts of giving and kindness. Performing such acts is their life's path. But not everyone is Mother Teresa, and not everyone is fit for sainthood or the convent. Helen wasn't. She needed to let down her armor of power and allow herself some vulnerability in order to give herself a better chance at a healthier life.

SHOW ME WHAT YOU'RE FEELING

Expressing emotions is healthy. Of course, it can also sometimes make your life more complicated. One thing about expressing your emotions is that other people then have to listen to them. Half the reason why we don't tell people our feelings is that we're afraid of their reactions. But then along comes your therapist, who says you *must* express your emotions. So you're a good little patient, and you pay attention to your therapist, who teaches you to put words to your feelings. Then you tell your husband that he's a slob and you're sick and tired of his always leaving the towels on the bedroom floor. But instead of running to pick up the towel he just dropped there after his shower, he gets angry and sulks for the rest of the day. (At least he's showing his feelings!) Now both of you are miserable, and you think maybe you might have been better off just picking up the stupid towel yourself and avoiding the whole drama. Remember, though: one towel a day leads to seven towels a week, which leads to 31 towels a month and 365 towels a year. If you make it through 25 years of marriage, that's 9,125 towels that you've picked up while swallowing your annoyance and resentment. Along the way, part of your soul learns that you're not in a partnership. You're worthy only of giving help and not getting it. You can only hide your feelings behind a brave face. Even in what is supposed to be the most intimate relationship in your life—marriage—you can't really express what you're feeling or get any nurturance. Then you realize it's not just a towel anymore. The towel is a symbol of the emotional health and the degree of reciprocity and intimacy you have in a key relationship in your life. After all, we all know about the relationships that break up over that last towel.

When you learn to express your emotions, your relationships may become somewhat more complicated. But the complications will be worth the trouble. Feeling the full range of emotions—happiness, joy, anger, grief, sadness, fear, and on and on—and sharing them with others in a balanced way will strengthen the health of your fourth emotional center and make your life the rich, rewarding adventure it should be.

TEN

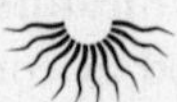

The Thyroid, Throat, and Neck: Communication, Timing, and Will

Listening to Frank Sinatra belt out "My Way" can make you feel strong and assertive. You get the clear idea that Frank's singing about a man who knew what he wanted, knew how to tell the world what he wanted, and had no problem believing that whatever came his way, he *would* get what he wanted. He was going to assert his will on the world, when and how he decided to, and he was going to get his way. Nothing was going to stop him from being true to himself.

"My Way" could be the theme song of the fifth emotional center. This is the center associated with issues in our lives having to do with communication, expressing who we are; timing, knowing when and how to go after our heart's desire; and will, the way we assert our own will or bend to that of others. This center is concerned with the stage of life where we declare "I will," and contend with the cycle of generativity versus stagnation," either continuing the life cycle through creation in the outer world or allowing things to stagnate and come to a stop.

Health in this center calls for a balance between expressing ourselves and listening to others; between pushing ourselves forward to fulfill our needs or waiting, when necessary, for things to come to us;

and between imposing our will on others or allowing others to impose their will upon us. The organs affected by our ability or inability to achieve this balance are the throat, the mouth, the thyroid, and the neck (see the following figure).

THE POWER AND THE VULNERABILITY

Some people are good communicators but terrible listeners. Do you know anyone who's really good at communicating his own point of view, but who turns a deaf ear when it comes to listening to yours? While you're talking, is he already planning what he's going to say next? What about people who absolutely hate to wait, who pass you in the right lane on the highway or whip around you with their shopping carts in the supermarket, vying for position at the checkout counter? My friends claim I'm in this category. I almost need to be medicated when I get one of those computerized messages on the phone: "All our operators are busy now. Please wait." If I hear the words "please wait," I just about go ballistic. I was always encouraged to be a go-getter and reminded that opportunities aren't salesmen who go from door to door. I don't hang around waiting for things to come to me. If I get a recording on the phone, I'll hang up a dozen times and keep dialing until I get through to someone rather than wait. Of course, I might get through *sooner* if I waited, but I've learned to push forward to get what I want and need instead of patiently waiting for someone to come to me.

Finally, how many people do you know who get an idea in their heads of what they want and need and who focus on this to such a degree that they'll stop at nothing to get it, regardless of what roadblocks stand in their way? In some instances, this is an asset; it shows determination, resilience, and stick-to-itiveness. But taken to an extreme, it can show willfulness and stubbornness. My friends say I fit right in here as well. "Wait" isn't the only word I'm allergic to; I also don't like the word "limitations," or being told "You can't do that; it's never been done before." I have a strong will and I often assert it. Sometimes this can backfire. Occasionally when I'm playing tennis, I'll find myself focusing on hitting the ball in a particularly determined way. And invariably I hit it way too hard and it goes right over the fence. You can overshoot with too much will the same way you can overshoot with a tennis racquet and a ball.

The kinds of people I've described are all too steeped in the power

Fifth Emotional Center

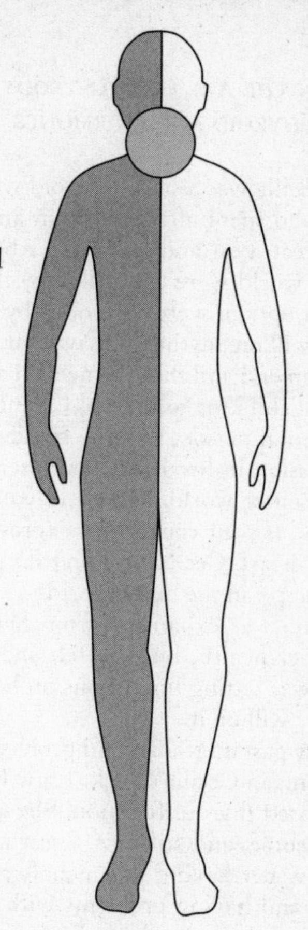

category of the fifth emotional center. Like the hero of "My Way," though admirable in lots of ways, they're a little too powerful in their willfulness. They barely ever acknowledge making any mistakes or having any regrets.

The organs of the fifth emotional center can be damaged by too much power in this area. They can also be affected by too much vulnerability—too great a fear of expressing yourself or an inability to communicate your own wishes and desires while always taking in those of others. If you're always waiting for things to happen to you and for the will of others to be asserted over you, your body will let you know this by setting the stage for illness in the fifth emotional center.

"HELLO, I'M ON THE AIR, CAN ANYBODY HEAR ME?" THYROID AND HORMONES

The Reading. Cecilia was a sixty-year-old woman who felt to me like someone who spent all her time in an intense struggle that was causing great wear and tear on her body. She believed that matters in her world were controlled by things outside her and that most of her options were controlled by other people. She couldn't assert her will on anything. I saw that something in her life was coming to an end and that she needed and wanted to get rid of an old way of thinking and an old identity. Cecilia, however, was a very mental person, and she could not connect what she wanted, the passion in her heart, with her mind's thinking and assert it in the outer world. What's in your fifth emotional center, or your neck, is your capacity to express what's below it, the passion in your heart. Cecilia couldn't do that. She couldn't communicate her desire in the outer world.

I saw that Cecilia was exhausted from her job. Something about it wore on her health, but she felt she couldn't leave it because the world was setting limitations on her and she had no capacity to exert her will on it.

In her head, I saw past migraines and problems with attention. I saw lots of problems in Cecilia's neck. I saw her primary problem as being decreased thyroid function. She also had problems with her neck vertebrae, and stiffness. I saw a subtle change in her heart rate. I saw her having melancholy and fatigue, being cold and lethargic, and having problems with her temperature-regulating system. I also saw her body having problems regulating fluids.

In her relationship with her husband, I saw problems with energy, libido, and fatigue. The stagnation at work was seeping into the energy in her relationship. I wondered whether or not someone had told her that her adrenals were exhausted.

The Facts. Cecilia used to love her work in a government agency. But lately it just wasn't fun anymore. She was getting more and more exhausted, and it wasn't really what she wanted to do. Her heart's desire was to open up a flower shop. She felt she couldn't do that, however, because she needed to continue at her job for five more years in order to get her pension and medical benefits. (How many people do you know like that, "dying for their benefits"?) Cecilia feared that if she left her job and lost her insurance benefits, she might get sick and not be able to afford to pay her medical bills. She preferred to stay put and be sick. So even though she had money set aside to support herself, Cecilia was afraid to risk leaving. She believed the world controlled her. She couldn't control the world, nor could she express herself in it.

Cecilia's primary problem was hypothyroidism, or decreased functioning of the thyroid gland. The thyroid is responsible for driving the hormone system, and, in a way, it times all the functions of the other organs in our bodies. Cecilia thus had problems with all her hormonal systems. She had insulin resistance and problems with blood sugar, and she had been told that her adrenal glands were shot, leading to decreased libido and energy as well as fatigue. Her immune system was also out of whack. Cecilia, in fact, had had multiple hormone failure, in the thyroid, adrenals, and ovaries, at an early age. She had gone through menopause at thirty-nine.

Cecilia had problems expressing who she is, as well as problems with will and creativity in the world. She couldn't assert her will, her drive to create in the outer world, nor could she communicate her heart's passion. Cecilia was stuck in one position. She was like a person playing Monopoly who ends up stuck in jail and can't get out no matter how many times she rolls the dice, so that after a while she just doesn't want to roll the dice anymore. Some people are able to assert their will in the world so strongly that they're unperturbed when they're told to "Go directly to jail, do not pass Go, do not collect $200." They have the attitude that they'll get themselves out of there in no time, pay the fifty bucks, and be off. They won't feel imprisoned by their circumstances or by a roll of the dice of life. But others, like Cecilia, won't trust that they can ever get out of jail. They won't feel that the attempt is worth the risk, and they'll just get stuck in jail because they don't feel that they can get themselves out. They feel they're prisoners to the dice of life.

Cecilia had saved money to make her dream possible, to get herself "out of jail" so she could open a flower shop. But when it came to actually expressing her desire and asserting her will, she didn't want to put fifty dollars of her hard-earned money in the center of the board, because she felt that one bad roll of the dice of life would land her in jail again.

Cecilia was stuck in the vulnerability category of the fifth emotional center. She was afraid, or unable, to express her desires and needs. She couldn't push ahead with her plans; she felt the need to wait in her existing job, to "die for her benefits," so to speak, in order to stay safe and secure. As a result, she was completely compliant to the will of others, to the world at large, in fact, in setting the course of her life. She didn't feel she could become who she wanted to be and assert her power in the world, because she was afraid that things would just happen to her and she wouldn't feel safe. Cecilia was convinced that she was at the mercy of the powers that be, that "they" were "doing it" to her. All of this hit her in her neck, affecting that area of her spine and disrupting the function of her thyroid.

The literature about thyroid disorders shows that people with these ailments frequently have issues associated with "I will," the ability to achieve some form of power in the outer world to express who you are and to change your environment. Future thyroid patients frequently have a pattern of precipitating factors.[1] They often find themselves in situations where they strive for self-sufficiency or freedom but can't achieve it.[2] They also often come from situations in which they can't take care of themselves and can't be independent. Faced with any kind of physical or emotional crisis, they become compliant, give way to the crisis, and are unable to assert their will to push through it. They frequently feel that they're getting beaten, that they're not able to assert themselves.

When scientists looked at what happens to the thyroids of rats who fight, they found that the thyroids of dominant rats, the ones who go out and assert themselves to the world, never changed in size. In contrast, the thyroids of the more submissive and compliant rats, who were not able to assert themselves and were thus beaten down by the dominant rats, became measurably smaller.[3] Cecilia was a person who felt beaten down by life. She was compliant and submissive and, like the weaker rats, unable to assert her will.

Although it's in remission, I have Graves' disease, a condition in which the body produces antibodies that stimulate the thyroid to action. The period of my life when I was diagnosed with this ailment was very significant. It was a time when my life was swinging back and forth between the power and vulnerability categories of the fifth emotional center. I was in medical school, in an M.D.-Ph.D. program. All that year I was stressed by the concern of whether I'd be able to pay for my education. I found that I was either constantly pushing, searching for the money to get me through, and asserting my will to get the funds I needed, or I was completely powerless, had to sit back, be compliant, and wait for the will of God and the heavens to act upon me and get me the money. What put me over the edge was discovering that two of my medical student loans had mysteriously defaulted, for no logical reason. I was still in medical school! I found myself talking to people on the phone till I was blue in the face, trying to straighten the mess out. I would scrub out of surgery while on a phone in the pre-op area, speaking to financial representative after financial representative trying to get to the bottom of things. But no matter how clearly I expressed myself or how firmly I asserted myself, no one would listen to me. I couldn't believe that I couldn't push my way through this situation and salvage it before somebody repossessed my cats. After all, I was a marathon runner. I knew all about pushing through the wall, forcing myself to keep going in spite of the pain. Push, push, push, even after you hit the wall of limitations. That could be the mantra of women of the nineties. We're told to be go-getters, not to sit around and let the will of God work on us. "If you sit around and do that," they tell us, "you'll be sitting at home, pregnant and on welfare." I wasn't going to do that. I wanted to be a go-getter.

Instead, *it* got *me*. One day a classmate looked at me and said, "You know, I think you may have Graves' disease. Your eyes look like Barbara Bush's." (This was not long after the former First Lady had been diagnosed with Graves' disease.) I scoffed at the idea at first. "We just have big eyes in my family," I said, laughing it off. But in truth, my classmate's observation made me uncomfortable. My intuition was telling me something. So I went and had a checkup, and sure enough, I was found to have the antibodies that indicated Graves' disease, although the condition was in remission.

I've always had problems related to communicating and expressing myself and advancing my heart's desire. I've never wanted to wait or to be compliant. All my life, my intuition has spoken to me through the organs of this center about my need to assert my will and about my impatience or inability to do so. In fact, I'm something of a poster child for the fifth emotional center. I'm usually swimming too much in the power column here. I have trouble with communication (especially writing, since I'm dyslexic); I'm impatient, especially in a car on the highway (I'm notorious at the Registry of Motor Vehicles in both Massachusetts and Maine); and I have a strong will and don't like limits even if I hit tremendous walls (or trucks). Where do you fit on the scale of expressing versus listening, pushing ahead versus waiting, being willful versus complying?

You might have difficulty with the emotions of the fifth emotional center if you find yourself saying things like "Where there's a will, there's a way." That popular old saying expresses the willfulness that can be a hallmark of problems in this area of your life. You're going to push through and assert your will. What about "I never have any say" or "I don't have a voice"? Do you have trouble expressing yourself and being heard and understood? Do you often say, "Oh, all right, we'll do it your way"? That's a sign of a compliant, unassertive nature. If you find yourself saying any one of these things too often, and if your body's weak link is somewhere in the neck, you could be setting yourself up for difficulties and disease in the fifth emotional center.

LISTEN TO ME: COMMUNICATION

Like lots of people, I'm terrified of speaking in public. The first time I ever spoke at a national conference, I was very nervous and I got mixed reviews for my performance. Some people thought I had passion and creative energy, while others noted that I had tripped over the lectern several times. Some people said they loved my unique way of talking and my energetic pace, but others hated the format I used and needed to use a much slower, more linear pace to make the information comprehensible. After that, I was *twice* as terrified of speaking. The next year, and the four years after that, when I was scheduled to speak at that same conference, I'd get a fever and a cough, which would blossom into full-blown bronchitis the day before my talk. I'd have to speak while nursing a cough drop in my mouth, so that I wouldn't break into fits of coughing. Then two people in the audience of 250 wanted to know if I had a speech impediment or whether I had gum or a mint in my mouth. And if I did, could I please tell the audience why this was necessary, since it was not proper in a formal presentation.

Losing one's voice is another form of stage fright and a part of speaking phobia from which many suffer. The vocal chords become dysfunctional in a manner similar to the symptoms of bronchial asthma attacks.[4] But it doesn't have to be the stress of lecturing that renders a person voiceless. A friend of mine is a famous speaker who travels around the country delivering brilliant, flawless lectures to audiences large and small. Prior to launching this career, she had worked at a law school, where she was mentored by a distinguished and well-known professor who was a leading authority in his field. When my friend decided to leave the university to pursue a different career path, this professor was extremely displeased and let her know of his feelings in no uncertain terms. My friend was deeply upset by his reaction. As it happened, her lectures sometimes brought her back to this same university. She found that whenever she had to give a talk in front of her former mentor, her voice would close off so that she could hardly speak. It was almost as though asserting her will to this man and then being criticized for it had caused a kind of posttraumatic stress disorder that led her to lose her voice and her will when she was in his presence.

My own speaking phobia, or fear of being on stage, stems from the memory of a trauma that continues to affect me and the function of the organs in my fifth emotional center to this day. When I was a girl, I studied piano, and once a year I auditioned for a piano educators' foundation. At the audition I had to play ten long and difficult piano pieces from memory before a judge. Every year I'd sit outside the audition room in a plastic chair, nervous and fidgeting. As I listened with terror to all the other contestants playing brilliantly, I grew more and more nervous about being able to do as well myself, about being able to express myself as brilliantly. I'd go in when it was my turn, hand the judge my music, sit down at the piano, and instantly discover that my mind had gone completely blank. I couldn't remember a note of what I was supposed to play. Every year I'd burst into tears and sit there, listening to my tears go *plink! plink!* on the ivory piano keys. And every year the judge, invariably a sweet, benign gentleman, would look up with alarm, exclaim, "Oh, my!" and hand me the music. And I'd proceed to play and earn a rating of superior, the highest score.

Why didn't everyone else cry and go blank every year the way I did? Obviously, I had a vulnerability about expressing myself, showing who I was, in a powerful way in the world. This was either genetic, empatterned in my brain, or environmental, due to experiences I'd had at home that were imprinted in my body. I had the feeling a lot of people have, that I was not competent, that I couldn't assert myself, that I wouldn't be good enough. And so I lost my voice—not my speaking voice but the voice that came through the piano. In the same way, your voice could consist in writing a book, presenting a report at work, or even just typing a report. It could be any form of expression of who you are in the world.

People who suffer from childhood sexual abuse frequently develop vocal chord dysfunction: they literally lose their voices.[5] (The poet Maya Angelou has written about this phenomenon.) Nothing makes more sense. If someone exerted his will over you at a time when you had no power in the outer world, he essentially took away your say as well as your ability ever to develop a say. He quite literally took away your voice.[6] In general, people who suffer from vocal chord dysfunction often have difficulty directly expressing emotions and problems related to leaving their families of origin—in other words, developing their own voice. Their voice loss is their intuition's way of telling them they need to develop a new way to approach the world and to express themselves in it.

All animals, and perhaps all living things, have the ability to express, in ways that are accessible to others what they think and feel. In humans, the vital capability to communicate through words makes it possible for all of us to move and develop through life, to succeed at our goals and fulfill our life wishes. Yet although most people have the mechanical capacity to speak and communicate, not all of us have the emotional ability to communicate what's most essential about ourselves in the most effective and positive way. When this ability is thwarted, the effects can surface in the form of problems in the organs of the neck.

LUMP IN THE THROAT

The Reading. Rita, at age forty-nine, seemed to be a very efficient person. I saw her as a teacher, working with groups of people and training them in public speaking. Although she was very good at what she did, I felt that she wasn't really fulfilled, that she had problems related to being who she really wanted to be and with her belief in her ability. She wanted to achieve more and more, but she felt that there were blocks before her, preventing her from becoming as successful as she wanted to be.

Her body seemed mostly fine to me, but when I got to her throat, I saw that she had difficulty swallowing. Her throat looked red and enlarged, as though the muscles in her throat had been tightened to resemble a rump roast. I saw no masses, and I even saw Rita going from medical center to medical center having a series of tests that all came back negative. But I saw that she sensed that she had a lump in her throat.

The Facts. Rita was a business consultant who taught corporations how to manage their affairs and worked to help execu-

> tives improve their communicating and listening skills. Although she was successful at her career, Rita felt she had never really gone as far as she wanted to go in a very competitive field. She craved more power and prominence, and although she kept trying to push herself forward, she had problems expressing herself and asserting her will. She felt she had a great deal more to offer her profession, but no one was listening. Instead, she was always listening to others and helping them to communicate and express themselves.
>
> Rita believed she had a mass of some kind in her throat. Although a number of tests had failed to show anything, she had difficulty swallowing, felt a constant lump in her throat and was full of concern.

Although Rita had no medically discernible disease in her throat, she was clearly emotionally focused on that area, and this emotional focus was related to her physical symptoms. She was like people who suffer traumatic sexual abuse and later develop chronic pelvic pain. They've suffered pain and trauma in the emotional center related to the organs giving them pain—the second emotional center: pelvis, uterus, ovaries. Despite the pain they feel, which can be utterly disabling, the medical tests and procedures frequently do not pick up any physical change in those organs that could be related to that pain. From my perspective, Rita's trauma, whatever it had been, had to do with communication and self-expression. Even though she taught communication to others, she felt that no one heard her voice, no matter how hard she tried to present herself to the outer world. Her problem wasn't in her head; it was in her neck. I validated that by perceiving it in a medical intuitive reading, knowing nothing but her name and age.

Rita had what is known in psychiatry as globus hystericus, a sensation of a lump in the throat that makes swallowing and breathing difficult. It's been described as the feeling of a hard ball pressing against the outside of the throat, a stick being thrust down the throat, or something rising up in the throat. Sufferers report difficulty breathing and a choking sensation.[5] It's now believed that the sensation is caused by the strap muscles in the neck contracting and pressing against the cricoid bone. In the past, however, because no physical cause could be found, globus hystericus was thought to be caused by a "wandering uterus" exerting pressure on the neck.[6] The Latin word for uterus is *hystera;* all our English words such as "hysteria" and "hysterical" derive from it, and refer to the old belief that women, who have uteruses, were much more emotional than men and prone to disturbing and irrational bursts of feeling accompanied by bodily symptoms. While Rita's uterus had hardly wandered into her neck, the old perception wasn't completely off the mark. Women, as I've said before, have greater access to the right hemisphere of the brain and so are more connected to their emotions at any given time. It's not surprising, therefore, that globus hystericus is found much more commonly in women than in men.[5]

People with globus hystericus are believed to be more anxious, depressed, and introverted than others.[5] An introvert is more likely to listen, like Rita, than to express himself to others. Globus hystericus has also been interpreted as a manifestation of repressed crying or repressed emotional expression, something you need to say, but can't.[5] In other words, it's a thought or emotion that can't be communicated.

The inability to communicate our thoughts, feelings, and selves to others can strike with even more serious consequences, however, and affect your entire quality of life.

SWALLOWING HER ANGER
SICK THYROID SYNDROME

The Reading. When I talked to Liz, age seventy, I could tell that she was a very emotional woman who had a deep desire to call out to others emotionally but had trouble doing so. She seemed to have a protective wall around her. I could see that she didn't want to express her anger directly because she was afraid she might have to pay a price for it. At the same time, she felt victimized by this state of affairs. I saw that she was in a relationship with someone who knew she was having difficulties, but ignored them because he didn't want to deal with them.

In her body, I saw sinus headaches and neck stiffness. I saw that women in her family had decreased thyroid function tests, and I saw inflammation in the thyroid area. In addition, I saw a capacity for inflammation in the area of her GI tract that straddled the fourth and fifth emotional center, from the esophagus to the throat and neck.

The Facts. Liz was an elderly woman who told me she had a history of depression and loneliness. She felt that her husband was cold and distant. She deeply wanted him to hear her, but she couldn't call out to him emotionally. She resented this, but she believed that it was a woman's duty to swallow her anger rather than express it.

Liz told me she had what we call sick thyroid syndrome. She was on a program of thyroid replacement.

Liz had problems with many of the organs in her fifth emotional center, having to do with communication and expression. She didn't believe that she had the right to communicate to the world who she was and what she was feeling, much less the ability to do so. She believed that women were supposed to swallow their feelings.

Not surprisingly, many more women than men have thyroid problems. It's far more common for women to go on thyroid replacement later in life. Women's thyroids appear to succumb to stress more readily than men's. This was illustrated by a study of men and women and how they react to the stress of taking exams. Women are known to have greater terror of exams than men and, generally, to score lower. Indeed, the study found that a hormone that stimulates the thyroid gland to produce its hormone (called TSH, or thyroid stimulating hormone) was slightly elevated in both men and women on the day of the exam, but the next day the women's values slumped down much more significantly than men's. This may indicate that the women were much more stressed by the exam than men.[7]

A test is a significant way for people to express themselves, to communicate who they are and what they know. Women have a harder time with exams because our society, at least until recently, has placed more limitations on women's freedom to express who they are and to assert what they know than on men's. In the past, women, like children, were expected to be seen and not heard. This is ironic, considering that women are superior in communication skills earlier in life.[8] Girls speak sooner, are more fluent, and have more grammatical accuracy. They use more words per phrase—that means we talk a lot—and they have fewer instances of stuttering and dyslexia. Girls, in other words, start out with a stronger voice than boys. Yet somewhere along the line, they lose that voice. Studies have shown that during adolescence boys begin to speak more in school while the girls fall silent. The girls' self-esteem plummets along with their teachers' willingness to listen to them.[9] In fact, this is the period when girls should start actually becoming more expressive. As their hormones kick in and their periods begin, their fluency should actually become even greater. Women are at their best verbally during their peak estrogen periods, midway through the menstrual cycle. Asked to repeat "A box of mixed biscuits in a biscuit mixer" five times rapidly, women can't say it as well after they get their periods, when estrogen dips, as they can mid-cycle.[10] However, they can almost always say it better than men, and this ability has nothing to do with kitchen or culinary skills; they're just better at speaking and communicating verbally. Yet the very thing women are gifted in is the very thing they've been least able to use.

Not all of this is the fault of society. There's also an innate difference in how the sexes express themselves. Most men (there are always exceptions) are prone to what I call the "seldom right, never in doubt" syndrome. Driven by androgens and testosterone, men react quickly and act fast. They don't hesitate to express themselves. In one scientific study (yet to be published)[11] men have been shown to make more so-called errors of commission. They're constantly releasing a lot of arrows into the air. Only a few hit the target, but those are the ones people notice. So men get credit simply for expressing themselves, whether or not they're right. Most women, by contrast, are more tentative about expressing themselves. They have a slower reaction time, and they consequently make more errors of omission. When they do shoot an arrow, however, they tend to hit the center of the target every time. But because the arrows come so rarely, the women don't get as much notice.

Women's biological predisposition to react more slowly, and therefore to talk and express themselves less, is then reinforced by culture and society. Studies of men and women in the same room have shown that when women talk even one-third as much as men, they're perceived by both men and women to be hogging all the space. What's the effect of such perceptions? If you have something in your throat calling, "Hear me, hear me," but no one listens, eventually it gives up, closes up shop, and goes away. It's been shown that when women in midlife feel they've lost their say, their thyroids atrophy and begin to give way.[9] That's the way biology is. If you don't use it, you lose it.

At some point, Liz stopped calling out to her husband, because he wasn't listening to her anyway. She received and internalized the message that no one could hear her, and so she didn't try to express herself. Like many women, she let herself fall into the vulnerability category of the fifth emotional center; she stopped trying to assert herself. When her thyroid gave way, her intuitive guidance system was trying to tell her that she needed to change, to find a way to express herself and begin a dialogue with her husband and the world. If she asserted her will and moved more into the power category of the fifth emotional center, especially in the area of communication, she might begin to find her way back onto the road toward health.

TIMING IS EVERYTHING

When people have problems with timing and balance in their lives, you can read it in their bodies. Their timing is off. Instead of ticking steadily onward, clocklike, they either start ticking at hyperspeed, like a metronome gone berserk, or they stop ticking altogether. They're either on or off, hyperactive or out cold. I'm probably one of the best examples you'll ever find of someone with problems of timing and balance. I'm usually either running around at 100 mph or I'm completely off, dead in my tracks, and out like a light, asleep. I'm notorious for the way I do hospital rounds. When medical students follow me, they have to wear sneakers so they can keep up with my sprint. On the other hand, I'm narcoleptic, and although I have this disorder under control now, I used to be capable of falling asleep while walking or riding a bicycle.

The thyroid is one of the body's timers. It helps regulate organ function and keep the body working smoothly and in balance. Very often, therefore, the thyroid is the place where the illness shows up. In that light, it's not surprising that I carry the antibodies for Graves' disease in my body. As I said, I don't like to wait. My friends joke that the only time I have any patience is when I'm working in the hospital as a physician. Otherwise, I can't wait for anything. While it may be an advantage to be a go-getter in some circumstances, there are many, many times and places where patience and a willingness to wait are clearly preferable. There's some truth to the saying that all things come to those who wait. At the very least, we should maintain a balance between pushing forward and waiting. (I confess that I have yet to know how to achieve this.)

When I lived in an apartment, I came home one night to discover that my bathtub drain was completely clogged. Now, somebody else might have noticed it was running a little slowly and might have solved a minor problem before it became major. Not I, though. I'm either on or off, remember? I tend to ignore things and ignore them until suddenly they're so big that I can't ignore them anymore; I wait until every drain in my house is clogged and nothing is moving. In any case, having discovered my drain was clogged, I was immediately impatient to unclog it at once. I went out to the grocery store, and, since I'm not prone to moderation and I wanted to be thorough, I bought three different drain cleaners. The instructions said to pour only a little down the drain and wait for fifteen minutes before flushing, but I ignored them. I didn't want to wait that long. I poured in an entire can of drain cleaner, heated some water in the microwave, and poured it in after. Then I watched as green smoke poured into the air and a green acid precipitate rose up out of the drain and collected on the bottom of the tub. This worried me a little. But the drain was still clogged, so I couldn't flush the stuff away. I decided to close the bathroom door and walk away.

I figured I'd watch *Seinfeld* and think about things for thirty minutes. As soon as the show was over, I quickly poured two more bottles of drain cleaner down the drain. I was worried at this point, but instead of moving slowly through this fear and anxiety, I figured I'd solve matters by speeding up my efforts. You see the problem with pacing and timing? Fear actually tells you to slow down; I was doing just the opposite. I did decide to let the stuff sit for two hours. Now I'd increased the amount to be used by 600 percent and left it in for four times the recommended time. But I figured that large problems require drastic measures, right?

Well, after a while the fumes from the chemicals were so strong they were making my eyes burn as I sat in the other room. I decided it was now or never. I went into the bathroom, turned the hot water on full blast, and kept my fingers crossed. Well, guess what? The drain opened up, all the water started running down, I reached over to turn off the water—and the hot-water faucet broke off in my hand. And the super was away for the weekend. The hot water ran for so long that it emptied the entire boiler and the whole building was without hot water for two days. You can imagine how popular I was.

In one moment, I'd gone from total obstruction to total flooding, from total constipation, metaphorically speaking, to total incontinence. It was a perfect illustration of my inability to regulate the rate and rhythm of activity in my life and in my body. In fact, I later had a very similar experience, having to do with plumbing, in my body. I had a simple operation recently, on an outpatient basis. After surgery of any kind, when you've been under general anesthetic, it's very common for the patient to be constipated for a few days before his bowels begin to work normally again. Quite simply, the plumbing and the drain in my own body were clogged. Being me, however, I couldn't wait for my bowels to assert their own rhythm and get back to work. I wanted to push forward, but I couldn't; I wanted to assert my will over my plumbing and get it flushing out and back to normal immediately. So I asked a doctor friend to give me some medication to help this happen. She handed me a packet of little red pills called Dulcolax. I glanced at the instructions, but being very impatient, I only looked at the first few words (I'd never do this with a patient, but when it comes to myself, I never exercise the same level of care and diligence). All that registered was "Take one." So I took one. I waited twenty minutes. Nothing happened. So I took another one. Waited another twenty minutes. Nothing. Took another one. Waited. Nothing. This went on for several hours. By the time I was finished, I had taken thirteen or fourteen of these little pills. I didn't think there was any harm; they just looked like red hots, the spicy red candies I used to chew on as a child. I figured I had to take a lot of them, because how could one or two little red hots get anything moving?

A couple of hours later my doctor friend dropped by to see how I was doing. When I told her how many of the pills I'd taken, she nearly fainted. "You took *how* many?" she cried. "*One* of those is like a bomb, and you took *thirteen*? You're supposed to take one and wait twelve to twenty-four hours!" Well.

About seven hours later I went to the mall with a friend. I was in the middle of the surplus store when it started. All at once, my bowels were making a low, steady gurgling sound. It was uncanny. It was the same sound my apartment drain had made when it came unclogged. Needless to say, at this point, I *couldn't* wait around. I had to move—and fast!

The drain in the bathroom was a metaphor for the drain in my body. In both cases I exhibited the problems with timing, will, and communication that can set the scene for illness in the fifth emotional center. In both instances I was willful rather than patient; I couldn't wait for the will of an outside force, the drain cleaner or the laxative, to work on me. I refused to listen, in the form of reading and comprehending the instructions on the packages. Most of all, I was off in my timing. I refused to wait for the appropriate moment to take the appropriate action, and insisted instead on pushing forward and ignoring all the warning signals, like green smoke and acid, that were telling me not to do that. As a result, I went from one extreme to the other, from complete constipation to complete incontinence.

This clogged-drain motif is very apt for people who have thyroid disorders. They often have problems with the timing of their bowels as well as the timing of other things. Constipation—the dam—is frequently a symptom of hypothyroidism, or an underactive thyroid gland, while diarrhea—the flood—frequently accompanies hyperthyroidism, or an overactive thyroid.

People with timing problems also lack a good sense of when to push themselves forward in the world. I have a friend whose husband always seems to pick the wrong moment to assert himself or make some request of others. My friend will be heading out the door for an appointment, and he'll come running up with the tax forms, insisting that's the very moment when they must go over them together. He's simply unaware of, or not receptive to, the emotional cues that are being issued in any given situation. Whenever this happens, when there's a disconnect between the emotional signals coming from the heart and the signals coming from the brain, the result can be an imbalance that can set the scene for physical problems in the organs and tissues of the fifth emotional center.

FORGING AHEAD
CERVICAL DISK DISEASE

The Reading. When I spoke with fifty-two-year-old Ellen I perceived that an important change had just occurred in her life. I saw her in a job where she received a lot of cooperation that gave her a good feeling. I saw someone in this job who was very focused and was instrumental in helping Ellen to put herself out in the world. This person acted as Ellen's announcer, a kind of Ed McMahon who introduced Ellen, communicated for her, and paved the way for her to come out and shine in the world. In fact, I saw this person as functioning as a kind of prosthetic will for Ellen. I could see, however, that some important part of Ellen's identity in her work was coming to an end. This was her primary emotional concern, and it was having an effect on her health.

I envisioned Ellen sitting down at a desk and writing a lot of notes. This activity was accompanied by severe neck pain. Indeed, in the vertebrae of her neck, I saw a large number of osteophytes, small bone fragments that can cause acute neck pain.

The Facts. Ellen had worked for many years as the director and administrator of a large social program. Although she was excellent at her job, she found it difficult to push herself forward and promote herself and her work in such a way as to get the attention and notice she deserved. In fact, Ellen told me that most of the time she felt timid, not heard, and almost invisible. She was highly fortunate, however, in that her immediate superior, a magnetic and dynamic woman, appreciated and prized her work. A master communicator, this woman served as Ellen's mentor and strongly promoted Ellen and her work within the organization.

Ellen had been happy at her job, but when her children all finally left home, she suddenly felt a yearning to change directions. She had spent her life raising her children, but now that she was alone, she felt the need to develop her own will and expression in the world. She decided to move out of the administrative arena and into clinical work more directly associated with her program's social concerns. When she made the job switch, however, her former superior was hurt, confused, and perplexed. Ellen hadn't discussed or explained her decision, and the woman didn't understand it. After having served so long as Ellen's voice, she no longer felt needed. She was so deeply wounded that she had stopped speaking to Ellen.

Although Ellen had always done a lot of sitting and writing in her work, she had never had problems with her neck. Soon after the job switch, however, she blew a disk in her neck. She now suffered from chronic neck pain.

Ellen's decision to change jobs, and thereby her identity, and the subsequent health problems she suffered can be seen as a result of timing. With her children gone, Ellen felt the need to express her own will. She then decided to push forward with this need, without taking into account any of the emotional signals that may have come her way as to the wisdom of making this move so precipitously. Rather than waiting, discussing her feelings with her superior, and listening to the woman's ideas and concerns, Ellen pushed ahead on her own. As a result, she all but irrevocably severed one of the closest and most important relationships of her life. She removed herself physically from the one person whose professional support was critical to her, and she also severed the strong emotional relationship that had sustained her and promoted her. She deprived herself of the voice that had spoken for her before she was able to develop and learn to use her own voice.

Ellen also clearly had difficulty communicating and expressing herself. Her timidity and her feeling of not being heard and being invisible indicate that she was deeply vulnerable in matters of both communication and of will. For most of her life she had needed someone else to speak for her, someone else to express and assert her will. She had spent most of her life on the vulnerability side of the fifth emotional center. When she realized she wanted to change this, however, she took a leap all the way over to the power side. Once again she was off-balance. Her intuition and her body knew this and, through the physical symptom of her neck pain, were sending her a signal to look for a more balanced approach to expressing and asserting her will.

WILL

God gave man free will. However you define "will"—as the power to make your own choices and assert yourself through your own actions, or as a strong purpose or a determined desire—will is essential to the makeup of every individual.

Like every gift we're given, however, will has to be used wisely and with a sense of responsibility, or there will be consequences. History is full of characters who thought they could impose their will on the rest of the world and who came to no good end because of it. A truly overpowering will can produce a Hitler or a Stalin, who will wreak havoc. One man imposing his will on millions of others necessarily deprives those others of their own will. Hitler crushed the will of millions of people. As many as he could, he killed; but even those who survived carry the scars of one man's willfulness through their lives.

Interestingly, those scars are often found in the fifth emotional center. A study of survivors of German prison camps found a high number of cases of thyroid toxicosis, a very serious disease in which the thyroid goes into overdrive and produces poisonous levels of thyroid hormone. I can hardly think of a situation where you'd be more obviously incapable of asserting your will and expressing who you are. We don't, of course, know whether such prisoners were getting sufficient amounts of iodine and other nutrients necessary for thyroid health; this could have been a contributing cause to the disease. But many other studies of prisoners, people deprived of the freedom to exercise their will, also indicate a high level of thyroid toxicosis.[1] The literature shows that the thyroid is often affected in situations where individuals feel a lack of control over their lives. Negative life events, as well as prolonged or severe life strain, have been tied to the occurrence of Graves' disease as well as to hyperthyroid developing into thyroid toxicosis.[2]

BATTLE OF WILLS
HYPERTHYROIDISM

The Reading. Irene, age thirty-six, seemed like a person of great determination. I saw that she was very focused in the world and didn't let others divert her from her purpose. However, she was involved with a group of people with whom she wasn't getting along well and from whom she received no cooperation. She no longer felt fulfilled where she was, and she wanted to end her affiliation with these people, but she wasn't being allowed to.

Although she looked big and strong, Irene felt weak to me. Her heart rate was faster than normal, and she had difficulty sleeping. In her neck, I saw a red and inflamed area at the base of the throat, where the thyroid would be.

The Facts. Irene was a sergeant in the U.S. Army. She had fought in Desert Storm, and had been decorated for heroism. She loved the military and her career in it, but recently, she had found herself in conflict with some of the people in her unit. She wanted to transfer out to a different unit, but her commanding officer was opposed to this and wouldn't approve a change.

Irene was experiencing muscle weakness, wasn't sleeping well, and had recently been diagnosed with hyperthyroidism.

Although she was a person of great will, Irene was finding her will thwarted in the place on which it was most focused, her work. Her will was thwarted within her unit, where she found herself in a battle of wills with her equals, as well as within the larger organization, where the will of her superiors was being imposed upon her. She felt trapped and out of control of her life.

Irene, in fact, was feeling vulnerable in all three areas of the fifth emotional center: she felt she had no say and wasn't being listened to, she was being forced to wait, and she was being forced to comply with the will of others. This emotional dilemma was showing its effects in her thyroid, which was part of her intuitive guidance system, telling her she needed to look for a way to cope with or adapt to her situation. Doing what she had probably always done in the past—expressing herself, pushing herself forward, and asserting her will—wasn't going to work in the place she now found herself. Like all of us, Irene needed to find a healthy midpoint between power and vulnerability in the fifth emotional center.

It's important to be true to yourself, to know what you want and to go after it in a fashion that doesn't betray your own soul and your life's path. It's just as important to know that you can't assert your will at the cost of mowing down others. You have to learn when to move forward and when to hold back and wait. Then the world will listen to who you are and allow you to do what you have to do in your own way.

ELEVEN

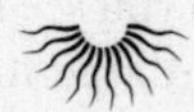

The Brain and Sensory Organs: Perception, Thought, and Morality

More than three centuries ago the French mathematician and philosopher René Descartes expressed what it meant to be human and to be alive. "I think," he said, "therefore I am."

The ability to think defines our very existence. How would we experience the world if we couldn't think about it? The idea's almost unimaginable—you can hardly *think* of it, can you? If we couldn't take what we perceive through our senses—what we see, hear, touch, taste, and smell on the outside—and form associations between that and what we feel and want on the inside, and then turn that into conscious thought and understanding, the world would undoubtedly have little meaning to us.

Perception and thought are at the heart of the sixth emotional center. Located chiefly in the brain, this center is constructed essentially along the lines of the brain's workings. Through the sensory organs of the eyes, ears, and nose, the brain first perceives the outer world, then attaches thought to these perceptions. Finally, we take our thoughts and compare them to our experience in order to form a series of codes of thinking and behavior that constitute our ethics, or morality, which is also seated in this center. How we see the world, then interpret it, and finally judge and act upon it, thus controls the issues that arise here, and helps to determine the degree of health or disease we may experience in the organs of this emotional center (see the accompanying figure).

THE POWER AND THE VULNERABILITY

How do you see the world? Do you see it clearly and insist that it must always be that way, or are you able to tolerate a blurry, ill-defined image and a world full of ambiguity. Are you always focused, or can you sometimes relax and become unfocused? Are you always protecting yourself by being unreceptive to input from others, or can you be receptive when the situation calls for it? Do you trust what you see and sense in the world, or do you tend to be distrustful, even verging on the paranoid? These are all powers and vulnerabilities of perception in the sixth emotional center, as illustrated by the figure.

We need to be able to balance wisdom and knowledge against ignorance, rational and linear thinking against nonrational, nonlinear thought, rigidity and obsessiveness against flexibility, and, in essence, the left hemisphere of the brain against the right hemisphere. What's your power-versus-vulnerability quotient? Do you believe you're usually right about things, or can you acknowledge areas of ignorance in your life? Are you educable and open to learning? Can you allow yourself to have a powerful way in the outer world with left-hemisphere, rational, and linear thought, but still acknowledge vulnerable parts of yourself and your right hemisphere and its nonrational, nonlinear thought style?

A couple of timeworn lines of the sixth emotional center are "I don't want to hear this" and "I'm not listening anymore." Have you ever said these things during an argument or heard the other person say them? Lines like these are a clear-cut warning that the receptors to the brain are shutting down. The outside world is being closed out, and a curtain is falling on perception. People who utter these lines are showing themselves to be out on the power limb of this emotional center, closed to new perceptions and thoughts. They are unreceptive to the opinions of others, sure of their own wisdom and knowledge, and rigid in their thinking. Here are some more lines: "Tell me what you think, not what you feel," and "I don't have enough information to make a decision." The person who makes remarks like that is rational, linear, left-hemisphere, unwilling to take into account the emotions of

Sixth Emotional Center

POWER

Perception
- Clarity
- Focus
- Acuity
- Lack of receptivity

Thought
- Wisdom
- Knowledge
- Rationality
- Linearity
- Rigidity and obsessiveness

Morality
- Conservative
- Law-abiding
- Judgmental
- Critical
- Conscientious
- Repressive

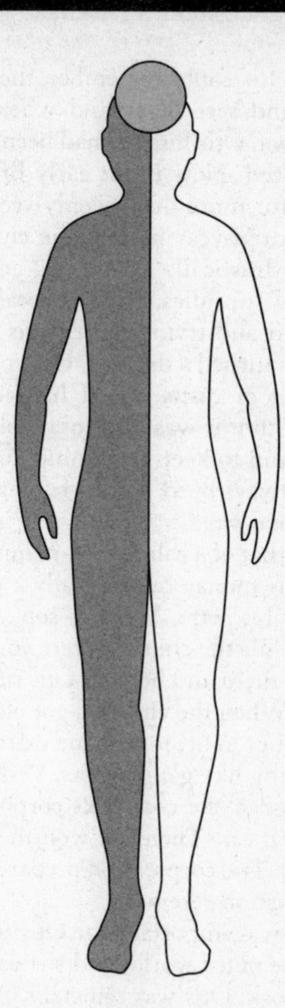

VULNERABILITY

Perception
- Ambiguity
- Lack of focus
- Blindness
- Receptivity

Thought
- Ignorance
- Educability
- Irrationality
- Nonlinearity
- Flexibility

Morality
- Liberal
- Risk-taking
- Guilty
- Available for feedback
- Uninhibited

the right hemisphere and its nonrational perspective. All these traits fit into the power column of the power-vulnerability chart. If they're leavened by a healthy dose of vulnerability in this center, they don't necessarily mean problems. But if the balance tips too far to the power side, a breakdown can occur in the very organs of perception that make knowledge, wisdom, and thought possible.

"I CAN'T HEAR THIS"
MÉNIÈRE'S DISEASE

For longer than Otis could remember, the men of his family had run the thousand-acre dairy and wheat farm the family owned in central Iowa. Otis himself had been raised to take over when his father retired. Now in his early fifties, Otis had been operating the farm for more than twenty years, but for the first time in its one-hundred-year history, the enterprise was struggling. Profits were drastically down, the government had cut back on agricultural subsidies, and the local real estate people were sniffing around and trying to get Otis to sell his valuable land. To all this, Otis turned a deaf ear. He wouldn't hear of shutting down the farm or disposing of his land. The very idea seemed immoral to him. It was his moral obligation to keep the farm in the family and to keep it running, to keep doing things the way they had always been done. He couldn't even think of things being any other way.

Otis's image was that of a calm, mild-mannered man who was a little tight with his money but basically a good provider. His family consisted of his wife, Verla; a son, Otis Junior; and a daughter, Eileen. While the children were young, Verla had concentrated on raising them and helping Otis run the farm by serving as bookkeeper. When the children got older, however, Verla began selling cosmetics to bring in some extra money. Very soon her business was going like gangbusters. Verla found herself flying to state meetings of the cosmetics corporation. She sold so much that she won a car. Then she won the award for highest sales in the Midwest. The corporation prepared to fly her to New York for the presentation ceremony.

Verla thought it was important for Otis to see what she was accomplishing in the outer world, and she asked him to accompany her to New York. Otis was reluctant. At first he had been pleased by Verla's business success, since it helped relieve the financial pressure. At the same time, though, he had no patience for listening to his wife talk about her work. A very rational man, he thought what Verla did was trivial and unimportant. Soon he began to feel a nameless discomfort growing inside him over his wife's success. She had a new car, but he was still driving the same old tractors. He became a bit resentful. At the same time, Otis had a conflict over information he was keeping from Verla. He had withdrawn money from their accounts and taken out a major loan without telling Verla. Now he felt pressure rising inside him, but he didn't share it with his wife because he had been raised to believe that men should handle such matters. He believed he knew best what was good for the farm and the family, and he didn't want to listen to anyone else's opinions. In fact, Otis Junior, who had recently graduated from college with a degree in agricultural business management, had been urging his father to make some changes around the farm to improve profitability. But Otis had refused to listen. He knew he was right, and nobody else could tell him anything.

Despite his misgivings, Otis decided to go to New York with Verla. On the return flight he became ill with dizzy spells so severe that he had to be brought home in a wheelchair. This was highly upsetting to him, since he'd always been a strong and strapping man, and couldn't perceive himself any other way. For a week and a half after he arrived back on the farm, Otis suffered periodic bouts of vomiting and was convinced he had caught some sort of intestinal bug. When the vomiting continued, however, he finally consulted a doctor. After a series of tests, he was diagnosed with Ménière's disease, a disorder in which fluid collects in the inner ear and affects the body's balancing mechanism.

It is very significant that Otis's illness had to do with balance, since he was clearly so out of balance in his sixth emotional center. Otis had always seen the world and his place in it with intense clarity and focus. His perception allowed for no ambiguity in the way life was or might be, but his clarity and focus always related only to his own point of view. He was unreceptive to others' perspectives, and he was rigid in his thinking, convinced that he could keep his farm working only by doing the same old thing. When his son tried to change the farm and the way it did business, Otis became judgmental and critical of him. Otis knew only one way of being: conservative, law-abiding, and conscientious, and determined to keep his feelings to himself. When the family met to urge changes, he would protest. "I can't hear this right now," he'd say. "I'm going to get better. I'm going to go back to running the farm, and things will be the way they were." Eventually, Otis's protests of not wanting to hear things became a self-fulfilling prophecy: the hearing in his left ear started to fail. The left ear, of course, is controlled by the right hemisphere, which, as we know, is the vulnerable part of the brain, associated with nonrational, nonlinear thinking, emotions, and connections to the body. And Otis's hearing loss was intricately intertwined with his psychological and emotional distress with the world and with his need for power in the sixth emotional center. One evening his wife and daughter were discussing the best-selling book *The Rules,* a rather retro manual for women on how to attract and keep a man. Glancing at her father, Eileen asked Verla, "Mom, was Dad your Mr. Right?" "Of course," Verla answered, but from across the room, Otis snapped, "It's not true. I don't always think I'm right." Otis was perceiving the world in distorted fashion as his power in this emotional center diminished.

Ménière's disease was a message from Otis's intuitive guidance system telling him that it was time to move out of the power category of the sixth emotional center and to listen to other people. His intuition had clearly spoken to him. Otis's unhappiness with Verla's success and the pressure he felt because of his bad business decisions had caused feelings to stir in him, suggesting something was wrong and that a change might be warranted. When he ignored his intuition, it decided to speak to him in a way that would get his attention: through physical symptoms. Otis's illness was a clear signal to him that the world was changing and that he had to see, hear, and accept this reality and learn to change with it. To do that, he had to relinquish some power and allow himself to be more vulnerable in the sixth emotional center.

It wasn't surprising that Otis should come down with a disorder of the sensory organs. Many studies have suggested that the eyes, ears, and nose—the organs through which we sense the outer world—are subject to our emotions. In fact, the nose and sinuses share with the stomach the distinction of being one of the body's main emotional targets.[1] A study of people with clogged sinuses—officially known as vasomotor rhinitis—showed that the mucous lining in the sinuses actually shrinks and expands in response to emotions. One part of the nervous system, the sympathetic system, causes the lining to shrink and open up the sinuses. By contrast, stress from the outside causes the other part of the nervous system, the parasympathetic nervous system, to increase the flow of mucus to the sinuses, closing things down and making breathing hard and life generally miserable.[1] Louise Hay hit on the same idea when she said that sinusitis is a physical manifestation of unshed tears, or some sort of emotional irritation.

As for Otis's affliction, numerous studies have noted that a certain personality type may predispose people to Ménière's disease. Otis himself had many characteristics of a type A personality, and type A's, as we know, like to wallow in the power category. Remember the type A's who refused nine out of ten messages that were sent to them by their partners?[2] Otis was certainly right up there as a message refuser. He also had an authoritarian personality and liked to control his partnership and other relationships. He was upset when his wife became more successful than he, and he couldn't deal with his son's management of the farm, especially after he himself fell ill.

Many people who develop Ménière's disease have type A personality traits. They tend to be more obsessive than other people and to have a ruminative thought pattern. This means they think about something over and over and over, chasing their thoughts in a circle, like a gerbil running endlessly in its exercise wheel. Their thoughts also tend to be overly detailed and very left hemisphere in orientation.[3] Other studies have noted that Ménière's disease patients are prone to anxiety, exhibit various phobias, and tend to suffer from depression,[4] all of which affects the extent of the hearing loss the patient suffers. One study put the number of Ménière's patients with major depression at 80 percent.[5] This is significant, because not all people who are ill are also depressed. Ménière's patients, however, are thought to have so-called masked depression, meaning that they hide their feelings and anxieties from the world and present an external appearance of calm and control.[6] Certainly, everyone had always thought Otis was calm and in control. That was his reputation, the calm, in-charge head of the household and good provider.

In fact, however, Ménière's patients have been found to have difficulty with loss of control. They're handicapped by their loss of hearing, which forces them to relinquish a lot of their responsibility. The more handicapped they are, the more responsibility they have to give up, and the more they believe the world is "doing it" to them and they have no control over the outer world.[7] They lose their "internal locus of control," the belief that they can affect things around them. This feeling of being out of control is reproduced physically in the nausea and dizziness they suffer.[8] In addition, Ménière's attacks have been associated with emotional stress and distressing thoughts.[9]

Otis was quite literally feeling his world begin to spin out of control as his farm failed and his wife superseded him in financial success and recognition. Moreover, Verla's accomplishment led to a conflict in their relationship. And conflicts in relationships are also believed to contribute to Ménière's disease.[10]

Otis's story is a perfect illustration of the consequences of an imbalance between power and vulnerability in the sixth emotional center. Marsha reflected a similar problem. She came from a large family with a very authoritarian patriarch and a somewhat meddling matriarch at its head who were overinvolved in their children's lives. Marsha herself had some major problems with rigidity and control. A librarian by profession, she was very rational and linear in her approach to life. As a housekeeper, she was a perfectionist; in her home, everything was in perfect order—every photo and knickknack in its proper place three and a half inches from the edge of the table or mantel, all the sofa pillows fluffed and aligned neatly, not a speck of dust on anything, and the carpets always vacuumed so that all the pile ran in the same direction. Marsha had serious problems with her mother, whom she considered controlling and meddling. She complained that her mother was constantly trying to tell her things she already knew, or knew better, and she considered her mother irrational and uninhibited, whereas Marsha always had her emotions under control—or even repressed—behind a calm, impassive exterior.

Marsha was prone to periodic bouts of tinnitus, or ringing in the ears, which is an element of Ménière's disease. She came into the clinic one day complaining of ringing and pain in her right ear. Earlier in the day her mother had urged Marsha to take a job she had been offered closer to home, listing all the reasons why it would be better for Marsha: it was more in keeping with the sort of work she thought Marsha really wanted to do; it represented a promotion from her current job; it paid more, had better benefits and an easy commute; and it would be closer to the family. Marsha felt she already knew all these things; she didn't need her mother to tell her about them, nor did she want to hear her mother's opinion. She worried that taking the new job would mean a risk, and she was by nature conservative, not a risk-taker. Marsha was trying to individuate from her family of origin and did not want to be closer to home, so her ears blocked out her mother's voice with the sound of ringing.

Marsha, like Otis, wanted to spend all her time on the power side of the sixth emotional center. She didn't like the feeling of vulnerability that came with being open to the other perspectives that come with being flexible and nonrational, with taking risks. When people like Marsha do eventually encounter challenges to their power and get hit in the sixth emotional center, they inevitably find themselves moving against their will to take risks, to be more vulnerable. Their intuition, whether they listen to it or not, signals and guides them toward making a necessary change in their lives. Otis and Marsha needed to find a new way of perceiving and thinking about the world, and they needed to allow other information and beliefs into their lives.

While Otis's and Marsha's problems centered largely on perception and thought, they also flowed over into the final emotional dimension of this center, which has to do with morality. In the sixth emotional center, we harbor our code of right and wrong. Our powerful attitudes include being law-abiding, conscientious, and analytical. More vulnerable attitudes are being willing to break rules, take risks, accept feedback from others, and be uninhibited. While being law-abiding and conscientious can be good, we've probably all known people who were extreme in these characteristics, who became rigid, moralistic, judgmental, critical, and repressed. These are the people you might call Mr. or Ms. Ideal Citizen or Teacher's Pet. Don't those people just drive you crazy?

On the other hand, it's possible to go too far the other way, into the vulnerability side, being excessively uninhibited, taking too many risks, and breaking too many rules. The current craze for political correctness, for example, reflects a rigidity of thinking, an excess of liberalism and guilt, that can become a kind of liberal fascism.

The ability to remain flexible in issues of morality, to balance power and vulnerability in this area of our lives, is vital to health in the organs of the sixth emotional center—the eyes, ears, nose, and brain.

CITIZEN OF THE YEAR
A CASE OF PARKINSON'S DISEASE

The Reading. When Paula, age forty-eight, called me for a reading, I immediately saw her working in a place with massive old stone buildings surrounded by leafy green shrubbery. I sensed that the people who worked there with her tended to be uptight types who had a lot of starch in their shorts. Paula herself felt to me like someone who wore thoroughly starched clothing in which she could never relax. Her idea of throwing caution to the wind consisted of buying weekender pants from L.L. Bean, which she'd wear on foliage-viewing excursions, but only in the first two weeks of October every year. Otherwise, she wore the same silk blouses, same narrow skirts, and navy blue blazers day after day, year in and year out. She'd even worn her hair in the same style for the last twenty years. She never followed fashion or wore makeup, considering both to be signs of self-indulgence. I could see that she was in a good relationship, but basically led a very calm, unexciting life. She came across as very conscientious, but unexpressive. Her face was like a mask.

In Paula's body, I saw rigidity in her left arm and leg, but couldn't tell what it was due to. I saw her having difficulty walking quickly. It didn't feel as if her problem was in her bones, but she had decreased mobility and looked to me like a statue in a wax museum.

The Facts. Paula taught ninth grade civics at an exclusive prep school for boys. Not long ago she had suspected one of the students of smoking a cigarette in the dorms, which was forbidden by school rules. Paula had reported the infraction to the dean's office and insisted that the student be suspended, as was required by the school's by-laws. The boy, however, happened to be the son of a prominent and influential local attorney who was an alumnus of the school and one of its largest donors. When the administration decided to soften the student's punishment and only issue a series of detentions, Paula was incensed. She went head-to-head with the school board, insisting that the proper punishment be meted out. Instead, Paula found herself on the outs with her superiors and was forced to take an unwanted three-month sabbatical.

Paula could be anyone's candidate for the citizen of the year award. She had operated according to a very strict moral code all her life. As a twelve-year-old, she had turned a schoolmate in for smoking in the girl's room during recess. She told me she always received high grades on her report cards for being conscientious and diligent. She was always the teacher's pet. Among her classmates, however, she was known as Stoneface, for never showing any feelings, and she had few friends. Paula had also always put a great emphasis on knowledge. She had been taught by her family that knowledge was power and that one should be a clear, rational thinker, and she had always worked hard to be just that. Although she was successful in her work, Paula had few adult friends aside from one or two teachers at the school. Her husband and daughter were the center of her life.

The issue over the delinquent student was finally resolved, and Paula was allowed to return to teaching. A week later she suddenly had trouble getting up out of her chair, and she had difficulty walking. Her body seemed to balk at the idea of moving. Concerned, Paula consulted a neurologist, who diagnosed her with Parkinson's disease, a degenerative disease of the brain.

Paula epitomized many of the problems that arise from an overemphasis on power in the sixth emotional center, especially those having to do with issues of morality. She would certainly have made a great candidate for citizen of the year, but she had a rigid sense of right and wrong. Convinced that she was right and everyone else was wrong, she refused to be flexible in her views. In all these ways, Paula was almost a poster child for Parkinson's disease. Parkinson's patients have been observed to possess very particular, lifelong personality characteristics: they're overly industrious, overly moral, they're stoic and serious, they emphasize work and productivity, they have stable marriages, they avoid risks and novelty, and they don't, as a rule, drink alcohol or smoke cigarettes.[11] Paula had never touched a drop of alcohol or smoked a cigarette in her life, and clearly she didn't believe anyone else should, either. It's funny, because scientists used to believe that smoking cigarettes had a protective effect against Parkinson's disease. This theory was advanced after research on pairs of twins, in which one had Parkinson's disease and the other didn't. The research showed that the twin who did develop Parkinson's had never smoked.[12] If genetic factors were considered solely responsible for the disease, this seemed to indicate that smoking might have helped prevent the smoking twin from getting the disease. Scientists are smarter about that today. They now believe that it isn't only genes that contribute to developing Parkinson's; they think personality traits might have a lot to do with it as well. So it wasn't that the one twin *didn't* get Parkinson's disease because he smoked. It was that the other twin *did* get it because he may have had the kind of personality that viewed smoking as somewhat immoral. Don't get me wrong. I don't smoke myself and never have, and I basically hate cigarette smoke. But I don't take the moral high road against people who do smoke.

Parkinson's patients also tend to be trustworthy, law-abiding exemplary citizens, whose home and family are at the center of their lives. They're successful at work because they're so diligent, resolute, and thorough. They tend to belong to a lot of organizations and to hold positions of trust and responsibility.[13] But they have few close friends with whom they share real emotional intimacy. All these descriptions fit Paula. She belonged to a number of volunteer boards associated with the school and the community and served on them diligently, but her family and home were the center of her world. While she had a few acquaintances at school and on her boards, she didn't share herself and her intimate emotions with anyone. The only people she had some relationship with were her husband and daughter.

In addition, Parkinson's patients have a lifelong pattern of repressing their impulses and their emotions, especially aggression and anger.[14] They have a lifelong history of "masked personality," hiding their emotions behind an impassive face as Paula did as a girl.[15] This emotional repression predates the onset of the disease itself, but in the illness, it's actually physically manifested by a "masked face"—in other words, the patient's face is blunt and flat, incapable of reflecting emotional expression. At this point, even if these patients tried to emote, they wouldn't be able to. That's because the area of the brain that initiates movement can no longer perform its function. Ironically, when they get ill or experience business problems, Parkinson's patients are actually extremely tense and anxious inside, even close to panic. But the world would never know that, because they control their feelings so well that others see them as calm, poised, and indifferent to the tension. Nor would the world ever know that they're actually complainers who make extreme demands on everyone they come into contact with, because they themselves are so overly conscientious.

What physical and biological mechanism is at work here? Parkinson's patients are very rigid. First they tend to be mentally rigid, and this is also physically expressed in their bodies.[15] Scientists believe the mechanism that causes this is tied to the brain chemical dopamine, which helps us experience pleasure, novelty, risk-taking, and thrills. It's possible that these people are predisposed to have lower levels of dopamine in their brains by heredity, and it's also possible that their lifelong pattern of rigidity and repression actually parallels the low level of dopamine in their brains.[16] If you take a very rigid schizophrenic and pump a load of dopamine into him, he drops his inhibitions and becomes very loose.

Parkinson's people, though, are anything but loose. Novelty and risks made Paula anxious. When her daughter had her ears pierced, Paula nearly had a fit. She furnished her house with the same plain Shaker-style furniture that had belonged to her parents. When she got anxious or fearful, she'd try to control her fear by doing the same things over and over again, obsessively. The effect could well have been to lower her dopamine levels, and then to make her even tighter and more rigid. This is not to say that rigidity causes Parkinson's disease, but it is notable that people with a lifelong history of psychological rigidity and obsessiveness tend to develop Parkinson's, which is characterized by rigidity in the body.[16] The only other type of illness where the person has similar personality characteristics of rigidity is rheumatoid arthritis.[17] The fact is that if you act in certain ways, then the biological machinery in your brain and body that's necessary to act that way is reinforced, and the machinery necessary to act in other ways atrophies. Dopamine helps to initiate movement in the body. If you're the kind of person who doesn't have a lot of initiative to try new movements or activities, then your biological machinery that initiates movement and action and flexibility may slowly disintegrate. This might explain why people with these characteristics have low dopamine levels.[16]

I told Paula it was important for her to try to decrease her overconcern about work and to try to increase her spontaneity by enjoying more recreation. She also needed to increase her emotional expression and try not to overcontrol her anger and aggression, or to mask her personality. Working with a therapist could help her stop repressing her impulses, allow more spontaneity into her life, and learn to be less cautious and overscheduled.

Paula's disease was her body-mind's way of telling her that she needed to learn to bend and be open to more messages and views from the outside world. She needed to allow more vulnerability into her life in the sixth emotional center for better health in her body and more happiness and pleasure in her life.

PERCEPTION AND PARANOIA

Perception can be tricky. After all, each of us sees the world in a different way, based on our unique personality and experiences. How do we know whose perception is more accurate? How can we trust what we're perceiving? Most of us find a way to do this that's in harmony with the context of the world we live in. Some people, however, can be so uncertain and distrustful of their own perception, of the images and messages coming from the outer world, that they distort them and are plunged into paranoia. When you're truly unable to see what's going on around you in the outside world, when your perception is blocked by unreceptivity and your inability to take in feedback from others, so that you can't trust what you're seeing and hearing, your brain begins to make things up about what's happening around you to fill in your vision. This can happen to you in the course of your life's experiences, or you may come into the world predisposed this way. The capacity to see and hear is in the brain's temporal lobe. Many people who have problems in that area are called schizophrenic. They have a developmental problem and come into this world with a predisposition to distrust what they see and hear. Paranoia is an extreme, and clinical, excess of power of the sixth emotional center. It's such extreme unreceptivity that it becomes pathological. Such a strong imbalance of the emotions can open the door to serious illness in the organs of this center.

Opening and Closing the Door to Reality
Paranoia

I was called in to consult on the case of Eunice, a fifty-two-year-old woman who'd been brought in to the hospital in a state of agitation, showing signs of psychosis and paranoia. When I went in to see her, I found that Eunice had clearly had a partial brain seizure, which was making part of her body, specifically the area of her face around the mouth and cheeks, twitch incessantly. As I examined her, she kept getting in and out of bed or toying with a slipper, putting it on and off her foot. When I questioned her, she made no sense. "Why are you here?" I asked. She replied, "It's Monday." When I asked again why she was in the hospital, she said it was Tuesday. She obviously thought I was trying to orient her, which is what psychiatrists called in for a consultation often do. This showed a high level of intelligence on Eunice's part, but far more striking was the fact that Eunice clearly was unable to take in any information. She could make no sense of anything she heard or saw. She couldn't understand any speech or language at all. She could make an educated guess at what I was saying, but she really had no idea what was going on. When I tested her specifically for language areas in the temporal lobe, she couldn't respond. The temporal lobe is essential to our ability to understand sight and sound. It forms memories and attaches emotions and feelings to them, including feelings of whether we can or cannot trust others. People who have seizures in this area have problems with memory and with trust. They hear things when nothing's going on outside them and see things that no one else can see.

I diagnosed Eunice with probable Wernicke's aphasia, which is an inability to comprehend verbal language. (The Wernicke's area is a small area of the temporal lobe that's related to the ability to understand language.)

Eunice, it turned out, had a history of paranoid schizophrenia. She was highly intelligent, a graduate of Stanford with a degree in biology. Since her college days, however, she had suffered from paranoia that had increased over time. She had married a fellow Stanford graduate, and they had lived for a time in California but then suddenly decided to pull up roots and move across the country to New England because Eunice couldn't trust the people they knew anymore. Suddenly her friends weren't her friends, she told me later. When her daughter was seven years old, Eunice was admitted to a mental health center, where she stayed for a month and was diagnosed with schizophrenia. Released, she appeared improved and continued to percolate through life, running a successful antiques business. Eunice's high intelligence helped her cover up her problem. Unlike a classic paranoid schizophrenic, she did have friends and was able to have a fairly normal life.

Then she went away on a buying trip to an antiques show in another state, and when she returned, she was changed. She wouldn't talk to her husband, refused to see her friends, and shut herself up in the house. The day she was brought to the hospital, a neighbor had approached Eunice after she had stood in her front yard for an hour methodically and ceaselessly opening and closing the door to mailbox and staring into space. It was as if she were opening and closing the door to reality.

In the hospital, Eunice was discovered to have a cancerous tumor in her breast that had metastasized, astonishingly, *to the Wernicke's area* of the left temporal lobe of her brain. The woman with the lifelong problem of paranoia, of not trusting or accepting what her senses perceived, now had a tumor in the very area of the brain that has to do with taking in what you hear.

All her life, Eunice's soul had told her that she had a problem with trusting and taking in everything she saw and heard. Yet Eunice had never quite learned to deal with or accept that. Instead, she had used her power of intelligence and knowledge to mask it from herself and from others. Now, though, her intuition was giving her a last chance to change. It wasn't even using a hammer anymore; it was using a Mack truck. It was speaking through the organs of her sixth emotional center, through the temporal lobe of the brain, to tell her that her life needed to be adjusted.

When I went in to see Eunice a second time, she'd been given some drugs that had shrunk the tumor in the Wernicke's area. She was competent, lucid, and able to talk normally. When I asked her if she could tell me what was wrong with her, she explained that she had a tumor in her breast that had spread to her brain and that if she didn't have it removed, she could die. Then she said something that nearly knocked me out of my chair. She began to cry. She looked at me and said, "You know, all my life, I haven't been able to trust anyone or trust anything I heard or saw. I don't know why that is, but it's so. And now people are telling me all kinds of things about what I should do for my health, and I can't get help from them because I don't trust anybody. But I trust you. What should I do?"

I was amazed, but Eunice's words gave me hope. A person with her lifelong problem with paranoia shouldn't have been able to trust anybody and should have been deeply incompetent. But here she was, opening up to me and trusting me with a problem she'd tried to hide from everybody for so long. She knew she had to make a decision about her health and her life. And she was opening up to her vulnerable side, allowing herself to get in touch with more of her vulnerability of being able to take in from the outside and from others.

Eunice's soul, through her intuition network, had attracted her attention to her problem by speaking through a physical symptom that was right smack in the place—and Wernicke's is not a very large area—that had to do with her ability to take in words from other people. Her words to me were an uncannily clear example of intuition speaking through the body's language. Eunice was being challenged to learn the lesson of her potentially mortal disease, the lesson of "Can I trust what I see and hear?" Now her fate was in other people's hands and in her ability to trust those people, to listen to them and hear them, to open up the vulnerable aspects of her sixth emotional center.

While Eunice's case didn't reflect this, people with paranoia and schizophrenia—with distorted perception—are also highly intuitive. Their problems are in the temporal lobe, which aids us in perceiving and understanding what we see and hear, and which also plays a role in intuition. When people can't see well in the outer world, they often have stronger psychic and intuitive talents in their inner world. Some of their delusions, the things they make up, may actually come from some remnants of truth to which they're able to gain access through intuition.

This came home to me very eerily in a recent incident. I have a schizophrenic patient with extreme delusions who believes that she's the illegitimate daughter of Zsa Zsa Gabor and Donald Trump, that she was given up for adoption because she had a serious disease, and that many of her major body organs were consequently removed. She believes that her heart is a clock and her liver's a metal box, that she has a metal shoulder like the Bionic Woman, and that surgery was performed on her in such a way that no X-ray could detect it, and no scars were left on her body. She's been telling me this same story for years. Then one day recently it suddenly changed. The patient came in with a totally new complaint. She'd had nose surgery, she claimed, and she was in pain. I was dumbfounded. I'd recently had some surgery on my own nose to repair an old break. But this patient couldn't possibly have known that, because I'd been careful to keep it private. I'd scheduled my appointments so that no one would even be aware that I was gone for the surgery and recovery period. I hadn't returned to work until my bruises had cleared. No one had an inkling I'd had any surgery. And yet suddenly here came this woman who was otherwise full of delusions but who had zeroed in on the very operation I had undergone.

While this patient had a problem with the thought receivers in her brain and their ability to make sense of the information she received from the outside world, she apparently had the ability to take in information in other ways. This story shows how close the connections are between intuition and the sixth emotional center, the organs of perception.

But the story tells us more than that. It underlines the truth that intuition is simply another form of perception. If we can learn to tap into it, take it in, and understand it, we can use it to help make positive changes in our lives that will affect the health of not only the organs of the sixth emotional center but our entire bodies.

TWELVE

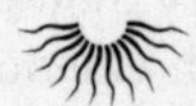

The Muscles, Connective Tissues, and Genes: A Purpose in Life

Why am I here?

This is the plaintive, fundamental question voiced by men and women since the beginning of time. What is our purpose for being? Why do we live? We want to know not only the collective purpose of the human race on earth but also the meaning and reason for each individual life, the purpose for which you and I and the man next door and the woman down the street exist. All of us, as we go through life, need a sense of our own life's purpose. The failure to connect with our purpose affects us profoundly in the seventh emotional center.

When I was a premed student at Brown University, I had a life-changing experience that brought this home to me vividly. This experience showed me that critical disease is a message we need to receive so that we can reevaluate some aspect of our lives and, most probably, change it. This is the message not only of the seventh emotional center but of this entire book.

As a premed student I was always on the run, living my life on fast forward and always focusing, like a horse with blinders, on the future that stretched before me. This was, in fact, pretty much the way I'd lived all my life. I was always studying and planning for the next stage of my life, always "pre" something. In grade school, I was pre–high school, planning my future as a physician and scientist and concentrating hard on earning good grades so I'd get into the honor classes in high school. In high school I was pre-university, focused on a level of achievement that would guarantee me entry into an Ivy League school, which in turn would ensure my entrance into medical school. I never lived in the now, in the present, in the moment. It was always tomorrow, tomorrow, I love you, tomorrow, like the song.

Then, during my junior year, my sleep problem escalated alarmingly. One day I was standing in line at the Ratty, the campus cafeteria. The next thing I knew, I was waking up to the sound of breaking glass. Looking around and hastily piecing the situation together in my mind, I realized that I had nodded off and dropped an entire tray. Food and broken glass covered the floor. A crowd of people stood around me, staring. I was shaken. This time I'd had absolutely no warning that I was falling asleep. After that, at the insistence of my friends, I took a bus to Boston for a medical evaluation. A physician examined me and then scheduled me to come back in a week for admission to the hospital for a battery of tests. As he booked the admission with his secretary, she asked him to put down an admission diagnosis. He glanced at me quickly, then said in a low voice, "Hypothalamic tumor."

At the sound of the word "tumor," I went into shock. I couldn't believe that I might actually have a brain tumor, for the hypothalamus, as I knew all too well, is in the brain. All at once, I was staring straight in the face of a possibility I'd never even considered before: the possibility of my own death.

Riding back to campus on the bus, I was full of anxiety and fear. But I also reached a decision about my life. It was as though a curtain had been drawn aside to reveal the world to me as it really was, and I knew what I had to do. No longer was I going to concentrate on the future, because the future was no longer certain. Instead, I was going to live in the present. I was going to savor every moment of every day, because every moment was precious and irretrievable. When I got off the bus and walked out onto the campus, suddenly everything looked different to me. I know what I'm going to say will sound a little corny, but it really happened. As if for the first time, I noticed the dazzling blueness of the sky, the shimmering green of the grass and leaves, and the splendor of the light that suffused everything around me. As I stood there, I could feel the life in everything—the trees, the grass, the wind, the sun—and I felt the oneness of the universe, how everything in the world was a part of me and I a part of everything. Waves of emotion and intensity swept over me. My facade, the shell we all wear as we navigate through the world, had fallen away, and I stood exposed to all the raw, throbbing reality of life around me and to all the knowledge available to me from the universe or the heavens or wherever it is that we believe it comes from.

I realized that my intuition network was turned on full blast. I was like any other person who'd been given notice of his or her mortality. All at once I knew many things, some of them quite paradoxical. I knew that there was a force in the universe—call it God or give it another name—that made things happen in my life in a way I couldn't control, but that I was simultaneously endowed with the power to influence what happened to me. I knew that my life contained an infinite variety of possibilities, but that there were limitations in the world that I would have to live with, too. I knew that I couldn't become overly attached to one certain identity, or it might be taken away from me. And I knew that I had to live more for the moment and, above all, to get in touch with my life's purpose to anchor me to the world and the life I loved and the universe that I now sensed as being of a whole, with all things in it part of each other and of me.

All of these issues are encompassed in the seventh emotional center. This is where we experience and express our oneness with God or the divine: God and I are one. The equation is simple: you have to have a sense of purpose in life, and you have to understand the locus of control, the degree to which you can control life and the degree to which its control is out of your hands. The seventh emotional center also deals with attachment and detachment, and with the question of our facades, the outer skin that separates us from the world and sometimes protects us from exposure to the blasts of life. Ultimately, the seventh emotional center deals with coming to a point in your life where your life might end. And because everyone eventually gets to that point, one way or another, everyone eventually—or suddenly—gets in touch with this emotional center.

The illnesses affecting this emotional center are multisystem disorders and disorders of the muscles, connective tissues, and genes. It's important to know, however, that any life-threatening illness and the end stage of any terminal illness can get you in touch very quickly with your seventh emotional center and the need to connect with a sense of your purpose in life and your reason for having lived (see the figure on page 294).

The Power and the Vulnerability

"I just don't know what to do with my life."

Have you ever heard yourself say that? Many people have felt this way at some stage in their lives, meaning that they have no clear sense of their reason for being, and aren't sure what to make of their lives or what life's path to pursue. They're consequently very vulnerable in the aspect of the seventh emotional center having to do with life's purpose. Power in this category of the seventh emotional center consists in defining or having defined a purpose and a clear sense of your path in life. Health in this emotional center requires that you balance the two: maintain a clear sense of purpose, but accept the uncertainty of some elements of your purpose and resign yourself to not knowing all the details of what will happen to you in life or how it will come about.

An overattachment to one particular path or identity can backfire on you. The universe is very quirky and seems to love irony. When people focus their entire lives and worlds on one skill, one identity, one way of being, or even one person, to such an extent that they exclude other dimensions of their personalities, the universe likes to play its little tricks: it may take away the very thing to which you have become attached in order to force you to develop other elements of your personality. When I was in my twenties, I used to run a lot. At first I ran to control my weight, but over time I became extremely attached to my identity as a runner and went on to run races and marathons. One day I said out loud, "As long as I can run for the rest of my life, I know I'll always be able to stay thin and happy." Not long after, I was hit by a truck while jogging and eventually had to quit running completely. It's important, in the seventh emotional center, to find a balance between attachment to some identity or calling and a certain necessary detachment to prevent setting the stage for illness here.

The seventh emotional center is also concerned with locus of control and creation. This has to do with who you think creates and controls your life. The power here is the belief that you have an *internal* locus of control. In other words, you create your life, you influence the events in your life. Your pilot is earthbound. The vulnerability is the sense that there's an *external* locus of control that directs your life and that you yourself have little or no influence over events in it. Your pilot is universe-bound—either God or the heavens or some other power. People who believe this tend to say things like "My life is doomed" or "It's out of my hands." Some think that either the heavens and the

Seventh Emotional Center

POWER

- **A clear sense of purpose in life**
- **A conviction that I create my life**
- **A belief that I can influence events in my life**
- **The capacity for attachment in my life**

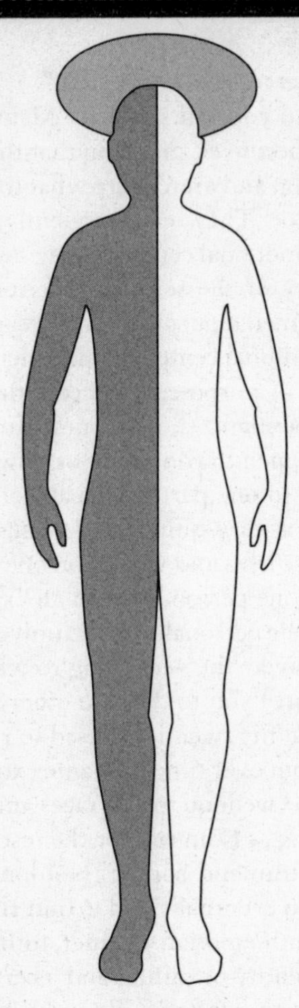

VULNERABILITY

- **An undefined purpose in life**
- **A conviction that the heavens direct my life**
- **A belief that things happen the way they should**
- **The capacity for detachment in my life**

world are doing it to them, or they're in charge of their life and no one else has input. This isn't the case. You can achieve a balance in this area by understanding a seeming paradox: that while the universe is in charge and events happen as they should, you are simultaneously in control and have input into charting your life's path.

Another paradox of this center consists of believing in unlimited or infinite possibilities while at the same time understanding that sometimes there are limitations on the directions in which you may go. I myself don't like limitations. When somebody says to me, "You can't do that," it's like putting gas on a match. I become determined to do whatever's necessary to make what I want happen. But as we grow older and go on in the world, we have to understand that we must accept some limitations. There are certainly momentary limitations. I've come to appreciate and work my way through these by saying, "This too shall pass." But there may be permanent limitations as well, decided by the will of the heavens, and you have to be open to that possibility.

Finding the right balance in all these areas can help to maintain our good health in the seventh emotional center. But if we tip the scales in one direction or the other, we can set the stage for illness and disease.

MY LIFE AS AN INVALID: I DESERVE TOTAL CARE
GUILLAIN-BARRÉ SYNDROME

Shirley was a sixty-year-old patient with Guillain-Barré disease whose husband, Fred, called the clinic one day with an unusual complaint. "My wife can walk again," he told me over the phone. I was stumped. "This is a problem?" I inquired. "She's getting better, she's healing, and you have a problem with this?" Fred brought her in for an evaluation. He told me his wife had contracted some virus when she was sixteen and had been paralyzed in the legs. She had been able to walk with crutches for a time. But three years after she had married Fred, she had taken to a wheelchair and had been in one ever since. She depended on her husband for total care.

Recently Shirley had begun to have trouble sleeping at night and had started taking Benadryl to help her sleep. Then one day she suddenly hoisted herself out of her wheelchair and walked into the kitchen, where she started cleaning. But she was clearly confused. She put her shoes in the oven and the phone in the freezer. That's when Fred called me.

Shirley was in a very early stage of dementia. She was also taking too much Benadryl, which was causing her confusion. But I was very excited by the fact that she had regained her ability to walk. I told her to stop the Benadryl and come back in two weeks. But when she returned, Shirley was back in the wheelchair, and Fred reported that she wasn't walking anymore. Shirley, meanwhile, was upset that she wasn't sleeping at night again, and demanded medicine to help her sleep. "But aren't you excited that you can walk again?" I asked. "Don't you want me to get you some physical therapy to help you get more func-

> tional?" Shirley looked at me for a moment. Then she said something amazing. "I can't walk," she said. "I'm an invalid, I need a wheelchair, and I deserve twenty-four-hour care." I couldn't believe it. I asked her again if I could help her become more functional and independent. But she only repeated, "I'm an invalid, I can't walk, and I need twenty-four-hour care." When I pressed her again, she said it again. I gave her a prescription and sent her home.

Shirley had a number of problems of the seventh emotional center. She was a woman without any purpose in life—unless you count being an invalid, and that doesn't count. In addition, she was a woman who not only accepted her limitations but defended them. She was an invalid, by God, and she was going to stay an invalid, and that was that. She was like the rats I described earlier in this book, who were given the chance to leave the box they'd always lived in, but chose not to. Even though they'd been shocked their whole lives in that box, they decided to stay put, because that was what they knew and felt comfortable with. They had accepted their limitations and could conceive of no other possibilities. Shirley had the opportunity to change her box, but she was too attached to it. Her case was almost a little cosmic joke. Through her dementia and subsequent confusion, the universe was trying to break down her attachment to her identity as an invalid and give her a measure of health. Yet Shirley chose illness as her life's path, and she chose it in the belief that she had no control over her own life and in fact needed complete care from the outside. Now she was becoming demented; a curtain was falling between her and the world, thickening the facade between her and the rest of life. Her intuition was speaking loud and clear of the need for change in her life and the need to get in touch with her life's purpose and to find a better balance between power and vulnerability in the seventh emotional center. Shirley preferred to cower in the vulnerability of her invalidism and the belief that she had no control over her life. Her case sadly illustrates the point that while our intuition may speak to us and urge us to take a different course, it can be effective only if we open ourselves to it and listen and heed the messages it brings.

The follow-up to Shirley's case is interesting. A month later her husband, Fred, contacted me. Fred told me that hearing his wife insist that she was an invalid had been a pivotal moment in his life. It had become clear to him then that he had a choice in how he could live his own life. On one hand, his life's purpose could be that of a primary caregiver for his wife, who insisted on being a total invalid, both physically and emotionally. On the other, he could choose to live in a way that more fully expressed his own potential. Fred decided that he could satisfy his wife's need for receiving total care by placing her responsibly in a good nursing home, and then he could pursue his own life goals. The last time I spoke with him, he said, "My life now has just begun."

A PURPOSE IN LIFE

When we think of people who really know what their purpose in life is, artists and poets may be among the first who come to mind. Some poets spend their whole lives exploring the meanings of life and our place in the universe. I personally learned a lot about the importance of having a sense of your life's purpose from the poet May Sarton.

After my diagnosis of a sleep disorder, and after the initial flurry of concern from friends and acquaintances passed, I found myself all alone in my struggle with my health. During the day I'd try to escape from it by keeping busy and active. But at night, I had to keep moving, because I dreaded falling asleep. As long as I was on the move, I'd stay awake, but I feared that the minute I stopped, I'd black out. So at night, after doing research in Boston (I'd taken a leave of absence from Brown), I'd ride around the city on the subway. Eventually, though, I'd have to go home to my studio apartment, close the door, and be alone with my problem. And this was very, very hard.

In the course of my efforts to start reading again, I found a book at the library called *Journal of a Solitude,* by May Sarton. Locked in my own solitude, I thought it might have something to say to me. It did. Sarton, a well-known poet, described her own struggles with living a solitary life. But she also wrote a lot about the search for creativity and how developing it had to do with going after your purpose and being in touch with the muse, the creative force in the world. Throughout *Journal of a Solitude,* Sarton writes about repeatedly waking up in the morning and being unable to write and feeling blue about that. But then she would glance at a vase of flowers on the table, and the simple sight of a shaft of light striking a rose petal in a certain way would suddenly put her in touch with the muse, and the poetry would pour out of her. I too was continuously looking for the light and joy in life in very simple circumstances, the light that would wake me up and make me feel more alive despite my sleeping disorder. I was so inspired by the book that I wrote Sarton a letter, telling her how much her book meant to me and how it had helped me find peace in the midst of my difficulties. I wrote that my illness had become a sort of muse to me, like the light on her rose petal. It had put me in touch with the importance of having a sense of purpose. It had made life seem different to me, more immediate, and made everything around me seem more alive. I said that it had put me in touch with the same sort of feeling you get when you create something. When you discover something in a lab, you feel as if you have touched the hand of God and had the electricity of life surge through you. Through my illness, I had learned how to touch life the way she, the poet, touched life, and then poured it forth in her writing, fulfilling her purpose in life.

Sarton wrote back and then called to thank me for the letter. Eventually I visited her at her home in Maine, where we talked more about these essential questions of life and its meaning. At one point she rose from the couch where she had been sitting and walked over to a bookshelf filled with beautiful leather-bound books. She gestured at the shelf with a sweep of her arm. "You know, Mona Lisa," she said, "whenever I feel that my own life is worthless, I just look at all these books I've written, and I know I've contributed something to the world." Our friendship continued for a decade and a half, until her death. It has always stood out for me as one of the most meaningful of my life. And it has always been tied in my mind to that significant time in my life when my intuition, through illness, opened my eyes to the truths of the seventh emotional center.

Having a purpose in life is central to health and well-being in everyone. What your purpose is depends on you. For some people, having children or dedicating themselves to others may be their life's purpose. For others, it may be work or career, a specific profession or art. Only you can know what your true life's purpose is. And you must be true to that purpose. Choosing some other path because it's what others want of you, or because it's convenient, doesn't really work. Its effects will show up in the organs of the seventh emotional center, or possibly in some life-threatening or critical illness.

On the other hand, you may pursue a path that you believe is your life's purpose, only to have the universe signal you, through your intuition, that this isn't the right path for you. Or a purpose you pursued for some period of your life may come to an end, and you'll need to find a new purpose. You have to be willing to detach yourself from an identity or a purpose if this happens. Being somewhat deaf to my body's intuition, I learned these lessons the hard way, through major illness, at the time when I wanted to continue pursuing neurology and kept blowing disks in my spine. My intuition was telling me that the universe didn't want me to go in that direction, and I kept ignoring it, because this was what I had always wanted to do and what I was convinced was my life's purpose and my identity. After I'd blown four disks I had to change my course.

It's not good or healthy to be attached to a purpose by your will (fifth emotional center) and your intellect (sixth emotional center) to such a degree that you create an overabundance in the power category. It's like standing on the railroad tracks saying, "I will stop this train, or the train will not come!" The only thing that will happen is that you'll get mowed down. The momentum of the seventh emotional center is such that it can impound every vehicle in all your other emotional centers. It doesn't matter if you have a whole committee of family members (support in your first emotional center) saying, "You will become a neurologist"; and a partner (support in your second emotional center) saying, "I will help you become a neurologist"; and professors who give you A's for your skills (third emotional center) in all your Ph.D. courses and say, "You will be a neurologist." And it doesn't matter if you have a passion in your heart for this (fourth emotional center), if you communicate this well to the outer world (fifth emotional center), and if your intellect tells you you can make it work (sixth emotional center). If it's not meant to be in the seventh emotional center, you must get a new purpose and start a new life.

The Stand-by-Your-Man Syndrome
Lou Gehrig's Disease

The Reading. When Irma, age seventy, called me for a reading, I immediately saw a woman who had no real reason to live. I couldn't see what kept her in her body, why she was here on planet earth. I saw that up to this point her whole reason for living had been a man. I saw a man who was her John Wayne on the noble horse. I saw that Irma had a supportive group of people, her family, all there for her, but they weren't a reason why she would want to stay here. The only member of the family who could have provided that reason was no longer with her, and that was it for Irma. I saw that it was very painful for other members of her family to see this. They would try to connect with her, to make her see that she was important to them and they were important to her, but their efforts did no good. It was almost as though Irma could hardly even see what they did, because she could only focus on this person who was no longer in her life.

When I looked at her body, I saw that her head tilted to the left. I saw her sitting down, and having a hard time getting up. Her body seemed constricted. I saw her as having rigidity and decreased motion in her extremities. Her right foot was in a clawlike position, turned inward and spastic. It didn't move. I couldn't understand what was wrong with Irma. I did know that she wasn't moving ahead in her life, and that her leg was literally cemented in that direction, never to move again.

The Facts. Irma had stayed home most of her life and raised her children. You could say that her children were her life, except that this wasn't quite accurate. Although she cared for all her children, her life really revolved around her eldest child, her only son. Along with Irma's husband, this son was the focus of Irma's existence and her reason for being. Irma lived, in short, for the men in her life. She bragged about her son and her husband to all her friends. When her son became a neurosurgeon, she nearly burst with pride.

Then Irma's husband died and her son accepted a job across the country at a prestigious university. Irma was devastated. In one sweep, both of the men in her life had left her. Irma's two daughters tried to make up for the losses to her. But Irma treated their efforts like the junk mail that you never really look at but just toss on the piles on the kitchen table. She wanted the real mail (and male). She wanted the letter you tear open before you even go back into the house, the one with the emotional charge in it. The daughters, in turn, felt devastated.

One day, Irma took a fall, and from then on she had trouble walking. She took to a wheelchair, and went from neurologist to neurologist seeking help. She was finally diagnosed with amyotrophic lateral sclerosis (ALS), a degenerative neuromuscular disease more commonly known as Lou Gehrig's disease.

Irma's problem was that she had lost her purpose in life, and she refused to find a new one to replace it. Her only previous purpose for living had been her men; she had existed for and through them. She was the original stand-by-your-man woman, and when she no longer had a man, she quite literally couldn't stand. Her case was very simple, as most cases are in this emotional center. If you try to make them complicated and go looking for more information, you start drifting down into the sixth emotional center, where you ruminate, think, and intellectualize.

Irma's lack of purpose in life meant that her level of psychological health was low. She was very much in the vulnerability column of the seventh emotional center, convinced that there was nothing she could do to change her life. Once her son left her, Irma began disconnecting from life. ALS is a disease, like multiple sclerosis, that can have a very variable course. Some people can live with it for years, while others die quickly. Studies of patients with ALS have shown that those with a low level of psychological health, an external locus of control, and a lack of a well-defined purpose in life have a greater risk of dying sooner than patients whose psychological health is good. In fact, those without a purpose lived an average of not quite one year after being diagnosed with ALS. By contrast, patients with an internal locus of control, who were less hopeless and less depressed, lived an average of nearly four years after diagnosis.[1]

This is an important finding for our victimization-crazed country, where most of us spend most of our time in the vulnerability category, believing that some unknown "they" are "doing it" to us and running our lives (external locus of control). Like the high-risk patients in this study, we believe that the rewards we receive in life have nothing to do with our actions but are controlled by fate, luck, and powerful others. Yet studies like this one suggest that if you try to acquire a better defined purpose in your life and if you perceive that you have more control over what's happening to you, you might improve your health and increase your survival time. In other words, if Irma had listened to the message her intuition was sending her—the message of necessary change, of a need to redefine her purpose—she stood a chance of changing the course of her illness to some degree. Another way of looking at it: Since so little mail was coming to her now, she needed to reexamine her perception of what she did have in her life, what she had so far always seen as junk mail. There were so many things she could still do, not the least being reconnecting with her daughters and finding meaning in the other relationships in her life.

Losing someone important to you in your life has long been recognized as a major factor in predisposing people to certain neurological diseases, including multiple sclerosis (MS), another disease of the seventh emotional center.[2] In a famous case in 1822, a young man named Augustus d'Este, the illegitimate son of the Duke of Sussex, was adopted by a surrogate father of sorts, who took the boy under his wing, gave him an identity and a reason for living, and raised him like his own son. This surrogate father died when Augustus was a young man. Immediately after attending his funeral, Augustus came down with multiple sclerosis.[3]

Many authorities have described similar cases in which the death or loss of a significant person causes the bereaved person to reassess and reevaluate his or her direction or purpose in life.[4] One woman found her beloved husband in bed with another woman and came down with MS the very next day.[5] Another woman got MS at age thirty-five after her husband died and her son was killed by a car,[6] leaving her bereft and searching for a reason for living. Still another woman developed MS at thirty-two after being notified that both her parents and her brother had died. In yet another case, a thirty-eight-year-old woman came down with MS after learning that she was sterile. Recently married, she had dreamed of having children all her life; it had been, she thought, her life's purpose.

All these people found that they weren't able to cope in a situation where they were suddenly responsible for creating their own lives. Persons or objects that had given their lives meaning and structure were suddenly removed, and they were forced to reevaluate and redetermine their purpose in life. When they couldn't do that, they succumbed to MS.[6] In fact, people with MS have been described as having a "giving up, giving in complex."[6] When they face emotional difficulties or an emotional shock, they give up. They disconnect from their reason for living and aren't able to move forward at all. Their ability to see their purpose in life is obliterated.[5] That's what happened with the woman in the following story.

THROWING IN THE TOWEL
MULTIPLE SCLEROSIS

The Reading. I saw Jane as a thirty-year-old woman who was clearly working at something that wasn't her heart's desire and that had no connection with her real purpose in life. In the work, she could not use her intellect and skills and was completely unrewarded. Jane was like someone treading water endlessly in the deep end of the pool, never getting into the race. In fact, she was treading water while waiting for someone else to complete his race. She was waiting for her turn. It was almost as though she and this other person were in a relay race, but he was doing his laps now, and she couldn't move until he had finished. But I could see that Jane was slowly getting very tired treading water.

In Jane's head, I saw white bits, like Q-Tips or little fuzz balls in her brain.

The Facts. Jane had always wanted to be a lawyer and had long planned to go to law school. As it happened, however, her husband had the same dream. In order to finance his studies, Jane had delayed her own plans and gone to work as a nanny. Her husband completed his course, and she prepared to apply to law school. But then her husband made a surprise announcement: he wanted to go on and get a Ph.D. in law in addition to his LL.D.

Once again Jane put her plans on hold. Soon she began to drop things at work. Her speech became garbled. Jane was diagnosed with multiple sclerosis.

Jane was unfulfilled and unhappy and wasn't living according to her purpose in life. She wouldn't consciously concede this, but her body, through intuition, was weighing in with the truth. When Jane agreed to let her husband continue his studies and postpone her own, she was giving in to someone else's desire to pursue his life purpose. That meant, however, that she wasn't pursuing her own. Jane might have been better off telling her husband that enough was enough, and it was her turn to do what she wanted to do. But Jane seemed to think she didn't have any control over what happened in her life. She was ruled by powerful others and had limited possibilities. She couldn't take responsibility for creating her own life.

The onset of MS was her intuition giving her another chance to get the message and assert her own purpose. Sad to say, however, Jane did the exact opposite. After discussing her diagnosis with her family, she decided not to hurry up and pursue her life's purpose with a vengeance but to give in to the wishes of others and *have a baby*. This, she thought, was all she could do for her family before her body succumbed to MS.

Jane not only gave in, she gave up. She thought, I have MS, I'm going to die anyway, I may as well give the world a child before I go. But this wasn't her true life's purpose, and it made for a poor prognosis. Studies have shown that people with a very malignant course of MS who become thoroughly disabled by the disease generally feel that they have little control over their lives.[7] They have an external locus of control and believe they have no say about what happens to them. It's not that they believe things are happening as they should or as the universe directs but rather that they're being victimized by forces beyond their control.

Like those people, Jane was living too extensively in the vulnerability category of the seventh emotional center. She was allowing herself to live too much with an undefined sense of purpose and felt there was little she could do to change her situation. When she felt victimized by the universe, she tried to change her purpose. But because she wasn't being true to herself, she was only making her situation worse. A move toward her true purpose, and toward a sense that she *could* influence events in her life would mean a move toward a better balance in this emotional center and thus a possible chance at better health.

MAINTAINING THE FACADE

When I told you about my brush with death at Brown, I said that the feeling I had was that of my facade falling away, so that nothing stood between me and the world around me and I could sense my complete oneness with the universe and all its beings. This, in fact, is a very common experience for people who've come close to death, whether through illness or accident or some other life-threatening event. They immediately get in touch with their seventh emotional center. They suddenly see life in a completely different way. They experience what's known as *primary intensity,* which means that they feel life in a particularly immediate and intense fashion. They feel things, hear things, and see things with great clarity. Nothing separates them from the raw energy of life around them. No veil obscures the harsh realities of human existence or cloaks the full exhilaration of passion and creativity. These people have no more facade.

As most of us go about the day-to-day business of living, our facade protects us from the more difficult, less pleasant aspects of the world and the human beings we share it with, such as all the constant, sometimes necessary hypocrisy that permeates human dealings. In fact, people who lose their facades find this very difficult to bear; they can't listen to others tell even little white lies, watch the games they play, or observe their manipulations and machinations without having a strong negative reaction. While this sort of greater honesty might seem like a good thing, it can actually make life in some ways more difficult and painful, because it sets you apart and can make you seem irritable and antagonistic.

Another consequence of not having a facade is that it also opens you up almost completely to intuition. When your facade is removed, nothing stands in the way of your feeling all the world and tapping directly into the pool of intuitive knowledge. That can be, of course, wonderful. But there's a danger in losing your facade. While it means that you can all at once hear or see or feel everything that's going on, you can go too far into the vulnerable aspect of this and begin to hear everyone's thoughts and feel everyone's pain, even literally, in your body. This can truly be extremely painful. You become like the empath on *Star Trek: The Next Generation.* Although I rarely watched the show because I could never tell the characters apart (they all wore the same suits), the empath impressed me. She was the opposite of Spock, the character on the original *Star Trek* series who was the epitome of cool, unemotional rationality. Deanna Troi was like a receiver with the volume turned way up, picking up every message that came along. She had trouble living her life "attached to the earth," grounded in her body, like a first emotional center person, because she was a seventh emotional center being. The empath is as overly vulnerable as Spock was overly powerful in the seventh emotional center.

Real humans can't live that way for long, of course. It's overwhelming to feel all that density of intuition. It's too much information to process without going mad. In fact, as I'll discuss in the last part of this book, most of us are more open to intuition at certain times than at others. During certain phases of the female reproductive cycle, for instance, because of the way the hormones work, women feel more electric, sensitive, and vulnerable, yet they can't stay in that state.

Surviving a near-death or life-threatening experience almost invariably changes people. A woman who comes close to dying from breast cancer but is pulled back by chemotherapy and radiation is changed, to a certain degree, forever. Such people commonly make a lot of external changes in their lives as a reflection of this. They may change their jobs, their relationships, and a lot of other things. After about four years, a degree of normality returns, some of their facade will come back, and they balance their seventh emotional center somewhat better between power and vulnerability, but they never completely lose that connection to the universe that has been revealed to them. They become a sort of combination of Spock and Counselor Troi. They can be sitting at the dinner table with you talking about drapes, but they can suddenly start discussing something incredibly crucial and existential. They never quite completely come back.

A normal, healthy facade keeps you in balance with the rest of the world. Having too strong a facade, being too powerful in your separation from the world, can cut you off too much from life and from your life's purpose. On the other hand, having little or no facade means you get every ripple of agitation from outside and you look at life differently from other people.

SHEDDING A SKIN
VITILIGO

The Reading. Carolyn, age fifty-five, seemed like a person of tremendous strength, a real powerhouse who liked to go out in the world and accomplish great things. Yet I could see that, for some reason, she wasn't able to do that much anymore. Her ability to accomplish in the outer world was diminished, and I could sense a great deal of disappointment in her. I could see someone near her who was sad and depressed. She wanted to teach him to focus on something other than his depression, but she wasn't able to do that. Her challenge was to know that she couldn't snap this person out of his problem; she couldn't teach him to look at life differently, even though she herself had developed the skills to do just that over the course of her life and now even taught others such skills in the course of her work.

In Carolyn's body, I saw multiple but minor problems in her pelvis, having to do with inability to hold urine. I saw potential problems in her lungs. But the major flags went up when I got to her skin. I didn't know precisely what the problem was, but Carolyn looked like someone who couldn't go out into the sun at all because it would expose her to the possibility of cancer.

The Facts. Carolyn was a therapist who was having problems with her son. Three years earlier he had retired from a career as an Olympic gymnast after suffering a severe injury to his knee, and this sudden loss in power had slipped him into a depression from which nothing Carolyn did could shake him. She tried to give him goals, involve him in her work or college, or find him an alternate occupation, such as real estate, but nothing worked. Her son resisted every effort on her part and clung to his depression. He had, in fact, a lifelong predisposition to depression, and Carolyn's efforts were in that sense futile.

Nevertheless, Carolyn couldn't accept her son's inability to change, to accept that his purpose in life had changed and that he could and should look for a new purpose. She couldn't accept it because she herself had faced that same challenge at a young age and had risen to meet it with all her strength. At the age of fourteen, not long after the death of her beloved mother, Carolyn had developed vitiligo, a rare condition in which the skin loses all its

> pigment. Carolyn's skin was an abnormal pure white, so that she looked like an albino. It was as though her skin had been stripped away, leaving Carolyn exposed to the world. In fact, she herself saw what had happened to her in precisely this way. She referred to the onset of the vitiligo as the time "when God took away my skin."

Carolyn's mother had been her hero, and she had been extremely attached to her. When she died, Carolyn lost a champion, and was exposed to the world. Then God took Carolyn's skin away, leaving her almost literally without a facade to protect her from the ripples and shock waves of the world. At fourteen this could be devastating, since this is an age when we're just presenting ourselves to the world, and our physical facade, or appearance, is vital. At the same time, Carolyn's condition took away her ability to play outdoor sports, which she had loved. When her skin was attacked, however, she could no longer expose herself to the sun.

Although Carolyn's vitiligo wasn't life-threatening, it did alter the way she lived. It forced her to look at herself and at life differently from the way she had looked at it before, and differently from the way that other people looked at it. The disorder put her in touch with her purpose for living. She said that her whole reason for being on earth had to change after that. She turned to her inner self, to her inner strength, to find new skills to meet the challenge of her intuition and forge a new path in the world. Carolyn became a therapist because she wanted to teach other people how to develop their own new skills to overcome adversity and obstacles. At the same time, however, she had a son whom she could never teach to do what she had done.

Carolyn still had problems with attachment and detachment, as well as with the consequences of having no protective mask. She couldn't detach from her son and accept him as he was, and she couldn't impart to him the feelings of intensity and immediacy that she had about life by virtue of her lack of facade and intimate contact with the world. She could see that her son needed to get in touch with a life's purpose, but she couldn't make him do it. The focus of your seventh emotional center can't become someone else's. Going on a crusade is not healthy here. Carolyn's son apparently had not yet reached the place in his life where he could see things the way she saw them or feel them the way she felt them. He couldn't experience or move with the same degree of passion and intensity as she.

THE MYSTERY OF IT ALL

Why are we here? Why does illness happen? Why to me?

Not all these questions can be answered. Some things will always remain a mystery. This is difficult for us to accept. The human tendency is to seek information, to grasp for the concrete, to fill in the details. Knowledge is power, after all, and if we have it, we can help ourselves.

Yet not all knowledge is accessible all the time. In the seventh emotional center, we have to confront the inherent mystery of our lives and learn to accept it.

If we wait long enough, the mystery is sometimes solved or at least explained. Some years ago I had a frantic call from a woman who begged me to do an immediate reading on her husband, who had just been taken to the hospital with multiple organ failure. He was in the intensive care unit, and he was dying. This is precisely the kind of situation that I, as a medical intuitive, do not get in the middle of. When people are in a crisis, they're not really available to hear about the emotions that may have helped to precipitate it or are affecting it. It would be the same as stopping in the middle of a raging fire to say, "Now, karmically, why did this fire break out?" First, you put out the fire. Then you do the investigation. In the same way, it was important for the woman's husband to follow his doctors' course of treatment and get stabilized. Then, if the couple still wanted a reading, they could turn to me or someone else to help them get in touch with their intuition network. Although the woman called me two more times asking for a reading, I regretfully had to decline.

About a year later I got a call for a reading from a woman whom I saw as having been completely uprooted, like a geranium taken out of its pot and planted in a new flower bed. I could see that something or someone in her life had died and that this death had created a new beginning for her, and put her on a life's path where she would contribute what she was supposed to contribute to the world.

This was the same woman who had called a year earlier from beside her husband's ICU bed. Her story was amazing. Her husband, who had been in his mid-fifties, had suddenly had a heart attack, and all his organs had inexplicably begun to fail. No one could understand it; no one knew why it was happening. His wife had called me, because she wanted to know why. When I declined to do the reading, she had called some friends who came to the hospital to administer therapeutic touch to her husband. Even as the priest was giving him last rites, the man's organs began to function, one by one, apparently in response to the touching therapy. The ICU staff and attending physicians at this major medical center could hardly believe their eyes. They were so impressed by what they had seen that they decided to launch a research project on therapeutic touch and how it might affect organ system function.

Although the man eventually died suddenly in the night, his response to the therapeutic touch marked a turning point in his wife's life. She found new meaning in her existence. She quit her job in real estate, which had been entirely meaningless to her, and became involved in the therapeutic touch research. She told me that despite the pain of her husband's death, she now believed that it had given her new perspective and that tremendous gifts had come from it.

The mystery of that man's death was thus explained, but it had to come in its own time. If I had done a reading on her husband and then tried to tell the wife that one possible reason, *in her life,* that her husband was dying was so that she could find more meaning in her life and find her true life's path, she would not have been very receptive. Nor should she have been. Often the mystery has to come to us. Only when it's ready to reveal itself will it be comprehensible and acceptable to us.

We need mystery in our lives. We have to have a kind of hole in our hearts that represents a need to know why. We need a hunger in our souls, a void that we strive to fill, because it helps to propel us forward in life. If we fill up the hole too soon, we lose the momentum that keeps us going, as in the homecoming queen syndrome. Certain girls and boys, like the homecoming queen and the football hero, peak in high school: They're popular and praised. They seem to have everything, but their lives may not develop much further. They've reached their full potential at seventeen or eighteen, their hungers have been satisfied, and they have nothing driving them forward.

When people call me or go to see a psychic, they may be looking for answers, but not all answers are ones they should receive. I once went to see a psychic, during the period when I was falling asleep unexpectedly, and she told me that she saw me having problems for the next eleven years. Not twelve, not seven, not seventy, but precisely eleven. Information like that just isn't helpful. Some people would take that information and essentially put their lives on hold for eleven years. They'd want to wait out their problems, and say, "Well, in eleven years my life will begin." I chose not to believe what the psychic had told me, and instead of giving up, I drove myself forward. Eleven years after I had visited her, I graduated from medical school.

People with issues in the seventh emotional center sometimes look to a belief in past lives to yield clues to the mysteries and difficulties of the present. This too can keep them from living in the present and keeping a balance in the seventh emotional center. Solving the mysteries of a past life—assuming that that can be done—won't necessarily give you the skills you need to live effectively in this one. Dealing with the issues in your life is like shoveling snow. There's enough snow for you to shovel and plow in your current life. Why would you want to go back into previous lives and plow out those lives as well? The chore is too overwhelming; it bogs you down so much that you can't deal with the problems in your present life.

Our culture is attached to information. We want to figure everything out. Even this book is designed to help you come to an understanding of the language of your body and your dreams and what your intuition is trying to guide you to do. In the end, however, there are some things we simply can never know. Even if you have highly developed intuitive skills, you will often not know why things are the way they are.

I once did a reading on a woman who represented the ultimate riddle of the seventh emotional center. When I read her, I felt as though some powerful force, like a tidal wave, had wiped her out. She was an educated woman who had her life set on course. She had married, bought a home, and was getting ready to have children. Her life was sort of artificially perfect, but still, everything was on course. And then one day it was all wiped out. Everything she had thought was important in life had changed. In her body, I saw that she had changes in her attention and memory. Her heart had a slightly irregular rhythm. Her skin seemed dry, and her whole body felt hot and electrical. I felt she had pain all up and down her left leg, as if it were on fire.

This woman had been hit by lightning. She'd gone for a walk up a mountain with her husband when a thunderstorm struck. She was holding on to a metal fence when a lightning bolt struck the fence and shot down her left leg, causing extensive nerve damage. After that, the woman's life changed completely. She dropped her postdoctoral studies and changed her career. Her relationship with her husband changed. The whole world seemed different to her. Matters that had seemed vital now appeared trivial. Her whole way of looking at things, thinking about life, and simply being would never be the same again. Even her body was forever different.

This woman could not understand why this had happened to her. Here was an event over which she had no control and which detached her from most of what she had previously known, stripped away her facade, and set her on a different life's course. Why me? she wanted to know. Regrettably, this wasn't anything I could tell her, either. Perhaps one day the meaning of her experience would be revealed. Or perhaps not. Perhaps it would forever remain a mystery.

Life itself is, of course, at its most fundamental, a mystery. The key to unlocking this mystery may lie somewhere in an inaccessible dimension of the universe or in the deepest unknowable recesses of our own souls. Until we find such a key, all we can do is embrace the mystery and immerse ourselves in it. This is what we learn, through intuition, in the seventh emotional center.

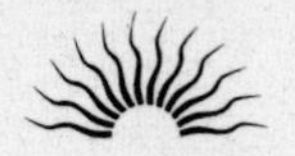

Part Three

Tuning in to the Network

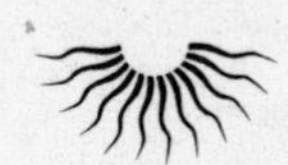

THIRTEEN

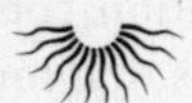

Your Intuitive Identity: Kinds of Intuitive Intelligence

"Find out who you are," Dolly Parton once said, "and do it on purpose." I love this quote, because it so concisely expresses the message at the heart of this book. If you can find out how your unique intuitive language expresses itself to you, and then use that knowledge purposefully and apply it deliberately, you can become a real body intuitive and know who you are. You can take steps to lead a healthier, happier, and more fulfilling life and help other people do the same.

The information about the intuition network, the body's seven emotional centers, and the emotionally charged memories of wisdom and trauma stored in the brain and the body together form a kind of instruction manual for the body. The language of intuition—the signs and symptoms by which your body signals that a certain emotion needs to be attended to in your life—is like an instruction manual for a car. It describes all the parts of the engine and the chassis, tells you how to operate the car, and explains the symptoms that may be signaling you about its soundness and ability to function. Reading an instruction booklet like this can give you a sense of safety and mastery over your vehicle. It is an invaluable and essential guide to the general rules of your automobile's operation, but there are a lot of variables that affect the functioning of any *individual* car, including its make, its age, the mileage you've put on it, any prior accidents, and any inherent quirks or flaws in the motor or the body.

It's much the same with our bodies and our intuition networks. We all possess the same basic elements, the same general parts that route intuition to us. As I said earlier, if you have a left brain, a right brain, and a body, if you have memories and emotions, if you sleep and therefore dream, then you have intuition—even if you think you don't. There *is* some way that intuition comes to you. What that way is depends on a string of variables that make you the individual you are: your sex, your age, your experiences in life, and the specific way your engine and your chassis are built, including any inherent strengths and weaknesses of brain and body. What this means is that you have to write your own addenda to the instruction booklet of your body intuition, using the vocabulary of your own unique intuitive language.

Who are you, in intuitive terms? Are you left-handed or right-handed? Male or female? Older or younger? Do you see yourself as logical, linear, rational, and intellectual? Or do you consider yourself emotional, nonrational, and creative? Are you comfortable being rational but uncomfortable in the world of feelings? Do you have an unusually short attention span? Are you disconnected from your feelings? The answers to these questions will help you discover your basic intuitive identity and apply this self-knowledge to your life and actions.

Even with the full instructional manual in hand, however, many of us may still have difficulty. Most of us can't fix our cars, for instance, without the assistance of a mechanic. In the same way, while we may now know what all the parts of the intuition network are and how they function and fit together, we may not always be able to read our own body intuition with accuracy and acceptance. That's because our rational, logical left hemisphere of the brain and its frontal lobe act as a censor and will always deny the validity of our intuition. Most of us don't want to believe the intuitive signals we get, either, because believing them would mean we'd have to change our behavior in some way, and change is frightening. Most of us tend to disconnect from our body intuition. When our hands go numb, we tell ourselves it's because our sleeves are too tight, not that we have a physical disk problem or a metaphorical emotional pain in the neck.

In fact, even the body itself conspires in this denial. The human body is designed to uphold the status quo through a process called homeostasis. The body is rigged to maintain its equilibrium even as the world around it changes. If something frightening happens, your heart races to let you know you need to be afraid. But it returns to normal as soon as possible. It wants to go back to its balanced state. In physics, a state of equilibrium equals inertia. But as Einstein said, nothing happens until motion occurs. So even though our signals are telling us, "Change! Emote!" the body is inclined to say, "No, calm down, it's okay. You're fine; everyone else has got a problem. Just get a Diet Coke, sit back in your chair, and watch TV."

This means that we'll probably have to get help from someone else to read ourselves, someone who can serve as a denial blaster. At the same time, however, we can serve as denial blasters for others. What you learn about your intuition and how to tap into it in this chapter and the next will help you apply your intuitive skills to reading your own body and the body intuition of others, as a means of illuminating the meaning of your own.

The intensity with which intuition speaks varies widely, as does its clarity. Some people receive intuition more strongly or directly, due to their mental, physical, and emotional makeup. To others, intuition comes more subtly and indirectly, and hearing or understanding it requires greater conscious effort. Wherever you fall on this spectrum, understanding your intuitive identity will help you make use of your own particular gifts to enrich your life and the lives of others in countless ways.

MALE OR FEMALE

In 1871, Charles Darwin wrote that "in woman, the powers of intuition…are more strongly marked than in man."[1]

The concept of woman's intuition probably predated Darwin, although he might have been the first to begin to quantify it scientifically. The idea that women have an innate ability to intuit, or sense, things in a manner that seems largely unavailable to men has been the stuff of folklore and folk wisdom in cultures all over the world. Think of all the stereotypical images we have of psychics and Gypsy fortune-tellers: they're invariably women in flowing skirts and beads, reading palms or tarot cards or tea leaves. Men intuitives do in fact exist, but they are scarcer.

The reason for this goes back chiefly, and not surprisingly, to the brain. In an earlier chapter we talked about the differences between the right hemisphere—the emotional, visual, and intuitive part of the brain—and the left hemisphere, which is the intellectual, verbal, and logical part. In our culture, people tend to be oriented dominantly toward one hemisphere or the other, but most women have more access to the right hemisphere more of the time than most men do.[2] This may be because women have a wider corpus callosum—the pathway between the two hemispheres—than men. This is true from infancy. As early as twenty-six weeks of age female babies exhibit a larger corpus callosum than males babies.[3] They therefore have more connections—telephone lines, if you will—between the two halves of the brain. In fact, women have denser connections between all the functional areas of their brains, even within one hemisphere. In scientific terms, women's brains have more connectivity and are less compartmentalized than men's brains, so that there's a lot of overlap in activity among the various areas.[3,4]

An apt metaphor for the typical male brain's organization might be a department store. Everything is neatly arranged and organized according to departments—men's wear on the left side of the aisle, women's cosmetics on the right, sporting goods in the basement, books and stationery one flight up, electronics at the back, and so on. You go from one department to another, finishing your business in each before moving on to the next. If you're a salesperson in men's wear, and the phone rings in cosmetics over on the other side of the store, you don't go to answer it until you've finished your current transaction. The traditional female brain, on the other hand, is more like your old-fashioned general store. You go in, and everything's a bit of jumble. Items are arranged according to general category, but there aren't the neatly separated departments, and items seem to wander out of their assigned spaces with regularity. Going over to the greeting cards, you're likely to trip over a mop, and you find a bottle of dishwashing liquid stuffed among the skeins of yarn in the crafts section. You wander aimlessly from section to section, picking up things as you need them and doubling back several times over as you remember additional items.

Women can structurally roam around all over the place inside their brains, shifting hemispheres at will at any given time. Men's brains, by contrast, are more lateralized and compartmentalized. Most men tend to use one area of the brain at a time and to stay in that hemisphere until a task is completed. They tend to stay more in the left hemisphere and shift less readily between the two. In fact, neuroanatomy shows that the way hormones affect certain areas of the brain, including the frontal lobe and the amygdala in the temporal lobe, tends to make women superior in tasks that require rapid shifts between the hemispheres, while men are superior at tasks that require the use of one hemisphere at a time.[5]

Women tend to be in their right hemispheres more than men. Because the right hemisphere is more closely connected to the body,[6] women are generally more in touch with their bodies. It also means they tend to be more in touch with their emotions and with intuition. In women, as a general rule, information tends to be processed by the left brain, the right brain, and the body, all as working together as a unit. The whole intuition network, in other words, is on-line and available to them all the time. A man, by contrast, is more likely to use a distinct and specific part of his brain to perform any given task. If the task is recognizing a familiar face, the right brain is mostly involved; if the task is speaking, the left brain tends to take over. What this means overall is that men may have less of their intuition network available at any one time to make a correct decision based on insufficient physical information.

There are probably very good evolutionary reasons for these differences between the sexes. Historically, men were the hunters and warriors of social units. This means they often had to function without feeling. The middle of the battlefield isn't the place to get in touch with your emotions. If you have to club someone over the head to survive and protect your family, you can't afford to be immediately crippled by your intuitive guidance system kicking in and telling you that you've just done something horrendous. You have to do it and keep going. On the other hand, women's historical roles as nurturers and caretakers required them to think and feel at the same time, to express emotion continuously in order to help their children develop, and to sense what their children were feeling as well.

Because women tend to use more connections between the right and left brain, they're also more able to communicate their intuition as it comes to them. They may have more activity than men in the cingulate gyrus, an area in the frontal lobe that plays a role in intuition and spoken language. This means they have better wiring between parts of the intuition network and the areas for speech. Men, on the other hand, have more activity in the temporal lobe, which prompts action and plays a role in receiving intuition but is unfortunately a step removed from spoken language. In other words, the temporal lobe is more important for receiving intuition, while the frontal lobe plays an important role in communicating it. If women, therefore, get intuition via the frontal lobe, which is right next to the communicating device, they tend to spit it out more readily. Men, on the other hand, get intuition through the temporal lobe, but in order to communicate it, they have to jump to another lobe. It's as though, after receiving intuition, men have to go over to another department in order to ship it out. As a result, they're more likely to *act* in response to intuition than to express it verbally.[7]

If you're a man reading this, you may be shaking your head and saying, "So that's it for me. It's hopeless. I can't be intuitive." Let me stress that *this isn't true.* Men can be and are intuitive in many ways. For one thing, no rule is hard and fast. Everything I've said here can be applied, in general fashion, only to *most* men and *most* women. Not all men and not all women, as we know all too well, are the same. There are right hemisphere–dominant men just as there are left hemisphere–dominant women. If you're a left-handed man, for instance, you may have as much ease of access to your intuition network as most right-handed women. Left-handers of both sexes have been shown to have a wider corpus callosum.[4] They have more connections to their right hemisphere, and thus to their body and emotions and therefore to more parts of their intuition network.

If you're a normal left hemisphere–oriented man, with nothing particularly unusual about your brain, you can certainly gain access to your right hemisphere. You just can't do it as quickly as many women, or recognize what's happening there with as much fluidity. You may have an intuitive hunch, but you can't name it. It is a challenge for you to connect with your intuition because the natural tendency is for the lines to get disconnected. When your intuition speaks, your left hemisphere—which as you'll recall, tends to deny the experience of the right—is likely to hang up the phone, the way you hang up on those telemarketing calls that always seem to come just as you're sitting down to dinner. You don't want to listen to them. You may have to reverse your thinking. Instead of receiving the calls, you may have to start making them, start dialing in to establish a connection with the right hemisphere, using the approach and techniques we'll discuss in the final chapter. You may find, in the beginning especially, that you have a lot of experiences that remind you of calling the Registry of Motor Vehicles. You're on the line for fifteen minutes waiting for someone to talk to, and then you get disconnected. It's maddening, but the best thing to do is to dial again and wait. You might get more hang-ups than women do, but if you keep calling and practicing, those hang-ups may decrease.

The bigger challenge in our society, from an intuition standpoint, is to keep everyone, female as well as male, more tuned in to the intuition network. With sex roles in society evolving and changing, men and women are now beginning to develop along more closely related lines. Unfortunately, however, women may be moving away from the right hemisphere and their traditional connectedness to emotions and intuition, which would be a great loss.

The Time of Your Life

Intuition isn't static. The ways and volume in which intuition speaks to us change at various stages of our lives. Where you are on the path of life may affect the way in which you can receive, understand, and express intuition.

Children have long been known to be more intuitive and often more observant than adults. I once walked into a crowded bookstore for a book-signing party for a friend, having just come from the hairdresser, where I'd had my hair subtly highlighted. There was the merest whisper of blond in it, making it just slightly brighter, and I was confident no one would notice anything. (You know how women are always trying to pretend that they don't do anything unnatural to their hair.) No sooner had I walked into the room than a colleague's eight-year-old daughter called across the room, her piping little voice cutting right through the conversational din: "Mona Lisa, why did you bleach your hair?" Two hundred heads swiveled as one to stare at me while I tried to shrink into the woodwork and fantasized about muzzling this normally adorable child.

Of course, she was only being her naturally observant self. Most of us have had some experience like mine, where you're sitting at a dinner table, perhaps, and little Johnny suddenly blurts out, "Mommy, why are Mr. Jones and Mrs. Smith doing that funny stuff with their feet under the table?" As children, we have the capacity to receive not only the maximum amount of information through our five senses but also the maximum amount of information through the intuition network. Even long before we obtain the power of speech, we get feelings about things, and we know things without really being able to name them. This may be because, developmentally, the right hemisphere comes on board before the left hemisphere.[9] Perhaps even more significantly, children's frontal lobes—those ever-present censors telling us, "You can't do that" or "Don't say that"—don't fully mature until later in life. It's as though some of the circuits haven't come on-line yet. While children know a lot of things, they don't know which of these things are essential or important and which are insignificant or even inappropriate for them to know or to say. As a result, children have insufficient social conditioning and poor social comportment, and they consequently have the "blurting out" tendency that can cause so many embarrassed silences among adults.

Nevertheless, children's access to their intuition is enriching to them and instructive to the rest of us. Watch children while they play, and see the free range they give their minds and their openness to the outer world. All this helps foster their intuitive gifts. Play encourages chance phenomena. In other words, when you're playing, you don't try to inhibit anything that might happen. You're open to anything that comes your way, and that includes intuition. We give up on that as we move into adulthood. We stop playing, and the world changes. Instead of a place marked by the unknown where fantastic things can take place, it becomes a familiar place where everything can be explained. We leave ourselves no room for intuition, that sudden spark that comes out of nowhere, often bringing with it new and creative possibilities.

Cultivating intuition in children, making them aware of this gift, is something we should do before their frontal lobes come on board to tell them not to listen to it anymore. Unfortunately, more often than not, adults end up acting as children's frontal lobes, inhibiting instead of encouraging their intuition. Children generally don't know they're being intuitive or that there's anything special about that. During a reading, I once spoke to a little boy who I could tell was very intuitive and who was fascinated with cars. I asked him to describe my car. His mother immediately took on the role of frontal lobe and tried to interrupt, saying, "Oh, he can't do that." But he could. He nailed my car. "A green Honda Civic hatchback," he said. I asked him to imagine me in the driver's seat and then to describe me, and his mother popped up as the frontal lobe again. But I assured her her son could do it, and he was right again: "Five-four, with straight hair to your shoulders, and thin." Calling me thin made me love him immediately. I thought this little boy had remarkable potential as a forensic intuitive, someone who could always pick out the vehicle at the murder scene. But unless his intuitive ability was encouraged, he stood to lose it or suppress it, the way so many of us do in our youth.

Children can be helped to focus on their intuition by drawing pictures, a right brain activity, relating their dreams and recording their actions. If a child spills a glass of milk, you might want to have him focus on why he did it, if there's some underlying current in the social order he's picking up on. And you can work with him in terms of symbols. If little Suzy says Uncle Martin reminds her of a porcupine, you might get the idea she's picking up the feeling that there's something painful about being with Uncle Martin.

Even if you strengthen a child's intuitive muscle, though, staying in touch with intuition throughout our lives can be difficult, as our intuitive identity changes with the life cycle. As we pass from childhood into puberty, everything in our world changes. Those infamous hormones come on board, and hormones really mature the brain. Now your frontal lobe locks into place, and you begin to hear more selectively, to filter out information that the frontal lobe is telling you it's not possible for you to know. You develop the capacity to inhibit yourself, and your attentiveness to the many intuitive signals coming your way recedes.

In women, puberty is the starting point for what can be called cyclical intuition, the intuition available to most women throughout their formative and reproductive years. This is intuition that ebbs and flows in rhythm with the menstrual cycle (see the following figure). In the days before ovulation, intuition is at a low ebb. But then, right before a woman gets her period, the intuitive flow begins, and a woman gains increased access to intuition. Christiane Northrup describes the premenstrual stage as the time when "inner wisdom," sensitivity, and awareness to emotions and their messages are most available to women.[10] This is the wisdom of intuition. Biologically, it appears to work this way. In the course of the menstrual cycle, levels of LH and FSH, the hormones that stimulate the ovaries to produce eggs, are low in the first half of the menstrual cycle. They gradually rise and then peak on day fourteen. Although we don't know where LH and FSH themselves bond to in the brain, we do know that estrogen, which is controlled by them and therefore also increases in midcycle, bonds to the limbic areas of the brain, which play an important role in intuition. Thus ovulation appears to prime the intuitive network and open up the channels so that women can hear more clearly.

Before ovulation, the left hemisphere of the brain is in control. Most

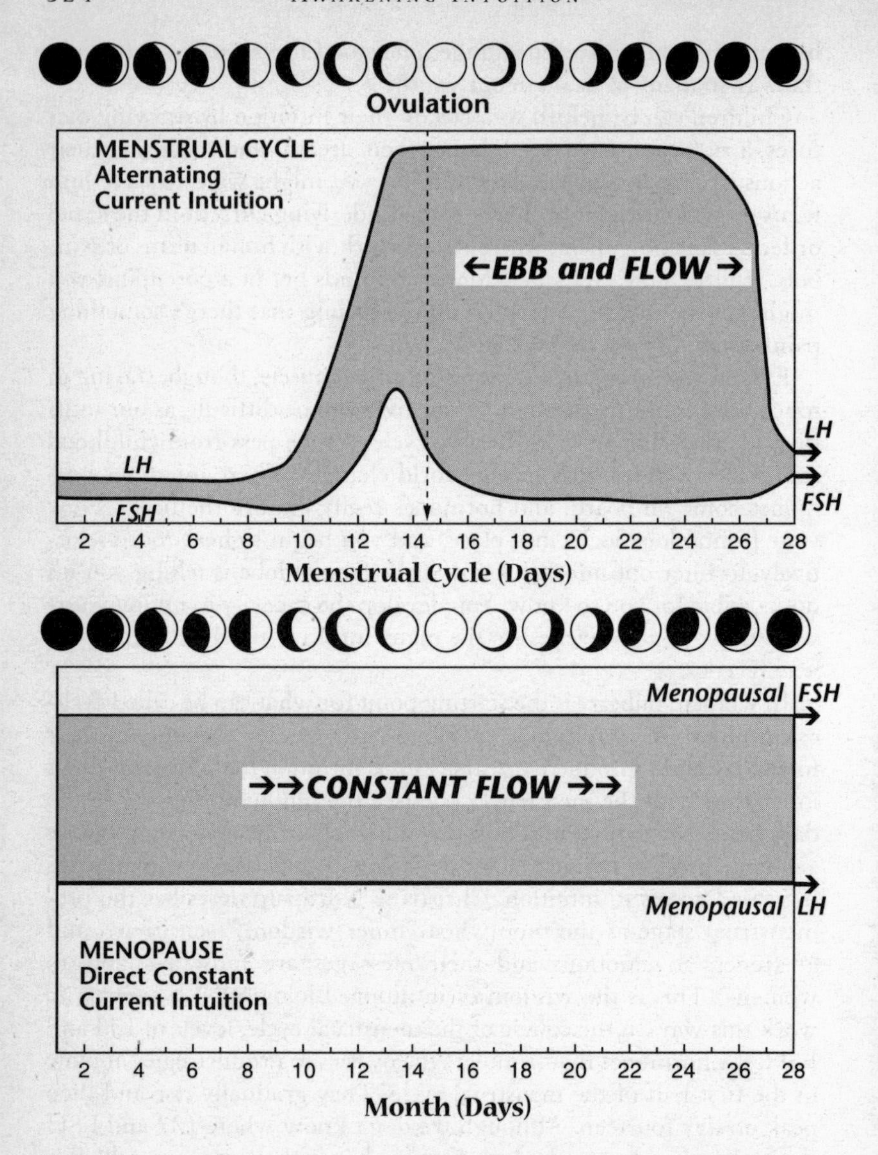

language function is supposed to be in the left hemisphere. But studies have shown that the left hemisphere is also chiefly primed to hear mainly *positive* words, such as "joy," "happiness," "love," and "cheer." After ovulation, however, the right hemisphere picks up the tempo and cycles into more control, while the left hemisphere goes into more of a down mode. In women, language can be in both hemispheres, but the language to which the right hemisphere is receptive is negatively charged words.[11] Women can hear words like "rage," "anger," "sadness," and "depression" more strongly premenstrually than the rest of the time. All at once, in this period, their brain allows them to hear things they don't usually allow themselves to hear. That's intuition at work; it makes us able to acquire information and knowledge that are not usually present in our external environment, knowledge we don't usually want to see, hear, or act on.

Dr. Christiane Northrup tells an illuminating story about a patient whose husband brought her in one day for an exam and said (and I'm not kidding): "Fix her, she's broken." What was the problem? Dr. Northrup asked, bemused. During the first half of her cycle, the man reported, his wife was normal: "She does whatever the family wants. She makes all the meals, does the laundry, darns my socks. And she does it all cheerfully. She's happy, she's content." Then, he reported, two weeks before she gets her period, everything changes. "Suddenly, she's not happy with her life, the ways things are around the house. She wants to go to college!" As an appliance repairman, the man was familiar with the concept of "fixing."

In her premenstrual period, this woman was hearing the wisdom of her intuition, telling her that her life needed to change, that adjustments had to be made. She repressed this the rest of the time, because her husband clearly didn't want to hear it, and she preferred not to hear it, either, because it caused an uproar in the household. After ovulation, her intuition slipped through the hole of the menstrual cycle and sent her signals she couldn't turn off.[10]

In a woman's reproductive years, she really needs to pay attention and tune in to her intuition network during the premenstrual period. As she enters into menopause and her menstrual cycles wind down and cease, another physical change takes place that affects her intuition. In the menopausal woman, FSH and LH levels stop fluctuating. As ovulations decrease, the FSH and LH levels gradually increase. Ultimately, they get stuck on high, as though the switch won't flip to turn them off anymore. Standard science will tell you that this happens because the brain keeps telling the ovaries to push out more eggs, but there are no more eggs to push. Because the usual ovarian signal telling the pituitary gland to decrease production of FSH and LH is no longer there, the pituitary is thought to keep blasting the bloodstream with high levels of FSH and LH in the vain hope that an egg will be produced anyway. Nature wouldn't do anything so wasteful.[10] Why would the brain continue making unnecessary FSH and LH, which are important, expensive neuropeptides, when it could be using the same energy to make nice strong protein for the thighs, for instance? The brain is producing FSH and LH for important reasons. It's not just talking to the ovaries and uterus, it's talking to itself and to all the other organs; it may be sending out intuition everywhere.

Christiane Northrup describes menopause as a change from an alternating current of wisdom to a direct current.[10] In menopause, instead of an ebb and flow of intuition, you now have a constant flow. In that light, it's not surprising that many cultures regard older women as wise women and celebrate the "wisdom of the crone." These women possess not only the wisdom of age and experience but also the wisdom of intuition. And they're not afraid to use it and act on it. It's a widely observed fact that many women, after menopause, become much more forthright and assertive than they were in their youth. Joan Borysenko puts it bluntly: in menopause, she writes, "Women get mouthy."[12] This occurs because there's a falling-away of the inhibitions that kept women from shooting arrows indiscriminately the way men do. This change may be a result of increased androgen production. The women who were more tentative in their youth, waiting a long time before even shooting at a target and thereby missing a lot of opportunities, in later life often assume more male patterns of processing. After menopause, they're more likely to see, shoot, and then score, as men did earlier in life.

All this should really give women something to cheer about and celebrate as they enter the age of menopause and beyond. Menopause is not a dead-end journey into decline and oblivion; it's an opportunity to tap fully into the intuition network and avail themselves fruitfully of all the wealth of insight and information that network has to offer.

Once again I can hear you thinking, "But what about men?" I certainly don't intend to give men short shrift. Unfortunately, however, very little is known about possible cycles in most men's brains that might correspond to those in women's brains and influence the flow of intuition. There is some evidence that as men get older, and after they go through their own change of life, or "testepause," there is a shift in their attentional mechanism, just as there is in that of women, which may affect the way they pay attention and react to intuition. Men who, in their youth, impulsively and wildly flung arrows into the air and missed the target most of the time now slow down, listen more carefully, and shoot fewer arrows but hit the target more often. In later life, therefore, most normal men now get a chance to experience what women experienced earlier in life. They now get a chance to shoot the puck, figure out the right thing to do, and then slap it in to the goal. They have a chance to open themselves more fully to intuition and apply it purposefully to their lives.

Scientists are just beginning to explore men's brain cycles and life changes. Greater research into this area may reveal that men have their own unique form of intuition.

THROUGH DISORDER INTO ORDER

Some people of both sexes have brains that are organized differently or function differently from those of the general population. Usually, these people are said to have a brain or mind disorder, which is a slightly different word for "disease." Very often they also have unusual gifts of intuition. In that light, the choice of the word "disorder" is interesting. You could say that disorder is what intuition creates. Intuition isn't like the more conservative members of England's royal family. It doesn't adhere to protocol or practice restraint. It tends to spill water, break cups, and blurt out comments that make everybody squirm. The disorder it creates is unsettling. But by working through disorder, we can often achieve a new, possibly better order.

Space Cadet Intuition: The Hypofrontal Brain

Has anyone ever called you a spaz? What about a space cadet? Do people say things to you like "Welcome to Earth?" If they do, it's probably because you're equipped with a slightly different type of attention mechanism than most people. You might be a bit more impulsive, you might like stimulus and find yourself drawn to it like a magnet, along with thrills and risk-taking. You have what I prefer to call an atypical way of being in the world and of paying attention to it. What's interesting is that one of the things intuition requires is that we change the way we pay attention to the world. Most of us pay attention predominantly to matters in the outer world. That means we're not paying attention to things in the inner world, where intuition comes to us. If you have an unusual way of paying attention, perhaps an *enhanced* way, then you probably have, by definition, interesting and enhanced intuitive gifts. What makes you different also makes you special. Your difference is your genius.

I can best describe this by using the example of people with extreme changes in how they process intuition, people with attention deficit disorder, or ADD. This is supposed to be a developmental problem, in which areas in the brain's attention network develop differently from normal. People with ADD (and others with different attention) are *hypofrontal*, which means that they have relatively unplugged frontal lobes, which consequently work less efficiently.[13] You'll recall that our frontal lobes act as censors and inhibitors and tell us when we can't know something or shouldn't do something. They're like the high school principal or the hall monitor, trying to inhibit excess activity and keep the noise down to a dull roar.

Since their frontal lobe censors are on siesta, people with ADD have difficulty paying attention for long periods of time. They tend to pay attention to several things at once. They have a poor ability to filter things out. If they hear leaves rustling outside the window, for instance, they can't filter that sound out, and it distracts them from what the teacher is saying. ADD people also exhibit excessively motor-driven behavior. They're always playing with a pen, twisting their hair, tapping their feet, getting in and out of their chairs. They're driven internally, and they can't stop. Like the Energizer bunny, they keep going and going and going. In addition, people with ADD are stimulus-bound. This means that if they see a stimulus of any kind, they bond to it like glue. I've been to Las Vegas a few times, and I remember that each time, I became simply mesmerized by the incredible flashing neon lights there. I'd find myself just staring and staring and staring, fixated on this stimulus, and having to be literally led in and out of the casinos. It's very common for someone with ADD to watch TV, listen to the radio over earphones, surf the Net, and talk on the telephone—all at the same time. Surrounded by all these stimuli, they're happy. Being stimulus-bound also means that people with ADD have problems with inhibition and blocking their impulses. They see the fire alarm on the wall, read the word "Pull," and automatically reach out and yank on the handle before they've read the rest of the message: "in case of emergency." I'm a poster child for ADD.

Because they're stimulus-bound, people with ADD have a way of blurting out the salient issue in any given situation. When I had to have my photograph taken, I arranged over the telephone to meet the photographer at a public location. I had seen him only once before, some time previously, and he asked if I would recognize him. I had a picture in my mind of that previous time, when he had arrived to take a friend's photos on a cold, snowy day. What I remembered was a man in a woolen hat with a runny nose. So that's what I said. "Sure, you're the guy in the woolen hat with the runny nose." There was a short silence. Then he gently reoriented my thinking. "No," he said, "I'm the guy who looks like Elton John, only with more hair." I had focused on the salient points about him on the day that I had seen him.

People with ADD have an exquisite ability to pay attention to many things everywhere, in the inner world and the outer world—everything but the one thing the scientists say they should be paying attention to: the sheet of paper in front of them and the boring lady by the blackboard. They look at anything in the world that stimulates them, and at the same time, they pick up innuendo in the air, which most people fail to notice because they're concentrating solely on the task at hand. They'll pick up things that others' frontal lobes are actively denying and suppressing. Because their own frontal lobes are underutilized, the ADDs frequently aren't up to society's par on the social comportment level, and will blurt out that innuendo even when it's inappropriate. A child with ADD will notice that every time Daddy comes home late from work, he smells like perfume. Mommy's frontal lobe, in the same instance, is busy blocking her intuition network, telling her "You don't want to think about that. That can't be." But every time his father comes in, little Johnny blurts out, "Wow, Dad, you smell good!" Each time, his father will rebuke him with a sharp, "Don't say that." But Johnny keeps saying it, because he can't stop himself. And what is he doing? He's focusing on the salient issue in the situation. Like a moth to the light, he picks up on the stimulus, and he goes unerringly to the area that needs to be paid attention to but that no one wants to look at.

If you take a group of people who are adhering strictly to protocol and plunk someone with ADD down in the middle of them, that person's going to read all the secrets underneath the surface of the situation, and he or she will voice them or act them out. The British royal family will all sit there stiffly and unexpressively during an uncomfortable discussion, but there at the end of the table will be the ADD kid, throwing objects and spilling things. People with ADD are often somatic intuitives, which means that they feel things in their bodies and act them out through movement. I do this a lot as well. If I'm in a business meeting where the surface is all smooth and civil but there's a lot of subterfuge going on, I'll invariably spill my water or shoot the ink out of my fountain pen across the table. I'll make some sort of mess that symbolizes the mess beneath the surface that everyone's trying to cover up. I have a friend who's somewhat obsessive (another "disorder" we'll be discussing a bit later). Obsessive people will try to order their environment in order to cover up the anxiety and chaos they feel underneath. But when I'm around them, I hear all that subterranean chaos. And because I have ADD and am a somatic intuitive, that chaos will come out. Unfailingly, whenever I'm at this friend's house, I'll spill something. I've spilled oil on her bed, dribbled orange soda on her brand-new rug, and burned holes in several objects. This happens at her house more than any other place I've ever been to, so much so that my friend started to get a little paranoid. I was simply responding to the undercurrent in her life, although this didn't absolve me from the responsibility of buying her a new rug and other furnishings on several occasions.

On a recent occasion I was having cappuccino with a colleague with whom I was supposed to have dinner that night at his house. I was feeling very unsettled and edgy, without knowing why, full of a jagged energy. Just as we got ready to leave, I somehow managed to drop or knock over one of those large cappuccino bowls. It fell to the floor, spilling cappuccino all over me and shattering into a million pieces. Drenched in coffee, I now had an excuse to beg off from dinner, which I had been wanting to do. As it turned out, my friend had had a fight with his wife, which I had been sensing all along. Once again, I had somatically and intuitively acted out the turmoil I had felt beneath the surface that evening.

Children with ADD often unconsciously act out any turmoil at home. Mom and Dad fight, then try to smooth the matter over. But Junior trips over the carpet and cracks open his head, because he knows that something's going on, and he acts it out physically. So now he's bleeding physically, because the family is bleeding internally, but no one is letting it on. Or, like the child in the Minuchin experiment discussed earlier,[14] he develops illnesses that are related to the memories and emotions going on in the family. He becomes the family's body intuitive.

You don't have to have full-blown ADD to have some of the same expanded sensitivity to your intuition. Lots of people have some elements of the ADD personality that help them get in touch with their intuition network in various ways. ADD itself is supposedly present in about 15 percent of the population. Since this is the same percentage of the population that's left-handed, which is considered a standard normal variant, I'd argue that ADD isn't a disorder or disease. It's an atypical way of being. Yes, it sometimes seems to make it harder to fit in with the rest of society, which still looks askance at the concept of intuition. This is the "devil" associated with this kind of atypical brain organization. But I prefer to appreciate the angels it brings—an openness to a sense that can help us achieve a new and different kind of order in our lives that can bless us with greater well-being.

Ziploc Intuition: The Hyperfrontal Brain

While attention disorders that unplug the frontal lobe help people to tune in to their intuition network more readily, there's another set of disorders, or brain organizations, that regrettably do the opposite. The hallmark of such syndromes is a powerful frontal lobe, the size of Arnold Schwarzenegger's biceps, that's always censoring and blocking intuition. These people have a figurative gerbil wheel in their frontal lobes, going around and around and around constantly. People who are obsessive-compulsive are also *hyper*frontal.[15] If you did a PET scan of their brains, the area of the frontal lobe would light up like a strobe. This means their brains are constantly telling them, You can't do this, what you feel in your body isn't right, don't move over there right now, it's not the right time, don't say that, people will think you're nuts. In these people, the temporal lobes with all their intuitive input are held at bay.

We all know someone with obsessive traits. They're the people who organize everything in their refrigerator in Ziploc bags. They're the ones who use the aluminum foil once, twice, three times, then fold it carefully and put it in the drawer after each use. These are people who give you the feeling that they never moan or groan, nor make any body sounds, or for that matter, even have bowel movements. Everything in their lives has to be orderly. They need all the facts, and they need a lot of time to make a decision. They usually like to sit on it for a long, long time. They worry and ruminate a lot.

The ironic thing is that underneath the nattering of their frontal lobes, obsessive-compulsives are actually very intuitive. Their disorder is highlighted by enhanced anxiety about very subtle things. This means that they're detecting and feeling those subtleties all around them, but before they can acknowledge or act on them, they start to obsess in an effort to order their environment and ease their anxiety. If they could stop their obsessiveness, they would have the potential to be very good body intuitives. But they would have to note when their frontal lobes, their censors, were coming on-line.

Say you're reading this, and soon you begin to wring your hands. Then you get up five times to wash your hands. And you're thinking that instead of reading this, you should be paying your bills or vacuuming the carpet. You haven't vacuumed in twenty-four hours, and there's a dog hair on the small rug; you must remove that right away. You must vacuum because you're feeling anxious. And as you vacuum, you're vacuuming away your intuitive guidance system, because you're using your compulsions and obsessions to cover up your body intuition. If you can note that moment when you start to wring your hands, you might be able to key into the body intuition that's expressing your anxiety, the emotions you're feeling in your body. You might need to record these notations in a journal. And then you might use this book as an instruction manual to translate the body language in which your intuition is being transmitted to you. If you notice that you get heart palpitations, you can go to the fourth emotional center and determine where you have an imbalance around issues pertaining to partnership or emotional expression. If you feel your stomach start to churn and you grow nauseated, you'd want to try to pinpoint the events that prompted the nausea, and then turn to the third emotional center and figure out any imbalance having to do with responsibility or competence. You can tap into what may be your dominant type of intuition and learn to be a good body intuitive.

"All Lines Are Down" Intuition: The Unconnected Brain

Another condition that presents a difficult challenge vis-à-vis intuition is called alexithymia. People with this condition essentially have brains in which all the various areas of the intuition network are disconnected. It's as though someone went in there with a pair of scissors and clipped all the lines. While these people have all the elements of the network, the various parts can't communicate with each other. They may actually have body intuition or somatic intuition, but they can't talk about it or express it. Indeed, they can't even recognize it, because of the lack of communication in their brains and, even more significantly, the dominance of the left hemisphere, which will deny the existence of any intuition at all.

I set out with some friends one day to go horseback riding. The day had started out sunny, but as we drove out into the country, clouds gathered. Soon it began to drizzle. Mary, the friend who was driving, switched on the windshield wipers. "Oh, no, it's starting to rain," another friend, Joan, lamented from the backseat. In the front, Mary shook her head. "No, it isn't," she said. "We'll have a fine day horseback riding. Everything will be marvelous." But she had just turned the windshield wipers on! It was remarkable. Her left hand had reached up and turned the switch for the wipers, but at the same time, her left brain was denying what her body had done. In a way, this woman was a somatic intuitive like an ADD individual, because her body reacted immediately to an intuitive message. The body, as this whole book has been designed to show you, always does the right thing, and it always wins. But it can't stop the left hemisphere from denying the truth.

The husband of another friend of mine is probably alexithymic. I was at their house one evening watching the Howard Stern movie *Private Parts.* Whatever you may think of Howard Stern, this is actually a pretty funny movie. My friend's husband, Mark, wasn't in the room at first. Being hyperrational and hypermoral, he doesn't really approve of Howard Stern's humor. At some point in the early part of the film, though, he wandered in. "I don't hear anybody laughing," he said, and sat down. The movie hadn't actually yet hit its stride. But after a bit, it began to get quite funny. And soon Mark began to laugh. Within a few minutes, we were all laughing. But Mark was laughing the hardest. He was actually rocking in his seat from laughter at times. The next day, Mark and his wife were driving to work, and she asked, "What did you think of that movie we saw last night?" And Mark replied: "I thought it was pretty primitive. I didn't think it was funny at all." My friend couldn't believe it. She'd watched him guffaw, watched his body move, watched him shake with laughter. And now he was denying that any of it had ever happened! He was denying that he'd felt any emotions, even though the rest of us had seen him expressing them openly.

Both Mary (who turned the windshield wipers on when it wasn't raining) and Mark (laughing at Howard Stern) had unconnected intuition networks. They felt emotions in their bodies and heard signals from their brains, but they couldn't recognize them. Their left hemispheres are so strong, and so disconnected from the rest of the intuition network, that they simply deny the network's existence. People like this can walk around feeling upset, their faces looking like Mount Saint Helens about to erupt. But if you ask them if something's wrong or how they feel, they'll insist, "Oh, I'm fine. Nothing's wrong." Their bodies are telling you one thing, but their mouths tell you another. Conversely, they may tell you that their dog just died, their father broke a hip, they need two units of red cells because they're anemic, and they're about to be audited by the IRS, but they do it with a smile, as if they don't have a care in the world.

In fact, however, their condition can make life very painful for them. Because they are as disconnected from other people as they are from parts of their own intuition network, they tend to be hypermoral and hyperrational as well as obsessive and ruminative.[16] They often have a history of depression and personal difficulties, because they may have a joyful experience, but they can't take in the joy, because their left hemisphere denies its existence. They always feel somehow separate from others and the rest of the world, and even from their own experience. This is regrettable, because underneath, they tend to be extremely nice, loving people, with good hearts, but they can't connect with others.

Alexithymia is a difficult syndrome. These people really do have a particular challenge in getting in touch with their emotions, their bodies, and their intuition. It may be that they can do it only through others. First, they have to come to the realization that they are so disconnected that they feel bereft, and they need help. Then they can reach out to others to provide the connection to the intuition network, to be their prosthetic telephone wires. And then they need to be available for feedback. The only way they can take in the experience of the right hemisphere and the body is to have someone reflect it back. When they say, "That movie wasn't funny," they have to be able to hear someone tell them, "Well, my experience of it was that you were really laughing and enjoying it."

If you're in this category, you may find that people will frequently think you're in a mood that you don't feel you're in. People will say to you, "Wow, did something bad happen?" And you'll say, "No, I'm fine," thinking that they're nuts. But if you find that you're surrounded by a lot of nuts and you're the only kernel of truth, you may have to ask yourself, "Is it possible my left hemisphere is hogging the show? Is it becoming like the loud soprano in the chorus, not letting anyone else be heard?" Then you'll have to ask people, "What was my face like?" You're going to have to tell them your dreams and let them help you understand them. You'll probably have a lot of nightmares, because your soul will have to use a megaphone to get through to you. It's going to send you terrifying images to get you to smarten up and change. It'll be difficult, but you can change. You can learn, with the help of others, to understand what your body and your emotions are telling you if you're willing to listen.

LEFT BRAIN, RIGHT BRAIN

Most people don't have any striking syndromes or atypical brain organization. Most people in our culture, men as well as women, tend to be left hemisphere–dominant, with strong, well-developed frontal lobes. Left-hemisphere people, as you know, put all their faith in intellect. They are very rational, linear, well organized, and verbal. They're the librarians, the William Safires of the world, to whom precision of language is important. They may not look like a whole lot of fun, but, boy, do they know language. If they see a leaf falling from a tree, they can go into rhapsodies describing that leaf, its color, the way it's falling, the swirls and spirals and eddies it makes in the air. They'd compose an ode to that leaf, because that's how they think—very precisely, in great detail, with the feeling submerged in verbiage. A right-hemisphere person, by contrast, would look at that leaf and say, "Wow, what a leaf."

The right hemisphere, you'll recall, provides a feeling, an instinct, an impression, or a general outline of a thought or an image—the gestalt of a situation. Intuition tends to come to us initially through the right hemisphere and the temporal lobe. The left hemisphere is very detail-oriented and focused: it has to fill in the details of the intuition we're getting. If we were making a cookie, the right hemisphere would provide the cookie-cutter configuration, while the left hemisphere supplied the sprinkles on the icing. Or it would work like something I saw in the news after Mother Teresa died. One of her nuns in India made a huge mosaic of Mother Teresa's face on the grass. From a distance, you could see the outline of the nun's face and features; but when you went in closer, you realized that the details were created by thousands of individual flower petals. The two together, the outline and the individual flower petals, made the portrait distinctive. In the same way, it takes both the right hemisphere and the left hemisphere working together to make our intuition intelligible to us.

The daughter of a friend of mine is distinctly left hemisphere–dominant. Maggie could drive you crazy buttering toast. She will put a pat of butter on a knife and proceed to smooth it meticulously into every corner and crevice of the bread slice, as though it were essential for her to cover every single individual grain. I, on the other hand, will be more likely to seize a knife, spoon, or any other handy utensil, including a finger, and slather the butter randomly over the surface, usually missing about half the piece of toast and losing some of the butter on the table. I get the general outline, however, while Maggie's missed her school bus because she's perseverated over the details of buttering her bread. Perhaps it would take both of us—Maggie the left hemisphere, and Mona Lisa the right hemisphere—to butter the toast properly.

The same is true of intuition. Maggie wants to be an actress. She is actually excellent at memorizing lines, because she has great strength in left-hemisphere analysis. Similarly, she's a very good singer, because she's able to analyze music in a left-hemisphere way and sing with accurate pitch, hitting all the right notes. On the other hand, no one would accuse her of being Ella Fitzgerald and putting a lot of soul into her songs. This is true of her acting, too. So much of acting is imagination, imagining what it would be like to be another person, to stand inside another person's skin. In fact, it's a lot like doing an intuitive reading of another person. Imagination, like intuition, is in the right hemisphere. Maggie, however, has difficulty tapping into her imagination. For me, that's no problem. I can put myself in someone's body and try to perceive how that person is feeling. On the other hand, I couldn't memorize lines to save my life. Once again, it would take two of us to make a complete actress, someone to whom the skill came naturally, with ease and brilliance. To help her get in touch with her imagination and her intuition network fully, I usually take Maggie through the exercise of an intuitive reading to help her learn how to be more aware of her right hemisphere and how to make use of the information coming from it instead of allowing it to be continually censored by her left hemisphere and frontal lobe.

This is the problem for people who live too much in the left hemisphere. Their powerful frontal lobes are always telling them to ignore what's coming from the right hemisphere. As they drown out any input from the right brain and the temporal lobe, these frontal lobes repeat, "You don't know that. You can't know that. That can't be." They thus inhibit the input of emotion, intuition, and body connection from the right hemisphere. Consequently, left-brain people believe they're not intuitive. The fact is that they simply have determined their intuitive strengths and learned how to use them to help overcome and shore up their intuitive weaknesses. This is what you'll learn to do in the next chapter. Left-hemisphere people, for instance, tend to think very symbolically, and they may get strong intuition through dreams.

Right-hemisphere people, meanwhile, have their own weaknesses. They may get strong intuitive images, but they're all cookie-cutter configuration and no detail. A right hemisphere doing a reading of someone would be able mainly to describe a scene: "Oh, this person looks like a real mother. She's ethereal and dreamlike. She loves pastels. Her work involves gardening and flowers." This is nice pictorial information, but it's not very analytical. It doesn't give you a lot of content. It requires a left hemisphere to come in and say, "She's about 5 feet 5, her left eye points in, and boy, does she have a pain in her left wrist." The left hemisphere puts a name to what you see or hear intuitively or to the emotions that you're feeling. It tells you, "That person is depressed," or "that person is lonely." Someone who's all right brain tends to express his or her intuition too impressionistically. This doesn't give you anything to sink your teeth into. Asked to describe someone, a right hemisphere will say, "Well, that person's, uh, kind of wavy, and um, you know, um, I can't really put my finger on what's going on with him." As a result, nothing ever gets done, because nothing is ever named, noted, felt, and resolved. In that sense, the left hemisphere gets a bad rap as not being very intuitive, but its input is very significant.

Both the left hemisphere and the right hemisphere play an important role in intuition. Where people might have gifts in one versus the other, both are needed to make your intuition useful and available for you to act upon.

Whatever your intuitive identity, you can figure out a way to awaken your intuition network. In all of us some parts of the network are strong and others are weak. It's important for you to know your intuitive identity in order to recognize those strengths and weaknesses and to be able to decipher the language of your intuition when it speaks to you. This is not to say that we should all try to determine what particular disorders or deficits we have. You shouldn't just ask yourself, "Am I more like a space cadet (hypofrontal) or are my thoughts more like Ziploc bags (hyperfrontal)? Are all of my lines down? Do my brain parts seem to be disconnected from each other as well as from my body?" That's a negative approach to intuition. You would be looking only at the vulnerability side of your intuition. You need to take a more positive approach. You need to look at the power aspect of your intuition. We all have areas in which we're gifted intuitively and other areas that are dark and less accessible. If we learn to understand and use our gifts, we can shine a light on the darker parts of our intuition network and bring them into play for a chance at a healthier, richer, more intuitive life.

FOURTEEN

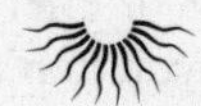

Your Intuitive Profile

When you first walk into a gym or health spa, the sight of the myriad machines and gizmos available to help you build your body and develop your muscles can be both bewildering and daunting. If you're like me, you're likely, at first, to gravitate toward the machines you find easier to use, because they work out parts of your body that are more developed. This makes sense, because it helps give you confidence and encouragement to keep working out. You might try some of the other machines later, but if you headed right for them in the beginning and found you could barely move them, your physical fitness career would probably be pretty short-lived. For my part, I don't have very good upper body strength, but I have strong legs, so I like to use the leg-building machines first. I'm trying to learn to use my arms more now, but if I had gone in using my arms alone, I might have been discouraged right away, felt like a failure, and quit.

This is exactly how it works with intuition. You'll find that you're already good at using some pieces of intuitive machinery. Other pieces, you won't want to try until later. If you go in determined to be a dream intuitive, but then find that you don't remember any of your dreams, you're bound to get frustrated pretty quickly. You may find there are parts you won't really be able to use at all, or very well. That's all right. Remember, we all have intuition, but we all have it differently, and the language it speaks to each of us is unique. Don't think that if you don't get intuition precisely the way I do, the way that an intuitive like Barbara Brennan does, or the way the person does who works in the cubicle next to yours, that you're not intuitive. Barbara Brennan's books are full of diagrams of chakras and energy fields and other images that I personally have never seen with my intuitive eyes. A lot of other intuitives speak in terms of chakras or energy fields as well. Some people see them, some people don't. If you don't see them, does that mean that you're not intuitive? No. It simply means that you have different muscles and your own language and mode of intuition.

MAPPING THE MUSCLES

When we look at an object, we all see it the same way: the light hits the retina of the eye, goes on to the optic chiasm, hits the visual cortex, and expresses the vision linearly across the surface of the brain. Physical vision follows the same distinct linear path in everyone. Intuition isn't processed this way. Intuition is more like passion. Everybody's experience of it is singular, not quite like anyone else's.

At the same time there are certain basic *types* of intuitives, which we discussed a bit in the first chapter. Some people are visual intuitives, receiving mental visual images. Some people are auditory intuitives; they hear thoughts, sounds, or messages that carry intuitive information. Some people are somatic intuitives, receiving somatosensory input, or body feelings about themselves or others. When people say to me, "I'm not intuitive. I can't see things," I ask them, "Then what do you hear?" or "What do you feel?" It's important to discover your own particular strength and to use the connections you do have instead of becoming blocked by the thought of the ones you don't have.

In getting in touch with their intuition network, people have to understand how they're *already using intuition,* perhaps in very subtle ways.[1] Once you recognize what you're already doing without being fully aware of it, you can work to build that muscle by exercising it more. I once gave a class on intuitive readings in which I had an interesting experience along these lines. One of the participants was a female surgeon at a large hospital who was obviously very left hemisphere–oriented, very rational and task-focused. She walked into the class and promptly announced: "I can't do this. I'm not going to be able to see bodies, I'm not going to hear sounds, I'm not going to be able to feel anything in my body about my patients. I don't have any dreams, and I'm not particularly intuitive. But I wanted to hear what you have to say." At which point I thought, "Well, at least her mind is still slightly ajar."

In the course of the class, it came out that this woman was already using her intuition in a very remarkable and singular way, even though she hadn't realized she was doing so. She told me that whenever she was on call in the hospital, getting some sleep in the doctors' lounge, she would unerringly wake up a few minutes before her beeper went off to summon her to attend to an urgent case. This happened every single time she had night duty. She had come to trust this instinct so much that as soon as she woke up she would automatically get up, get dressed, and start downstairs, not waiting for the beeper to go off, which it invariably did. I asked her *where* she felt this intuition. She said she didn't know; she just got a "gut feeling." She was clearly clairsentient, a somatic intuitive or body intuitive, which was a good thing, after all, since she was a surgeon who operated on bodies. She was getting a feeling in her body, and her body was responding and acting on it, the way my body responded to the woman having a heart attack in the ER. The important muscle in this surgeon's intuitive network seemed to be her stomach. It sent the signal to her body to start warming up to the task at hand, to get ready to move, like the cars in the old VW Rabbit commercials that would go up the ramp from zero to 60 mph in just a few seconds.

It was interesting that this surgeon acted on her intuition. The biggest problem most people have with getting in touch with their intuition is that even when they get a sense about something, they don't or won't act on it. I've talked throughout this book about the warning lights and buzzers we ignore until some vital piece of body machinery falls out. Not only are we opening ourselves up to problems, but when we fail to act on our intuitive hunches, we don't get reinforcement or reward for being intuitive. Such reinforcement helps bolster your confidence and keep you working on that muscle and developing it further. Acting on her intuition was really an important thing for the surgeon to do, not just for the sake of her intuition network but for the sake of her patients as well. If doctors don't act on their intuition—which means, as we know, acting without sufficient information—then patients could die. Because she had acted intuitively so many times, the other staff members had come to trust her intuition; they knew she always had an accurate sense of when something was going on that required attending to.

The surgeon, however, had never thought of her experiences on call as intuitive experiences. She had to be taught to pay attention to them in a new way before she could recognize their nature and their value and begin to build on them to develop more intuitive skills.

I was once interviewed by a network TV producer for a documentary on intuition. From the beginning of the telephone conversation, the woman sounded very closed off, and her voice was like cold steel. I felt she didn't like me and was very wary of me. She asked me to do a reading of her over the phone. I said no. I felt it would only reinforce her belief that I was like some sort of fantastical creature with horns. This in turn would only strengthen her sense that she and other "ordinary people" aren't intuitive and couldn't do what I do. Her voice became even more steely once it became clear that I wasn't going to give her something she wanted. Interestingly, her intuition began to communicate her discomfort with the fact that she wasn't getting what she wanted out of our interview. As I started instead to tell her about some other readings I had done, she suddenly began to make choking and coughing sounds. Excusing herself, she said she'd call me back later.

The next morning, when her call came, her voice was completely different—all the steel was gone. "I have to tell you what happened yesterday!" she said excitedly. "The moment I got on the phone with you, I started to feel pressure in my neck. My muscles started to tighten, and by the end of the conversation, I could barely breathe. When we hung up, the feeling went away." She hesitated a moment, then continued tentatively: "I have to ask you this. Do you have neck problems?"

It was amazing. This woman was clairsentient, a body intuitive who had picked up on my neck problems. In fact, I had just recently blown two disks in my neck—an incredibly painful experience. She was floored when I told her this. "So now you know, in your own body and soul, that intuition exists," I said to her. "Now you have a show." The woman agreed. "Yes, but I was afraid to tell you this," she said. And then she said something that I hear all the time: "I felt foolish."

How many times do people stop themselves from saying something they know to be true, from expressing their intuition, because they feel foolish? How often do you do it? That's the frontal lobe again, saying you can't possibly know what you think you know, and for goodness' sake, don't *say* it, because people will think you're crazy. In the intuition gym, while we're trying to build our intuitive muscle, we'll also try to reduce that frontal lobe a little bit. Look what wonderful things happen when the frontal lobe is even temporarily quieted. When the surgeon described above slept, her frontal lobe became unplugged from the intuition network. Consequently, when she got an intuition, her body was able to feel the impulse to jump up and select a motor routine that got her dressed and moving before her frontal lobe could fully wake up, plug back in, and tell her she shouldn't do that. Who knows how many patients were saved as a result?

Think about your own life. Do you have, or have you ever had, experiences like the women described above? Do you have vivid dreams, full of distinct and interpretable symbols? Do your dreams sometimes seem prescient? Have you ever had a feeling about someone that turned out to be true? Have you ever had a sense that you should do something, not done it, and then paid the price and kicked yourself for not acting on your gut instinct? If your answer to any of these questions is yes, then you know you have intuition. Now you need to pinpoint the area of the intuition network through which it reaches you most strongly.

To help you map the strengths and weaknesses of your intuition network, try the following. Take two felt markers, one black and one yellow. Turn to the diagram of the intuition network that follows. Now, thinking about your intuitive identity, go through and mark off the areas of your network that are strong and weak. With the black pen, put a big *X* on the area that doesn't work well for you, the muscles you're going to avoid for now in the gym. With the yellow pen, highlight the areas that are dominant in your intuition network. The following guide will help you:

- If you're a very left hemisphere–oriented person (think in words, usually right-handed, majored in English lit, liked courses that involved lots of reading and papers, love details, and probably can't draw to save your life), you'll cross out, with black, the right brain and probably the body. You'll highlight in yellow all of the left brain and, most likely, dreams. Left brain–dominant people are often particularly good at dreams. With their left hemispheres unplugged, they can get access to intuition that's symbolically represented in their dreams by images, including body images. This may mean you'll have to read a lot of books on interpreting dreams and delve into a lot of Jungian analysis, but that should be right up your alley. Keeping a journal will help you decode your dreams more accurately.

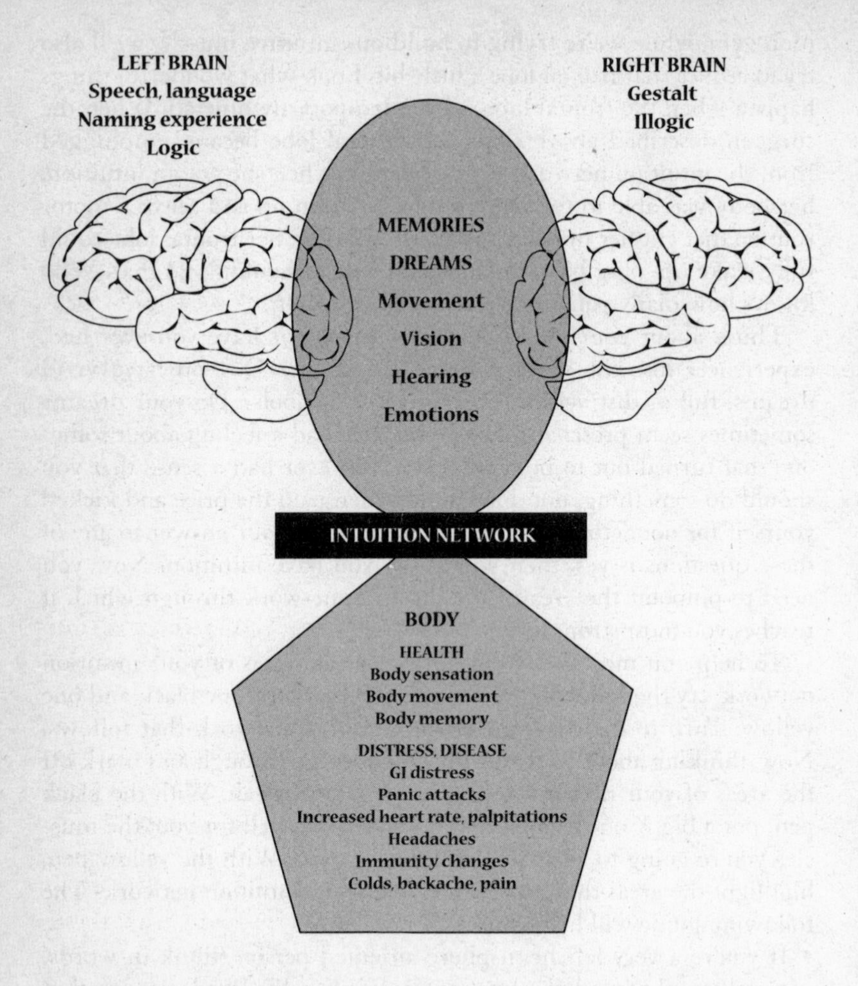

- If you're a right hemisphere–oriented person (think in pictures and images, could be either right- or left-handed or ambidextrous, avoided classes that required reading and writing papers, love art, hate structure), cross out the left brain. Highlight the right brain, the body, and dreams.
- If you're hypofrontal, like someone with ADD, who experiences things through movement and the body, cross out the left frontal lobe. Highlight the right brain and the body.
- If you're hyperfrontal, like someone with obsessive or compulsive qualities, cross out the right brain. Highlight the left frontal lobe and the body.

- If you're a young child, highlight the right brain.
- If you have PMS, highlight the right brain and the body.
- If you have lots of illnesses of any kind, highlight the body.
- If you've never had an orgasm, cross the body out.
- If you're a woman, highlight the connective areas between the left and right brain and between the right brain and the body.

Now you should have a diagram of your intuition network. You know the places into which you can probably go easily and the locations that are less accessible to you at present. With this map of your intuitive musculature in hand, you can embark on the process that will help you build on these areas of strength and then use that strength to help open up and build up your less developed areas. You can learn to do an intuitive reading.

THE INTUITIVE READING

To learn the language of each emotional center, you learn to listen to the little brain inside each one that speaks to you through its unique, emotional language of thoughts, and through its physical language of body symptoms and disease. It's easier to begin to pay attention to the physical language first. What are your specific physical symptoms? Do you have a specific disease or condition? In what part of your body does it reside? Do you have any frequent pains or complaints?

To begin to isolate where in your body and life your intuitive messages speak to you, go through the following summaries of the emotional centers and the symptoms or issues associated with them. Whenever you are reminded of a physical symptom that you have or have had, make a note of it in a notebook or journal. Remember that you need to pay attention to the area of your body where a symptom occurs—this is a part of your body-mind you will need to refer back to repeatedly for information and guidance. Explore the emotional issues associated with each emotional center and symptom to begin to read the life messages that your body-mind is trying to transmit to you in your own intuitive language.

FIRST EMOTIONAL CENTER
PHYSICAL BODY SUPPORT, BONES, JOINTS, SPINE, BLOOD, IMMUNITY

Look at the illustration of the first emotional center (page 141) and assess what imbalances of power or vulnerability you have with regard to:

1. **Trust.** The ability to know when to trust or to mistrust someone.

2. **Dependency.** Do you have a family that supports you? Can you depend on someone when appropriate but also stand on your own, independently, when necessary?

3. **Sense of safety in the world.** Do you feel the world is not a safe place? Do you feel helpless or fearful in general or in certain situations? Do you lack the capacity to cope or adapt to changes in your environment?

- Do you feel like The Lost Sheep (Lucy Graham, page 146), having lost contact with your family or homeland? Do you feel like Bambi (Vanessa, page 149), having lost members of your family? Do you believe that you are alone and don't belong to a truly supportive family of some kind?
- Are you similar to Mark, with all his Eggs in One Basket (page 155)? Is your social network of support limited to only a few close friends?
- Do you experience, like Martha and her son, the Ziploc Syndrome (page 161), believing that the world is basically an unsafe place and inescapably stressful?
- Do you find yourself frequently making statements like the following?

"You can't trust anyone but yourself." (Excessive mistrust)
"It's okay, I'll do it myself." (Excessive independence)
"If you want it done right, do it yourself." (Excessive independence)
"No one's ever there for me. No one cares." (Poor sense of belonging)
"No one's helping me here." (Excessive helplessness)
"The world is a dangerous place." (Excessive fearfulness)

Second Emotional Center
Uterus, Ovaries, Cervix, Vagina, Prostate, Testes, Bladder, Large Intestine, Rectal Areas, Lower Back

Turn to the illustration on page 169 and assess imbalances in power and vulnerability you have with regard to your personal drives. How do you go after what you want?

1. **Drives.** Do you go after what you want actively or passively? Directly or indirectly? Are you shameless or ashamed of your urges and desires?

2. **Relationships.** In relationships, do you tend to be excessively independent or dependent? Do you characteristically take more or give more? Are you overly assertive or submissive? Do you always protect others or do they always protect you?

- Are you like Marcy (The Rolling Stone Gathers No Moss, page 172), always driving relentlessly toward what you want in life?
- Are you similar to Harriet (Holding On for Dear Life, page 180)? Do you become so attached to or dependent on someone in a relationship that you can barely let go even when it is obvious that the relationship no longer serves you?
- Are you like Donna (The Golden Handcuff Syndrome, page 181), passively staying in a dead-end job because you are too frightened to figure out what else you could do or because you think you can't figure it out?
- Are you like Ruth (Relationship on Ice, page 187), who gives and gives to her partner but receives little in return?
- Are you like Sandra (The Praying Mantis Syndrome, page 190), having difficulty maintaining boundaries in a relationship?
- Are your experiences similar to Katrina's (Traumatic Memories, page 191)? Have you experienced traumatic sexual relationships or physical or emotional abuse?
- Are you like George (Rooster without a Henhouse, page 193), who lost everything in love and money? Have you ever suffered a reversal of fortune in relationships and work?
- Do you find yourself making statements like the following?

"I'll do anything for you." (Excessive giving)
"I can have it all." (Excessive independence)

"No one will ever love me. Everyone always leaves me." (Excessive dependence)

THIRD EMOTIONAL CENTER
ABDOMEN, MIDDLE DIGESTIVE TRACT, LIVER, GALLBLADDER, KIDNEYS, SPLEEN, MIDDLE SPINE

Take a look at the illustration of the third emotional center on page 199 and assess imbalances in power and vulnerability that you may have with regard to:

1. **Adequacy.** Do you feel competent and skilled in what you do for work in the world or are you constantly plagued with feelings of inadequacy and incompetence?

2. **Responsibility.** In work and in relationships, are you hyperresponsible? Are you irresponsible? Do you often find yourself caught in the middle in an argument between two friends, family members, or colleagues?

3. **Aggression.** Do you have frequent issues about territoriality? Do you often get involved in turf wars? Do you use intimidation to get what you want or are you easily intimidated by others?

4. **Competition.** In competitive situations, do you always have to win? Are you always losing or conceding points?

- Are you like Peter (The Corporate Takeover, page 198), who is always aggressively competing with others, whose main source of responsibility and feeling good about himself is conquering others in the business place?
- Like Marshall (You're on My Turf, page 205), do you have difficulties with territoriality at work? Do you base your self-esteem on the approval of others?
- Are you like Felicia (Caught in the Middle, page 208), always feeling it's your responsibility to settle conflicts, always putting out fires at home or at work?
- Do you share with Maureen (Drowning Her Sorrows, page 211) or Andrea (Food Is Love, page 212) an addiction to alcohol, food, or work to cover up emotions, especially feelings of inadequacy over responsibilities?

FOURTH EMOTIONAL CENTER
HEART, BLOOD VESSELS, LUNGS, BREASTS

Turn to the illustration on page 218 and assess imbalances in power and vulnerability that you may have with regard to emotional expression and partnerships. In relationships, are you able to experience a full range of emotional expression? Are you able to cycle freely in and out of passion, love, anger, resentment, courage, anxiety, grief, abandonment, and forgiveness? Or do you tend to get stuck in one emotion? In partnerships, can you balance isolation and being alone with intimacy? Do you nurture others more than they nurture you?

- Are you like Mike (The Great Imposter, page 221), Frances (Carrying a Grudge, page 227), or Fred (A Rock Feels No Pain, page 232), who are not able to experience, express, or resolve a full range of emotions?
- Perhaps, like Violet (The Smothered Sparrow, page 236), you are in a relationship that is uneven, where one person is always the giver and the other always the taker? Does one partner have more authority than the other?
- Are you like Samantha (The Ambivalent Mother, page 241) or Helen (No Way Out, page 248)? Do you have extreme, life-long ambivalence about being a parent and immense insecurity about your capacity to nurture another individual? Are you prone to self-sacrifice and martyrdom?

FIFTH EMOTIONAL CENTER
NECK PAIN, THYROID PROBLEMS, TEETH AND GUMS

Take a look at the illustration on page 253 and assess imbalances in power and vulnerability that you may have with regard to communication (speaking and listening), timing (pushing forward or a holding back), or willfulness.

- Are you like Cecilia ("Hello, I'm on the Air, Can Anybody Hear Me?," page 254), who has difficulty expressing who she is in the world? Are you unable to exert your will or assert yourself at work and in relationships?
- Are you like Liz (Swallowing Her Anger, page 262)—afraid to

express your desires and needs? Do you feel that people don't hear your point of view?

- Like Ellen (Forging Ahead, page 268), do you have difficulty with timing—knowing when to push forward or when to wait to express yourself?

SIXTH EMOTIONAL CENTER
BRAIN, EYES, EARS, NOSE

Turn to the illustration on page 275 and assess imbalances in power and vulnerability that you may have with regard to perception, thought, or morality. Do you always need to be focused or do you always end up being unfocused in your thinking and activities? Are you excessively receptive or unreceptive? Are you overly rational? Are you overly rigid or overly flexible? Do you tend to be critical? Can you accept criticism? Are you overly cautious or can you throw caution to the wind when appropriate?

- Perhaps, like Otis ("I Can't Hear This," page 276), you have had difficulty being receptive to others' perspectives.
- Are you similar to Paula (Citizen of the Year, page 281), sometimes overly moralistic and somewhat rigid in your views?

SEVENTH EMOTIONAL CENTER
GENETIC DISORDERS, LIFE-THREATENING ILLNESS, MULTIPLE ORGANS INVOLVED IN ANY CONDITION

Look at the illustration on page 294 and assess imbalances in power and vulnerability that you may have with regard to your purpose in life. Do you know why you are on the earth? What is your authentic work or true calling? Do you believe that you alone create your life or that you submit to life as it occurs to you? Can you balance your attachment to the fruits of your labors with a healthy detachment and an attitude of blessing?

- Are you like Shirley (My Life as an Invalid, page 295), who has never known what her purpose in life is?
- Are you like Irma (The Stand-by-Your-Man Syndrome, page 299), whose only purpose for living was to exist for and through her husband and son?

Remember, if you have a body, a right brain, a left brain, and you dream at night, you are intuitive. Your body expresses the symptom, your right brain attaches emotion or meaning, and your left brain puts the emotion into words and analyzes it. Your dreams may present you with images, sights, or sounds relating to the health or disease of the organs in your body.

Let me stress once again that *you can do an intuitive reading.* You can read your own and others' bodies.

Don't let your frontal lobe tell you you can't. Don't let it elbow out all the other parts of your intuition network and take center stage. You'll learn how to quiet your frontal lobe in a moment, but first look at the intuitive data practice sheet on the following page. This will guide you through the intuitive reading process. You've figured out your intuitive identity and highlighted the strong muscles of your intuition network. Those strong areas should correspond to one or more of the boxes on this chart. In these boxes you'll write down anything and everything that comes to you about the person you're reading. It's important to write everything down, whether it makes sense or not, because every piece of information is potentially valuable.

When I conduct intuition workshops, I have people pair off with a partner. This helps people integrate their various strengths and come up with a more complete reading in the early stages, when their muscles still need developing. Partner A gives partner B the name and age of a real person. Then, as partner B begins to recount whatever thoughts or sensations or emotions come to him or her, partner A records them on the intuitive data practice sheet.

Very often the best way to start is to perform a visualization or relaxation exercise. In my workshops I usually hire someone to conduct a special visualization exercise, conducting the attendees down an imaginary road through a tranquil landscape and relaxing you so that your frontal lobe quiets down and recedes from center stage. Most people think you have to sit in a chair and calm down—get in the mood, so to speak—before you can do a reading. Actually, sitting in a chair and calming down are not in my repertoire. I don't need to set a special mood to do a reading. But most people, with their big frontal lobes, need this to unplug those censors. I work with a lot of physicians, who are, as a group, among the most left hemisphere–oriented, rational, organized people you could ever hope to meet, with powerful frontal lobes telling them that they can't do this. If you're the kind of person who ruminates a lot, has insomnia at night, the chances are you're somewhat hyperfrontal, too, and have a gerbil wheel in the

Intuitive Data Practice				
Client	Intuitive Data			
	Auditory and Visual	Body Sense	Emotion	Dream/Other

front of your head. So you will have to do something to stop it for a while. At home you can use a relaxation tape to calm you down, mute your frontal lobe, and put you in the mood for the reading.

Once you've begun the reading, tell your partner everything that comes to you. You might hear words; write them down. You might see the person or aspects of his or her life. You might see a bicycle. You won't understand what that is, but write it down. You might get a feeling in your body. You might be overcome by an emotion; perhaps you feel dread or worry or euphoria. Maybe you find yourself thinking, "This person makes me so angry that I want to bash him and leave him by the side of the road!" Write it down. You might get an image of a television show or a movie. Write it down. Everything is data; later you'll figure out the language that your intuition is using and what it's imparting to you. If you get nothing, write that down as well. Nothing can be information, too. Above all, don't feel foolish.

It's vital that you stay in the flow and that you don't judge what comes to you. This is where you need to exercise what I like to call windshield-wiper cognition. If you're very frontal, your mind may start to roam and try to distract you. You may notice that your pen is running out of ink, that you need more paper, or that there's no ice in your water. That's your frontal lobe trying to squelch the fear you feel at performing this reading. In workshops I always know when people are fearful, because they (or their left brain frontal lobes) start asking me very specific questions: Do you have to have the full name or will just a first name do? Married or maiden name? What if the person changed his or her name to Cloud or Sunshine? Will that work? What if the person is adopted? Does being an identical twin confuse the issue? And so on. Or they fixate on how I do readings over the phone, asking me what kind of phone I use. Is it cordless? Can you do a reading from a cellular phone? Forget all that. When distracting thoughts like these come to you, turn on your mental windshield wiper and just imagine it pushing all these concerns aside. Say to your left hemisphere and frontal lobe, "Thank you for sharing that. Now let's get back to the task at hand."

After you've finished, you and your partner will go over the information that you've recorded and decipher the symbols and images you've picked up. At this point, you'll also have to determine what images or sensations came from the life of the person you were reading and which came from your own life. If you felt tremendous rage, was it related to the person you were reading? Or were you suddenly reminded of that tax bill you recently received?

To give you an idea of what you might get in a reading, depending upon your intuitive strengths and weaknesses, let's look at some sample readings done by four different people with four different areas of intuitive strength. Each reader was given a name, age, and location: Mary, thirty-eight, of York, Maine. Here are their readings:

1. **Right hemisphere–dominant individual.** "Wow, it's like putting my finger in an electric socket. I feel all this electricity. She runs all over the place all the time. Why do I want to go shopping? Let's go to the mall!"

2. **Individual with ADD.** "Oh, she reminds me of when I was four years old, and I had really blond hair, and I was always at the Y in the pool. Boy, has she got blond hair, wow, the blond hair, it's like, it reminds me of bleach. Oh, you know, that reminds me, I've got to clean my kitchen floor, it's so dirty, you know what it's like when those workmen come in and they track mud all over the place, and— What was I saying? Oh, yes, Mary, okay. So maybe the blond hair, I'm not

sure. But, boy, is she— Why am I thinking of the shopping network on TV? Oh, you know, just the other day they were selling these dolls from Afghanistan. Hold on a second, I've got to write that down. So what were we talking about? Oh, Mary. Oh, yeah, the shopping network. What is it about the shopping network? So I think she has a little boy. Why do I see a little boy in the Y pool? She has a little boy in the Y pool. Oh, wow, does this burn your nose...."

3. **Left hemisphere–dominant individual.** "I can't do this." So you ask him to take the name and go home and get a good night's sleep and write down anything he dreams. The next day he comes back with this report, typed neatly, single-spaced, and placed in a binder with metal clips: "I had the most remarkable dream. It was mythical, something about a Greek myth, or a Grecian urn, and a woman like one of those goddesses on the urns, with flaxen hair. And she had a beautiful, perfect life, with everything in its place and absolutely wonderful. And then the dream shifted. I was sitting at work—I'm a librarian, you know—and people would come up to my desk and ask me where a particular book was. I'd tell them it was on the second shelf in the fourth row, and they'd look at me and ask, 'Why?' [Y] Everyone who came up to me asked me 'Why?' This bothered me tremendously."

4. **A body intuitive.** "Oh, my hands and arms feel so tense. Very tense. Why am I thinking about cranberry juice? I just want to drink cranberry juice. Why am I drinking cranberry juice? I don't know. I can't focus, can't focus at all. All I want to do is move around, move around, move around. It reminds me of going shopping at the mall when everyone's there on Christmas Eve and there's such a rush. Why am I thinking of that blond actress, what's her name, the one who was in *French Kiss*—Meg Ryan?"

Who is Mary, thirty-eight, of York, Maine? She's a woman with bleached blond hair who works at the YMCA teaching young children to swim. In her private life, Mary wants to be Martha Stewart. She wants everything in her life and her house to be and look perfect, in a Martha Stewart way. Mary has a shopping addiction. There's a bumper sticker on her car that says, "When the going gets tough, the tough go shopping." And she suffers from repeated bladder infections, for which her alternative physician gives her cranberry juice.

Each of these people did a correct reading of Mary Brown. Each one hit on elements of the truth. Yet taking each of their readings separately, you might not be able to understand it, the symbolism in it, or who Mary was. The left-hemisphere person's dream of people running around asking "Why?" may not be immediately recognizable as a symbol for the Y in Mary's life. The ADD person needs to be constantly redirected to the subject at hand. There are a lot of irrelevant references in her reading, to Afghan dolls and dirty kitchen floors.

All of these people would have to work at understanding the particular symbolism in their reading and figuring out the language in which their intuition comes to them. As they become better and better acquainted with that language, they'll find it easier and easier to decipher their readings, and they may find that the readings flow more easily. This isn't any different from working out a muscle in a gym. Or think of it as practicing the piano. If you perform your finger exercises over and over, you not only strengthen the muscles in your hands, you also wear a kind of groove in your brain that automatically conducts the necessary signals to your fingers that direct them to play accurately and with more polish.

I know this works, because I've seen it happen time and time again at conferences and workshops. At most workshops I've held, nearly everyone in the room comes up with something in a reading. Occasionally I even get a real stunner, which confirms for me, once again and incontrovertibly, that all of us have access to intuition if we only learn to listen to it.

Not long ago I conducted a workshop at which one of the participating physicians and her partner came up to the stage. After a visualization exercise, the partner gave this physician the name of a two-year-old girl. As we all watched, the physician suddenly changed in her appearance, adopting the seating posture and mannerisms of a two-year-old child. She began to twirl her hair, and her feet turned inward. You could almost see her wearing patent leather Mary Janes. Then she began to speak, and her voice was that of a toddler. "I'm here in the doctor's office, and my mommy and daddy are talking to the doctor," she said. "They're very worried. I'm having a hard time breathing"—at this point, her breathing actually became labored—"and it's been going on for a long time, and I'm getting tired. They put a plastic worm in my heart. But I'm getting ready to pass [die], and it's gonna be okay. My mommy and daddy don't want me to pass to the other side, but it's okay. I feel pretty good about it. I figure I can play wherever I am."

The whole room was stunned. We had just watched something truly astonishing. The little girl the physician had just read was a child with cystic fibrosis. She had recently had an artificial pulmonary artery placed in her heart. This is a tubelike device, which the physician decoded using a description a child would use: she saw it as a worm. The physician gave a strongly accurate description of the child's physical ailment. But what was most significant and extraordinary about this reading was the way the physician went straight to the heart of the matter, to the salient issue involved—the emotional ambience of the child's life and condition.

This woman had never done a reading before. Yet she was obviously an amazing, exceptional intuitive. She was truly able to put herself inside another person's body and not only adopt that person's mannerisms and gestures but also imagine how that person would think and feel. She really could have had a marvelous career as an actress.

This particular experience was so moving to me that it actually brought tears to my eyes. Seeing someone get so thoroughly in touch with her intuition network is tremendously fulfilling. While not everyone demonstrates such exceptional gifts from the outset, it's always exciting to me when people in my classes find that they can indeed "get" something when they attempt a reading. Usually, everyone in the room has some success. And afterward people come up to me and say, "Wow, I can do this! I really believe in intuition now!"

Occasionally one or two people do not succeed at a reading. Yet I've found that they *are* in fact getting something, receiving some kind of information. It just happens that what they're getting isn't directly related to the matter at hand. It is actually useful information; it's just not useful at that particular time. In one class a woman complained that she simply wasn't having any success with a reading. Nothing was coming to her. "I don't see anything, I don't hear anything, I don't feel anything," she said. "Nothing." She felt left out, shorn from the bunch. It was a difficult situation, and I felt sorry for her.

Then she looked at me. "But you know," she said, "I do worry about you." She commented on how, despite all my spine problems, I was running around the room and tripping on microphone cords. "I'm afraid you're going to fall and get hurt," she said.

My response to this was to become defensive. After all, *I* was the medical intuitive and the instructor in the room. I didn't like feeling vulnerable and being told about *my* problems. I was supposed to do that for other people. Whenever I feel vulnerable, I tend to spout data, so I assured the woman that studies on people with back problems showed that walking confidently and quickly tended to reduce the risk of reinjury. She just gave me a look. "I think you're going to get hurt," she repeated, shaking her head.

Two weeks later I arrived at my home to find an upsetting letter in the mail. I was looking at it when the telephone rang. I dropped the letter and set off for the phone. Along the way, I stepped on a set of keys I'd let fall to the floor—and broke my foot.

I now have a picture of me in a foot cast that I display at lectures. That incident taught me a valuable lesson. The woman in that class, far from being the failure she felt herself to be, was actually a very insightful intuitive. Instead of reading the person she'd been assigned to read, however, *she was reading me!* The trouble was that I was too defensive, and my left hemisphere leaped up to deny the woman's intuition. I should have been tabulating it on a data sheet instead.

This is why it's so important that you take note of *any* information that comes to you in a reading. You'll have to sort out what's intuition and what's projection, what has to do with your own life and what is related to the other person's. Some of the information you get may not seem relevant at the time, but it may have value in the future. Take note of it all.

Remember that hearing your intuition really requires little more than simply *paying attention,* even to seemingly random, insignificant, irrelevant thoughts, ideas, sensations, and emotions. Intuition comes to us from unexpected sources at unexpected times. Choosing to hear it or choosing to ignore it can make the difference between health and disease, happiness and unhappiness, a richer or an emptier life.

LANGUAGE LESSONS

Very often the intuitive muscle you develop most fully is related not only to your intuitive identity but also to your occupational identity. Or you may have a kind of intuition that expresses itself in terms of a particular hobby or interest in your life. Your intuition takes on a very specific language from your life, expressing itself in terms that are intrinsic and individual to you. Learning to pay attention to this kind of intuition, if it operates in your life, can help you appreciate the intuitive gifts you possess and work on developing your intuition further.

Intuitive identity frequently helps to determine a person's occupation. I've observed, for instance, that many psychiatrists are left-handed, which sometimes means that they're right hemisphere–dominant. This means they're more readily in touch with their intuition. Since intuition and the ability to read people is a very useful tool in psychiatry, it makes sense that people with this capacity should be drawn to a career in psychiatry.

But while a certain type of brain organization or intuitive identity may draw a person to a specific field, it also happens that a chosen field of endeavor or occupation can then help to predispose a person to develop intuition in a certain area. In other words, a given job or profession can help you develop strong intuitive muscle in that field. Some people are business intuitives. Others are forensic intuitives, people who know where the body's buried. We talked earlier about nurses and how heeding their intuition helped set some nurses above the average in their profession. I know a woman who's a brilliant fund-raiser and obviously has a strong intuitive capacity for her work. She told me a story once about calling a major donor to solicit funds for a project. She succeeded, as usual, in eliciting a large pledge from him and ended their conversation with a sense of accomplishment. Yet no sooner had she put the phone down than she had an overwhelming urge to call the donor back and ask for more money. After a few moments she gave in to the feeling, placed another call to the man, and asked him for an additional contribution. Can you imagine what had happened in the five minutes between their conversations? The donor had received news of a windfall for his company. Feeling in a generous mood, he immediately pledged another large sum of money to the fund-raiser's cause!

Another woman I know, an executive in a publishing company, got in touch with her intuition by doing "readings" on promotional materials for various projects. Looking at one package, she said that it should be like "*Life* magazine after President Kennedy died." Based on that intuitive vision, she went on to design the layout, color package, and emotional tone of the publication in question and to issue it with confidence that it would be successful. And it was.

Think about your own life. Is there an area or a field for which you have an affinity? Do you tend to think in terms of certain kinds of symbols? I have a friend whom I'd call a movie intuitive. When she gets intuitive hits, they come to her in terms of movies and movie symbols. I asked her to try to read someone in my apartment building. She immediately said, "He reminds me of Norman in *On Golden Pond.*" Using movie symbols, she was describing someone who's dementing. In fact, the person I had asked her about did have memory problems.

I know a pediatrician who hates his work but loves to draw and do cartooning in his spare time. By day, he appeared to be a typical left-brained physician. I tried to get him to do a reading on someone, and he kept coming up blank. He couldn't see, hear, or feel anything, he said. Finally I handed him a pen and a pad of paper and said, "Maybe you could draw something." He immediately began to draw a tall man with curly hair, standing on the beach with a German shepherd at his side. The man I had asked him to read was tall, curly-haired, lived on the beach, and had a German shepherd. Moreover, the physician had gone into exquisite detail on the dog, even more so than on the man. This inclined me to think he was probably in the wrong profession. I believed he could have been a wonderful veterinary intuitive, working with animals. Or perhaps he could have been a forensic intuitive, drawing artist's sketches for law enforcement organizations.

The most notable aspect of his reading, however, was that he was able to demonstrate exceptional intuitive gifts even though he couldn't talk about them. His intuition was visual, right-brain. But the connection between his right brain and his left brain was evidently clipped, so he couldn't give a name to what he saw. That didn't mean that he didn't have intuition. He simply had to learn the language his intuition spoke. In his case, it spoke the language of drawings.

Once again, the key is to focus in on the intuition you do have, to pay attention to ways that you may be using it in your life, in your profession, in your interests, in your dreams, in ways of which you aren't presently aware. If you can do this, you can use that knowledge and build on this muscle to provide a foundation for strengthening other muscles of your intuition network.

WAKING UP TO YOUR INTUITION

We all make good decisions every day based on inadequate facts. That's using intuition. At this point, I know no other way of living than by using my intuition. When I walk around my house, I know when the phone is about to ring; a lot of times I even know who it is. So I know when I want to pick it up and when to let the answering machine get it. Sometimes I can even tell about the caller by the way the phone rings. When an old friend of mine is having an argument with her husband, I know it because I get a headache. I know when the argument is over, because suddenly the headache goes away! I know just the right amount of time to wait before I call her. A mother knows the same about her daughter or her son, so I bet you have had similar experiences.

Finally, I know when the patients on my schedule are going to be particularly difficult, because my body feels as if a storm is coming. You probably have had the same experience on the way to work—a feeling that tells you absolutely that you are going to have a bad day. Intuition is like an internal pilot telling you that turbulence lies ahead, so fasten your seat belt and make the necessary mental and physical adjustments. Intuition provides us with direction in our lives. It is a key point on an internal compass. Living without intuition is like living without the east point on your compass. Can you imagine traveling in life without ever going east? You could go in only three out of four possible directions, only north, west, or south.

While I know now how my body talks to me through health, symptoms, or disease, I still get feedback from other people, who often notice my symptoms before I do and tell me.

"Mona Lisa, did you realize you were asleep during the first two acts of the play tonight? Are you worried about a work deadline or something?"

"Mona Lisa, does your neck hurt? You're walking funny. Are you still worried about that job offer?"

"Mona Lisa, do you have bronchitis again? You must be getting ready to give a talk soon."

My friends always remind me that the emperor has no clothes. Ask your friends to do the same for you. Input from people who care for you about the symptoms in your body can help you trace them back to the emotions that are associated with the symptoms.

Health or disease, happiness or dissatisfaction, pleasure or pain: the degree to which we experience each of these depends upon the choices we make in each moment whether or not to heed the messages that are continuously broadcast through our intuition network. This network tells us what is right and wrong in our lives. It tells us what we need to change and where we need to make adjustments.

My friends make fun of me because the TV is always on at a low volume in my home. I find the background noise soothing. The intuition network exists within all of us, like a television that is always on. Whatever your source of intuition, be it your body, your right or left brain, or your dreams, there is always a transmitter buzzing with information within you. Tune in to your unique intuitive network.You have various ways to change stations until you find the clearest signal, where you can turn the volume up or adjust your reception as needed.

Notes

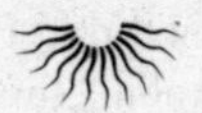

One. The Commonest Sense

1. M. R. Westcott, *The Psychology of Intuition* (New York: Holt, Rhinehart, 1968); U.S. Department of Health, Education and Welfare, M. R. Westcott, *Antecedents and Consequences of Intuitive Thinking, Final Report* (Poughkeepsie, N.Y.: Vassar College, 1968).

2. B. D. Schraeder and K. K. Fischer, "Using Intuitive Knowledge to Make Clinical Decisions," *Am. J. Mat. Child Nursing* 11 (1986): 161–62; J. E. Bogan, "The Other Side of the Brain. II. Appositional Mind," *Bull. L. A. Societies* 34 (1969): 135–62; A. Baldwin, "The Development of Intuition," *Learning about Learning* 6 (1966): 84–92; B. Fallik and J. Eliot, "Intuition, Cognitive Style, and Hemispheric Processing," *Perceptual Motor Skills* 60 (1985): 683–97; J. Levy-Agresti, "Cerebral Asymmetry and the Psychology of Man," in M. C. Wittrock, ed., *Brain and Psychology* (New York: Academic Press, 1980), 295–321; I. Page, "Science, Intuition and Medical Practice," *Post Graduate Medicine* 64, no. 5 (1978): 217–21; L. Rew, "Intuition: Concept Analysis of a Group Phenomenon," *Adv. Nursing Sciences* 8, no. 2 (1986): 21–28; R. B. Fuller, *Intuition* (San Luis Obispo, Calif.: Impact, 1983); R. Assagioli, *The Act of Will* (New York: Penguin, 1976).

3. S. P. Gott, "Technical Intuition in System Diagnosis or Accessing the Libraries of the Mind," *Aviat. Space Environ. Med.* 59, no. 11 (1988) suppl.: A59–A64.

4. P. Brenner and C. Tanner, "How Expert Nurses Use Intuition," *Am. J. Nursing* (Jan. 1987): 23–31; B. D. Schraeder and K. K. Fischer, "Using Intuitive Knowledge in the Neonatal Intensive Care Nursery," *Holistic Nurse Practice* 1 (1987): 45; H. Dreyfus and S. Dreyfus, *Mind over Machine: The Power of Intuition and Expertise in the Era of the Computer* (New York: Free Press, 1985).

5. R. Sheldrake, *A New Science of Life: The Hypothesis of Formative Causation* (Boston: Houghton Mifflin; Los Angeles: Tarcher, 1981); C. J. Jung, *The Portable Jung,* R. F. C. Hall, trans. (New York: Penguin, 1971), 223–25, 261–67; Jung, *Psychological Types* (New York: Harcourt Brace, 1923); Jung, *Analytical Psychology: Theory and Practice* (New York: Pantheon Press, 1964).

6. R. A. Coster and J. C. Aplin, "Intuition and Decision Making: Some Empirical Evidence," *Psychol. Rep.* 51 (1982): 275–81; D. Kahnemann and A. Tuersky, "On the Study of Statistical Intuitions," *Cognitions* 11 (1982): 123–41; S. Ostrander and L. Schroeder, *Superlearning* (New York: Dell, 1979).

7. H. R. Jacobs, "Intuition, the Welcome Stranger," *Perspectives in Biology and Medicine* 24, no. 3 (1981): 457–66; R. Davis-Floyd, "Intuition as Authoritative Knowledge in Midwifery and Homebirth," in R. Davis-Floyd and Carolyn Sargent, eds., *Childbirth and Authoritative Knowledge: Cross-Cultural Perspectives* (Berkeley: University of California Press).

8. J. Salk, *Anatomy of Reality, Merging Intuition and Reason* (New York: Columbia Univ. Press, 1983).

9. T. Bastick, *Intuition: How We Think, How We Act* (New York: Wiley, 1982).

10. T. Sugrue, *Edgar Cayce: There Is a River* (Virginia Beach: A. R. E. Press; New York: Holt, Rinehart, 1973).

TWO. WHEN THE GODS COME CALLING

1. Aristotle, "De Somniis" and "De Divinatione per Somnum," in W. S. Hett, trans., *On the Soul* (London: Loeb Classical Library, 1935); Hippocrates, in W. H. S. Jones, trans., *Ancient Medicine and Regimen,* vols. 1 and 4 (London and New York: Loeb Classical Library, 1923); L. Strümpell, *Die Natur und Enstehung der Traume* (Leipzig, 1877), 107; J. A. Hobson, *The Dreaming Brain* (New York: Basic Books, 1988).

2. S. Freud, *The Interpretation of Dreams,* standard ed., vol. 4, J. Strachey, trans. (New York: AVM, 1965).

3. A. Rechtschlaffen, "The Singlemindedness and Isolation of Dreams," *Sleep* 1 (1978): 97–109; H. W. Gordon et al., "Shift in Cognitive Asymmetrics between Waking from REM and NREM Sleep," *Neuropsychologica* 20, no. 1 (1982): 99–103; M. J. West-Eberhard, "Adaptation: Current Usages," in E. F. Keller and E. Lloyd, eds., *Keywords in Evolutionary Biology* (Cambridge, Mass.: Harvard Univ. Press, 1992), 7–18; O. Flanagan, "Deconstructing Dreams: The Spandrels of Sleep," in S. R. Hameroff, ed., *Toward a Science of Consciousness* (Cambridge, Mass.: MIT Press, 1996), 67–88; F. Crick and G. Mitchison, "The

Function of Dream Sleep," *Nature* 304 (1983), 111–14; P. Garfield, *The Healing Power of Dreams* (New York: Simon & Schuster, 1991), 108–9; J. M. Calvo et al., "The Role of the Temporal Lobe Amygdala in Pontogeniculo-occipital Activity and Sleep Organization in Cats," *Brain Res.* 403 (1987): 22–30; C. Smith, "Sleep States and Memory Processes," *Behav. Brain Res.* 69 (1995): 137–45.

4. A. Maeder, "The Dream Problem," *Nerv. Ment. Dis. Monograph,* series 22 (1916); E. A. Erikson, "The Dream Specimen of Psychoanalysis," *J. Am. Psychoanal. Assoc.* 2 (1954): 5–56; T. M. French and E. Fromm, *Dream Interpretation: A New Approach* (New York: Basic Books, 1964).

5. P. Maquet et al., "Functional Neuroanatomy of Human REM Sleep and Dreaming," *Nature* 383 (1996): 163–66.

6. A. Lehrman, *Aberglaube und Zanberei von der Ältesten Zeiten bis die Gengenwart* (Stuttgart: 1908).

7. F. Seafield, *The Literature and Curiosities of Dreams,* 4th ed. (London: Lockwood, 1869), 270–71.

8. Van de Castle published an excellent book on prodromal dreams and the function of dreams in creating health. R. Van de Castle, *Our Dreaming Mind* (New York: Ballantine, 1994), 364–69; P. M. Simon, *Le Monde des Rêves* (Paris: 1888); K. A. Scherner, *Das Leben des Traumes* (Berlin: 1861); A. Krauss, "Der Sinn in Wahnsinn," *Allg. Z. Psychol.* 15 (1859): 617; J. Volkelt, *Die Traume Phantasie* (Stuttgart: 1875); P. Tissié, *Les Rêves: Physiologie et Pathologie* (Paris: 1898); P. Tissié, "Les Rêves: Rêves Pathogènes et Therapeutiques," *Journ. Méd. Bordeaux* 36 (1898): 293–320; E. Hartmann, *The Biology of Dreaming* (Springfield, Ill.: Charles C. Thomas, 1967), 116; E. G. Mitchell, "The Physiological Diagnostic Dream," *N.Y. Med. Journal & Med. Record* (Oct. 3, 1923), 416–17; D. E. Schneider, "Dreams of Flying and Dreams of Weightlessness," *J. Hillside Hospital* 9, no. 3 (1960): 171; A Ziegler, "A Cardiac Infarction and a Dream as Synchronous Events," *J. Analytical Psychology* 7 (1962): 142–43.

9. A. Schopenhauer, "Essay V: Versuch über des Geisterschein und was damit Zusammenhängt," *Parerga und Paralipomena,* 2d ed., vol 1 (Berlin: 1862), p. 213, cited in S. Freud, *The Interpretation of Dreams,* standard ed., vol. 4, J. Strachey, trans. (New York: AVM, 1965).

10. C. Winget and F. T. Kapp, "The Relationship of the Manifest Content of Dreams to Duration of Childbirth in Primaparae," *Psychosom. Med.* 34 (1972): 313–20; H. Deutsch, *The Psychology of Women,* vol. 2 (New York: Grune & Stratton, 1945), 126–201, 202–58.

11. R. C. Van de Castle and P. Kinder, *The Content Analysis of Dreams* (New York: Appleton-Century-Crofts, 1966); R. C. Van de Castle, "Dream Content during Pregnancy," *Psychophysiology* 4 (1968): 375.

12. R. A. Lockhart, "Cancer in Myth and Dream: An Exploration into the Archetypal Relation between Dreams and Disease," *Spring* 1 (1977): 1–26.

13. B. Siegel, *Peace, Love, and Healing* (New York: Harper & Row, 1989), 64–65.

14. D. Schneider, *Revolution in the Body-Mind. I. Forewarning Cancer*

Dreams and the Bioplasma Concept (East Hampton, N.Y.: Alexa Press, 1976); L. H. Bartmeier, "Illness Following Dreams," *Int. J. Psychoanal.* 31 (1950): 8.

15. H. Warnes and A. Finkelstein, "Dreams That Precede a Psychosomatic Illness," *Canad. Psychiatr. Association J.* 16 (1971): 317–25.

16. V. N. Kasatkin, *Teoriya Snovidenii (Theory of Dreams)* (Leningrad: Meditsina, 1967), 352, cited in R. C. Van de Castle, *Our Dreaming Mind* (New York: Ballantine, 1994).

17. E. G. Mitchell, "The Physiological Diagnostic Dream," *N.Y. Med. Journal & Med. Record* 118 (1923): 416–17.

18. D. E. Schneider, "Dreams of Flying and Dreams of Weightlessness," *J. Hillside Hospital* 9, no. 3 (1960): 171; E. Hartmann, *The Biology of Dreaming* (Springfield, Ill.: Charles C. Thomas, 1967), 116–17; E. G. Mitchell, "The Physiological Diagnostic Dream," *N.Y. Med. Journal & Med. Record* 118 (1923): 417.

19. A. Mandel and M. Mandel, "Biochemical Aspects of REM Sleep," *Am. J. Psychiatr.* 122 (1965): 391–401.

20. R. Armstrong et al., "Dreams and Gastric Secretions in Duodenal Ulcer Patients," *New Physician* 14 (1965): 241–43.

21. P. H. Knapp, "Sensory Impressions in Dreams," *Psychoanal. Quart.* 25 (1956): 325; E. Jones, *The Theory of Symbolism in Papers on Psychoanalysis* (London: Balliere, Tindall & Cox, 1923); R. E. Mason, *Internal Perception and Bodily Functioning* (Int. Univ. Press, 1961); R. Smith, "The Meaning of Dreams," *Psychiatry Research* 13 (1984): 267–74.

22. D. M. Connelly, *Traditional Acupuncture: The Law of the Five Elements* (Columbia, Md.: Center for Traditional Acupuncture, 1979).

23. E. Hartman, "Dreaming Sleep (The D-State) and the Menstrual Cycle," *J. Nerv. Ment. Dis.* 143 (1966): 406–16; E. M. Swanson and D. Foulkes, "Dream Content and the Menstrual Cycle," *J. Nerv. Ment. Dis.* 145, no. 5 (1968): 358–63; T. Benedek and B. Rubenstein, "Correlation between Ovarian Activity and Psychodynamic Processes: The Ovulatory Phase," *Psychosom. Med.* 1, no. 2 (1939): 245–70.

THREE. EAST SIDE, WEST SIDE, ALL AROUND THE BRAIN

1. B. Fallik and J. Eliot, "Intuition, Cognitive Style, and Hemispheric Processing," *Perceptual Motor Skills* 60 (1985): 683–97; E. Kaplan, "A Process Approach to Neuropsychological Assessment," in *Clinical Neuropsychology and Brain Function* (Washington, D.C.: APA Press, 1988), 127–67; E. Zaidel, "Hemispheric Monitoring," in D. Ohoson, ed., *Duality and Unity of the Brain* (New York: Plenum Press, 1987); J. Sargent, "Human Perception and Performance," *J. Exper. Psychol.* 8 (1988): 1–13, 253–74; S. J. Luck et al., "Independent Hemispheric Attentional Systems Mediate Visual Search in Split Brain Patients," *Nature* 342, no. 6249 (1989): 543–45; M. S. Gazzaniga, "Consciousness and the Cerebral Hemispheres," in *The Cognitive Neurosciences* (Cambridge, Mass.: MIT Press, 1995), 1391–400; J. Semmes, "Hemispheric Specialization: A Possible Clue of Mechanism," *Neuropsychologia* 6 (1968): 11–26; H. Goodglass and

M. Calderon, "Parallel Processing of Verbal and Musical Stimuli in Right and Left Hemispheres," *Neuropsychologia* 15 (1961): 397–407; D. Kimura, "Cerebral Dominance and the Perception of Verbal Stimuli," *Canad. J. Psychol.* 15, no. 3 (1961): 166–71; R. C. Gur and I. K. Packer, "Differences in the Distribution of Gray and White Matter in Human Cerebral Hemispheres," *Science* 207 (1980): 1226–28.

2. B. Fallik and J. Eliot, "Intuition, Cognitive Style, and Hemispheric Processing," *Perceptual Motor Skills* 60 (1985): 683–97; R. W. Thatcher et al., "Human Cerebral Hemispheres Develop at Different Rates and Ages," *Science* 236 (1987): 1110–13; R. C. Gur et al., "Sex and Handedness Differences in Cerebral Blood Flow during Rest and Cognitive Activity," *Science* 217 (1982): 659–60; J. McGlone, "Sex Differences in Human Brain Asymmetry: A Critical Survey," *Behav. Brain Sci.* 3 (1980): 215–63.

3. B. Fallik and J. Eliot, "Intuition, Cognitive Style, and Hemispheric Processing," *Perceptual Motor Skills* 60 (1985): 683–97; G. Rizzolatti and H. A. Buchtel, "Hemispheric Superiority in Reaction Time to Faces: A Sex Difference," *Cortex* 13 (1977): 300–305; J. L. Bradshaw and E. A. Gates, "Visual Field Differences in Verbal Tasks: Effects of Task Familiarity and Sex of Subjects," *Brain and Language* 5 (1978): 168–87; R. Graves, T. Landis, and H. Goodglass, "Laterality and Sex Differences for Visual Recognition of Emotional and Nonemotional Words," *Neuropsychologia* 19 (1981): 95–102; D. A. Lake and M. P. Bryden, "Handedness and Sex Differences in Hemispheric Asymmetry," *Brain and Language* 3 (1976): 266–72; W. F. McKeever and A. D. VanDeventer, "Visual and Auditory Language Processing Asymmetries: Influences of Handedness, Familial Sinistrality, and Sex," *Cortex* 13, no. 3 (1977): 225–41; D. Kimura, "Sex Differences in Cerebral Organization for Speech and Praxic Functions," *Canad. J. Psychol.* 37 (1983): 19–35.

4. R. Doktor and D. Bloom, "Selective Lateralization of Cognitive Style Related to Occupation as Determined by EEG Alpha Asymmetry," *Psychophysiology* 14 (1977): 385–92.

5. D. M. MacKay and V. MacKay, "Explicit Dialogue between Left and Right Half Systems of Split Brains," *Nature* 295 (1982): 690–91; E. Zaidel, *Cerebral Correlates of Behavior. Cerebral Correlates of Experience* (Amsterdam: Elsevier, 1978); D. Zaidel and R. W. Sperry, "Performance on the Ravens Colored Progressive Matrices by Subjects with Cerebral Commissurotomy," *Cortex* 9 (1973): 34–39; R. D. Nebes and R. W. Sperry, "Hemispheric Disconnection with Cerebral Birth Injury in the Dominant Arm Area," *Neuropsychologia* 9 (1971): 247–59; J. E. Levy, C. Trevarthen, and R. W. Sperry, "Perception of Bilateral Chimeric Figures Following Hemispheric Disconnection," *Brain* 95 (1972): 61–78; T. M. Landes et al., "Semantic Paralexia: A Release of Right Hemisphere Function from Left Hemisphere Control," *Neuropsychologia* 21 (1983): C359–64; D. Henninger, "Inkblot Testing of Commissurotomy Subjects: Contrasting Modes of Organizing Reality," in S. R. Hameroff et al., eds., *Toward a Science of Consciousness: The First Tucson Discussions and Debates* (Cambridge, Mass.: MIT

Press, 1996), 203–21; B. I. Belyi, "The Role of the Right Hemisphere in Form Perception and Visual Agnosis Organization," *Int. J. Neuroscience* 40, nos. 3–4 (1988): 167–80; E. A. Phelps and M. S. Gazzaniga, "Hemispheric Differences in Mnemonic Processing: The Effects of Left Hemisphere Interpretation," *Neuropsychologia* 3 (1992): 293–97.

6. C. Armengol, personal communication.

7. R. A. Drake, "Familiarity and Linking Relationship Under Conditions of Induced Lateralized Orientation," *Int. J. Neuroscience* 23 (1983): 195–98.

8. N. Geschwind and A. M. Galaburda, "Cerebral Lateralization: Biological Mechanisms, Associations and Pathology. I. A Hypothesis and a Program for Research," *Arch. Neurology* 42 (1985): 428–59; H. W. Gordon, "Learning Disabled Are Cognitively Right," in M. Kinsbourne, ed., *Topics in Learning Disability,* vol. 3 (Gaithersburg, Md.: Aspen Systems, 1983), 29–39; B. Rimland, *Infantile Austism* (New York: Appleton-Century-Crofts, 1964); B. Rimland, "The Autistic Savant," *Psychol. Today* 12 (1978): 69–80.

9. M. A. Denkla, "The Child with Developmental Disabilities Grown Up: Adult Residua of Childhood Disorders," *Neurologic Clinics* 11, no. 1 (1993): 105–26.

10. R. Gur, "Left Hemisphere Dysfunction and Left Hemisphere Overactuation in Schizophrenia," *J. Abnormal Psychology* 87 (1978): 226–38; I. A. Smokler and H. Shevrin, "Cerebral Lateralization and Personality Style," *Archiv. of Psychiatry* 36, no. 9 (1979): 949–54.

11. The corpus callosum shrinks as men age but does not shrink in women. S. F. Witelson, "The Brain Connection: The Corpus Callosum Is Larger in Left-handers," *Science* 229 (1985): 665–68; S. F. Witelson, "Hand and Sex Differences in the Isthmus and Genu of the Human Corpus Callosum," *Brain* 112 (1989): 799–835; C. De La Coste-Utamsing and R. L. Holloway, "Sexual Dimorphism in the Corpus Callosum," *Science* 216 (1982): 1431–32; S. F. Witelson, "Structural Correlates of Cognition in the Human Brain," in A. B. Scheibel and A. F. Weschsler, eds., *Neurobiology of Higher Cognitive Function* (New York: Guilford Press, 1990); S. F. Witelson and D. L. Kiger, "Individual Differences in Anatomy of the Corpus Callosum: Sex, Hand Preference, Schizophrenia and Hemispheric Specialization," in A. Glass, ed., *Individual Differences in Hemispheric Specialization* (New York: Plenum Press, 1987).

12. H. S. Bracha et al., "Rotational Movement (Circling) in Normal Humans: Sex Difference and Relationship to Hand, Foot, and Eye Difference," *Brain Research* 411 (1987): 231–35.

13. N. Linchan, *Skills Training Manual for Treating Borderline Personality Disorder* (New York: Guilford Press, 1993).

14. M. W. O'Boyle and C. P. Benbow, "Enhanced Right Hemisphere Involvement During Cognitive Processing May Relate to Intellectual Precocity," *Neuropsychologia* 28, no. 2 (1990): 211–16; M. Annett and M. Manning, "The Disadvantage of Dextrality for Intelligence," *Brit. J. Psychology* 80 (1989): 213–16.

15. R. Klein and R. Armitage, "Rhythms in Human Performance: 1½-Hour Oscillations in Cognitive Style," *Science* 204 (1979): 1326–28.

16. M. Altemus, B. Wexler, and N. Boulis, "Neuropsychological Correlates of Menstrual Mood Changes," *Psychosom. Med.* 51 (1989): 329–36; H. A. Sackeim et al., "Hemispheric Asymmetry in the Expression of Positive and Negative Emotions: Neurologic Evidence," *Arch. Neurol.* 39 (1982): 210; R. Davidson and N. Fox, "Asymmetrical Brain Activity Discriminates Between Positive and Negative Affective Stimuli in Human Infants," *Science* 218 (1983): 1235–37; H. A. Sackeim and R. C. Gur, "Lateral Asymmetry in Intensity of Emotional Expression," *Neuropsychologia* 16 (1978): 473.

17. D. M. Tucker, S. L. Shearer, and J. D. Murray, "Hemispheric Specialization and Cognitive Behavioral Therapy," *Cognitive Therapy & Research* 1, no. 4 (1977): 263–73.

18. U. Mittwoch, "Lateral Asymmetry and Gonadal Differentiation," *The Lancet* 1 (Feb. 15, 1975): 401–2; C. Overzier, ed., *Intersexuality* (London, 1963), p. 182; C. Overzier, "The Classification of Intersexuality," *Triangle* 8, no. 2 (1967): 32–41.

19. K. S. F. Chang et al., "Scrotal Asymmetry and Handedness," *J. Anat.* 94 (1960): 543–48.

20. U. Mittwoch, "Lateral Asymmetry and Gonadal Function," *The Lancet* 1 (1975): 401–2.

21. J. Howard, N. L. Petrakis, I. D. Bross et al., "Handedness and Breast Cancer Laterality: Testing a Hypothesis," *Human Biology* 54 (1982): 365–71; M. A. Kramer et al., "Handedness and the Laterality of Breast Cancer in Women," *Nursing Research* 34, no. 6 (1985): 333–37.

22. A. Lewinski et al., "Unilateral Post-Deafferentation of the Hypothalamus and Mitotic Activity of Thyroid Follicular Cells under Conditions after Hemithyroidectomy," *Endocrinol. Exp.* 16 (1982): 75–80.

23. I. Gerendai et al., "Unilateral Ovarectomy–Induced Luteinizing Hormone-Releasing Hormone Content Changes in the Two Halves of the Mediobasal Hypothalamus," *Neurosci. Letters* 9 (1978): 333–36; I. Gerendai, "Lateralization of Neuroendocrine Control," in N. Geschwind and A. M. Galaburda, eds., *Cerebral Dominance: Biological Foundation* (Cambridge, Mass.: Harvard Univ. Press, 1984), 167–78.

24. I. Gerendai, "Lateralization of Neuroendocrine Control," in N. Geschwind and A. M. Galaburda, eds., *Cerebral Dominance: Biological Foundation* (Cambridge, Mass.: Harvard Univ. Press, 1984), 167–78; H. Merskey and G. D. Watson, "The Lateralization of Pain," *Pain* 7, no. 3 (1979), 271–80.

25. K. Hoppe, "Split Brains and Psychoanalysis," *Psychoanalytic Quarterly* 46 (1977): 220–24.

26. M.-M. Mesulam, *Principles of Behavioral Neurology* (Philadelphia: F. A. David, 1985), 35–40.

27. M. A. Persinger, "Psychological Phenomena and Temporal Lobe

Activity: The Geomagnetic Factor," in L. A. Henkel and R. F. Berger, eds., *Research in Parapsychology* (Metuchen, N.J.: Scarecrow Press, 1988), 124–25.

28. P. Gloor et al., "The Role of the Limbic System in Experiential Phenomena of Temporal Lobe Epilepsy," *Ann. Neurol.* 12 (1982): 129–44; D. M. Bear and P. Fedio, "Quantitative Analysis of Interictal Behavior in Temporal Lobe Epilepsy," *Arch. Neurol.* 34 (1977): 454–67; D. M. Bear, "Temporal Lobe Epilepsy—A Syndrome of Sensory-Limbic Hyperconnection Hypothesis," *Cortex* 15 (1979): 357–74.

29. J. R. Stevens, "Sleep Is for Seizures: A New Interpretation of the Role of Phasic Ocular Events in Sleep and Wakefulness," in M. B. Sterman and M. N. Shonse, eds., *Sleep and Epilepsy* (New York: Academic Press, 1982), 249–64.

30. M. A. Persinger and G. B. Schaut, "Geomagnetic Factors in Subjective Telepathic, Precognitive, and Post-mortem Experiences," *J. Am. Soc. Psychiat. Res.* 82 (1988): 217–35.

31. H. Klüver and P. C. Bucy, "'Psychic Blindness' and Other Symptoms in Rhesus Monkeys," *Am. J. Physiol.* 119 (1937): 352–53; H. Klüver and P. C. Bucy, "Preliminary Analysis of Functions of the Temporal Lobes in Monkeys," *Arch. Neurol. Psychiatr.* 42 (1939): 979–1000.

32. W. Penfield and B. Milner, "Memory Deficit Produced by Bilateral Lesions in the Hippocampal Zone," *Arch. Neurol. Psychiatry* 79 (1958): 475–97.

33. A. Z. Spilken and M. A. Jacobs, "Prediction of Illness Behavior for Measures of Life Crisis, Manifest Distress, and Maladaptive Coping," *Psychosom. Med.* 33, no. 3 (1971): 251–63; D. Mitchell et al., "Habituation under Stress: Shocked Mice Show Nonassociative Learning in a T-Maze," *Behav. Neurol. Biol.* 43 (1985): 212–17; M. E. Seligman and J. M. Weiss, "Coping Behavior: Learned Helplessness, Physiological Change and Learned Inactivity," *Behav. Res. Therapy* 18 (1980): 459–512.

34. D. C. Poskanser, "Hemiatrophies and Hemihypertrophies," in P. J. Vinken et al., eds., *Handbook of Clinical Neurology,* vol. 22: *System Disorders and Atrophies* (North Holland, 1975), 545–54; A. Gesell, "Hemihypertrophy and Twinning," *Am. J. Sci.* 173 (1927): 542–55.

FOUR. REMEMBRANCE OF THINGS PAST

1. F. W. Putnam, "A Brief History of Multiple Personality Disorder," *Child Adolescent Psychiatr. Clinics of North America* 5, no. 2 (1996): 263–71; F. Putnam et al., "The Clinical Phenomenology of Multiple Personality Disorder: Review of 100 Recent Cases," *J. Clin. Psychiatry* 47 (1986): 285–93.

2. K. Shepard and B. Braun, "Change in Visual Function of the Multiple Personality Patient," paper presented at the 1985 Conference on MPO and Dissociative Disorders (Chicago, Oct. 1985); S. Miller, "Optical Differences in Cases of Multiple Personality Disorder," *J. Nerv. Ment. Dis.* 77 (1989): 480–86.

3. C. Alvarado, "Dissociation and State Specific Psychophysiology During the Nineteenth Century," *Dissociation* 2 (1989): 160–68; K. Lamore et al., "Multiple Personality: An Objective Case Study," *Brit. J. Psychiatry* 131 (1977):

35–40; P. Coons, "Psychophysiologic Aspects of Multiple Personality Disorder," *Dissociation* 1 (1988): 47–53; R. Loewensten and F. Putnam, "The Clinical Phenomenology of Males with Multiple Personality Disorder," *Dissociation* 3 (1990): 135–43.

4. L. Valzelli, "Serotonergic Inhibitory Control of Experimental Aggression," *Psychopharm. Res. Communication* 12 (1982): 1–13; M. L. Laudenslager and S. M. Ryan, "Inescapable but Not Escapable Shock Suppresses Lymphocyte Proliferation," *Science* 221 (1983): 568–70; D. Mitchell et al., "Habituation Under Stress. Shocked Mice Show Non-Associative Learning in a T-Maze," *Behav. Neurol. Biol.* 43 (1985): 212–17.

5. B. A. Van der Kolk, "The Psychobiology of PTSD" and "The Body Keeps Score: Approaches to Psychobiology of Post Traumatic Stress Disorder," in B. A. Van der Kolk et al., eds., *Traumatic Stress: The Effects of Overwhelming Experience on Mind, Body, Society* (New York: Guilford Press, 1996); B. A. Van der Kolk, "Inescapable Shock, Neurotransmitters, and Addiction to Trauma: Towards a Psychobiology of Post Traumatic Stress," *Biol. Psychiatry* 20 (1985): 314–25.

6. C. C. Chen et al., "Adverse Life Events and Breast Cancer: A Case Control Study," *Brit. Med. J.* 311 (1995): 1527–30; D. H. Wiesel and T. N. Hubel, "Binocular Interaction in Striate Cortex of Kittens," *J. Neurophysiol.* 29 (1965): 1041–59; W. M. Jenkins et al., "Behaviorally Controlled Differential Use of Restricted Hand Surfaces Induces Changes in the Cortical Representation of the Hand in Area 3b in Adult Owl Monkeys," *Soc. Neurosci. Abstr.* 10, no. 1 (1984): 655; T. Wiesel, "Postnatal Development of Visual Cortex and the Influence of the Environment," *Nature* 299 (1982): 583–91.

7. C. N. Shealy and C. M. Myss, *The Creation of Health* (Walpole, Mass.: Stillpoint, 1993), 98–100; C. L. Northrup, *Women's Bodies, Women's Wisdom* (New York: Bantam, 1994), 151–54.

8. C. E. Wenner and S. Weinhouse, "Diphosphopyridine Nucleotide Requirements for Oxidations by Mitochondria of Normal and Neoplastic Tissues," *Cancer Research* 12 (1952): 306; Horace White, trans., "Appian of Alexandria, The Syrian Wars," in *The Roman History XI,* chap. X, vol. 2 (Cambridge, Mass.: Loeb Classical Library, 1962); M-M. Mesulam and Jo Perry, "The Diagnosis of Lovesickness: Experimental Psychophysiology without the Polygraph," *Psychophysiology* 9 (1972): 546–51.

9. R. L. Moody, "Bodily Changes during Abreaction," *Lancet* 2 (1946): 934–35; R. L. Moody, "Bodily Changes during Abreaction," *Lancet* 1 (1948): 964; I. Stevenson and D. J. Graham, "Disease as Response to Life Stress. I. Obtaining the Evidence Clinically," in H. I. Lief, V. F. Lief, and N. R. Lief, eds., *The Psychological Basis of Medical Practice* (New York: Harper & Row, 1963), 137–53.

10. D. P. Agle and O. D. Ratnoff, "Purpura and Psychosomatic Entity," *Archiv. Int. Med.* 109 (1962): 685–94.

11. R. F. Q. Johnson and T. X. Barber, "Hypnotic Suggestion for Blister

Formation: Subjective and Physiological Effects," *Am. J. Clin. Hypnosis* 18 (1976): 172–81.

12. G. F. Powell et al., "Emotional Deprivation and Growth Retardation Simulating Idiopathic Hypopituitarism," *NEJM* 276 (1967): 1271; R. C. Patton and L. I. Gardner, *Growth Failure in Maternal Deprivation* (Springfield, Ill.: Thomas, 1963); J. B. Reinhart and A. L. Drash, "Psychosocial Dwarfism: Environmentally Induced Recovery," *Psychosom. Med.* 31, no. 2 (1969): 165–71; N. B. Talbot et al., "Dwarfism in Healthy Children: Its Possible Relation to Emotional, Nutritional, Endocrine Disturbances," *NEJM* 236 (1947): 783; R. Fried and M. F. Mayer, "Socioeconomical Factors Accounting for Failure in Children Living in an Institution," *J. Pediatri.* 33 (1948): 444; E. M. Widdowson, "Mental Contentment and Physical Growth," *Lancet* 1 (1951): 1316.

13. L. M. LeCron, "Breast Development through Hypnotic Suggestion," *J. Am. Soc. Psychosom. Dent. & Med.* 16, no. 2 (1969): 58–61; R. D. Willard, "Breast Enlargement through Visual Imagery and Hypnosis," *Am. J. Clin. Hypnosis* 19, no. 4 (1977): 195–200; A. R. Starb, "Hypnotic Stimulation of Breast Growth," *Am. J. Clin. Hypnosis* 19, no. 4 (1977): 201–8.

14. S. Minuchin, B. L. Rosman, and L. Baker, *Psychosomatic Families* (Cambridge, Mass.: Harvard Univ. Press, 1978), 23–29.

15. L. Dossey, "Running Scared: How We Hide Who We Are," *Alternative Therapies* 3, no. 2 (1997): 8–15; L. Dossey, *Healing Words* (San Francisco: Harper, 1993), 50–53; B. E. Schwarz, "Possible Telesomatic Reactions," *J. Med. Soc. N.J.* 64, no. 4 (1967): 600–603.

16. J. H. Rush, "New Directions in Parapsychological Research," Parapsychological Monographs 4 (1964): 18–19; L. E. Rhine, "Hallucinatory Experiences and Psychosomatic PSI," *J. Parapsychol.* 29 (1967): 88–111.

17. I. Stevenson, *Telepathic Impressions: A Review and Report of 35 New Cases* (Charlottesville, Va.: University Press Virginia, 1970), 144; I. Stevenson, *Reincarnation and Biology: A Contribution to the Etiology of Birthmarks and Birth Defects,* vol. 1, *Birthmarks* (Westport, Conn.: Praeger, 1997), 33–88.

FIVE. BODY LANGUAGE

1. J. E. LeDoux, "Sensory Systems and Emotions: A Model of Affective Processing," *Integrative Psychiatry* 4 (1986): 237–43; L. R. Squire and S. Zola-Morgan, "The Medial Temporal Lobe Memory System," *Science* 253 (1991): 2380–86.

2. L. S. Sklar and H. Arlsman, "Stress and Cancer," *Psychol. Bulletin* 89 (1981): 369–406.

3. G. Ironson et al., "Effects of Anger on Left Ventricle Ejection Fraction in Coronary Artery Disease," *Am. J. Cardiol.* 70 (1992): 281–85; R. G. Traxler et al., "The Association of Elevated Plasma Cortisol and Early Atherosclerosis as Demonstrated by Coronary Angiography," *Atherosclerosis* 26 (1977): 151–62.

4. C. C. Cupps and A. S. Fauci, "Corticosteroid Mediated Immunoregulation in Man," *Immunol. Reviews* 65 (1982): 133–55.

5. Beijing College of Traditional Chinese Medicine, *Essentials of Chinese Acupuncture* (Beijing: Foreign Language Press, 1980).

6. L. L. Hay, *You Can Heal Your Life* (Santa Monica: Hay House, 1984).

7. S. Kasl, S. Gore, and S. Cobb, "The Experience of Leaving a Job: Reported Changes in Health, Symptoms, and Illness Behavior," *Psychosom. Med.* 37, no. 2 (1975): 106–22.

8. G. W. Paulson and N. Dadmehr, "Is There a Premorbid Personality Typical for Parkinson's Disease," *Arch. Neurol.* 41, no. 2 (1991): 73–76.

9. D. M. Connelly, *Traditional Acupuncture: The Law of the Five Elements* (Columbia, Md.: Center for Traditional Acupuncture, 1989).

10. G. A. Bachman et al., "Childhood Sexual Abuse and Consequences in Adult Women," *Obstetr. Gynecol.* 71, no. 4 (1988): 631.

11. C. L. Bacon, R. Renneker, and M. Cutler, "A Psychosomatic Survey of Cancer of the Breast," *Psychosom. Med.* 14 (1952): 453–60; M. Wirshang et al., "Psychological Identification of Breast Cancer Patients before Biopsy," *J. Psychosom. Res.* 26, no. 1 (1982): 1–10.

12. M. Koskenhuo et al., "Hostility as a Risk Factor for Mortality and Ischemic Heart Disease in Men," *Psychosom. Med.* 50 (1988): 153–64.

13. M. Friedman and R. H. Rosenman, "Association of Specific Overt Behavior with Cardiovascular Findings," *JAMA* 162 (1959): 1286–96; J. Denollet, S. U. Sys et al., "Personality as Independent Predictor of Long-term Mortality in Patients with Coronary Artery Disease," *Lancet* 347 (1996): 417–21.

14. C. L. Northrup and M. L. Schulz, "Empowering the Patient," letter to the editor, *Casco Bay Weekly,* December 5, 1996.

SIX. BLOOD AND BONES

1. A. Z. Spilken and M. A. Jacobs, "Prediction of Illness Behavior for Measures of Life Crisis, Manifest Distress, and Maladaptive Coping," *Psychosom. Med.* 33, no. 3 (1971): 251–63; K. Goodkin et al., "Active Coping Style Is Associated with Natural Killer Cell Cytotoxicity in Asymptomatic HIV-1 Seropositive Homosexual Men," *J. Psychosom. Res.* 36, no. 7 (1992): 635–50; K. Goodkin et al., "Life Stresses and Coping Style Are Associated with Immune Measures in HIV Infections—A Preliminary Report," *Int. J. Psychiatr. Med.* 22 (1992): 155–72; L. Temoshok et al., "The Relationship of Psychosocial Factors to Prognostic Indicators in Cutaneous Malignant Melanoma," *J. Psychosom. Res.* 29 (1985): 139–53; J. M. Weiss et al., "Effects of Chronic Exposure to Stressors on Avoidance-Escape Behavior and on Brain Norepinephrine," *Psychosom. Med.* 37 (1975): 522–34; M. E. Seligman and J. M. Weiss, "Coping Behavior: Learned Helplessness, Physiological Change and Learned Inactivity," *Behav. Res. Therapy* 18 (1980): 459–512; A. H. Schmale, "Giving Up As a Final Common Pathway to Changes in Health," *Adv. of Psychosom. Med.* 8 (1972): 20–40; J. K. Kiecolt-Glaser et al., "Psychosocial Modifiers of Immune Function in Medical Students," *Psychosom. Med.* 46 (1984): 7–14; M. L. Laudenslager et al., "Suppression of Specific Antibody Pro-

duction by Inescapable Shock: Stability Under Varying Conditions," *Brain Behav. Immunity* 2 (1988): 92–101; M. L. Laudenslager et al., "Coping and Immunosuppression: Inescapable but Not Escapable Shock Suppresses Lymphocyte Proliferation," *Science* 221 (1983): 560–70.

2. S. Cobb, "Social Support As Moderator of Life Stress," *Psychosom. Med.* 38 (1976): 300–314; J. K. Jackson, "The Problem of Alcoholic TB Patients," in P. F. Sparer, *Personality Stress and Tuberculosis* (New York: International Universities Press, 1954); I. G. Sarason et al., "Life Events, Social Support, and Illness," *Psychosom. Med.* 47, no. 2 (1985): 156–63; M. L. Laudenslager, M. Reite, and R. J. Harbeck, "Infant-Mother Separation in Bonnet Monkeys," *Behav. Neurol. Biol.* 136 (1982): 40; S. Cohen and J. A. Wills, "Stress, Social Support, and the Buffering Hypothesis," *Psychol. Bull.* 98 (1985): 310–52; S. Cohen, "Social Support and Physical Health," in A. L. Greene et al., eds., *Life Span Developmental Psychology: Perspectives on Stress and Coping* (Hillsdale, N.J.: Erbaum, 1991); G. W. Brown et al., "Social Class and Psychiatric Disturbance among Women in an Urban Population," *Sociology* 9 (1975): 225–54; G. Bennette, "Psychic and Cellular Aspects of Isolation and Identity Impairment in Cancer: A Dialectic Alienation," *Ann. N.Y. Acad. Sci.* 164 (1969): 352.

3. G. G. Luce, *Biological Rhythms in Psychiatry and Medicine* (Washington, D.C.: Public Health Service Publication No. 2088, 1970); M. A. Hofer, "Relationships as Regulators: A Psychobiologic Perspective on Bereavement," *Psychosom. Med.* 46, no. 3 (1984): 183–95; R. Wever, "Zur Zeitgeber-Starkke eines Lichtdunkelwechsels Fur die Circadiane Periodik des Menschen," *P. Flengers Arch.* 321 (1980): 133–42; J. Vernikos-Danellis and C. M. Wingest, "The Importance of Social Cues in the Regulation of Plasma Cortisol in Man," in A. Reinberg and F. Halbers, eds., *Chronopharmacology* (New York: Pergamon, 1979), 101–6.

4. J. Mason, "Psychological Influence on Pituitary Adrenal Cortical System," *Recent Progress in Hormone Research* 15 (1959): 345–89.

5. M. K. McClintock, "Menstrual Synchrony and Suppression," *Nature* 224 (1971): 244–45.

6. M. K. McClintock, "Estrous Synchrony and Its Mediation by Airborne Chemical Communication," *Human Behav.* 10 (1978): 269–76.

7. M. C. Moore-Ede, F. M. Sulzman, and C. A. Fuller, *The Clocks That Time Us* (Cambridge, Mass.: Harvard Univ. Press, 1983).

8. E. Lindemann, "The Symptomatology and Management of Acute Grief," *Am. J. Psychiatry* 101 (1944): 141–48; P. Solomon, P. E. Kubzansky et al., eds., *Sensory Deprivation* (Cambridge, Mass.: Harvard Univ. Press, 1961).

9. L. LeShan, "An Emotional Life History Pattern Associated with Neoplastic Disease," *Ann. N.Y. Acad. Sci.* 125 (1966): 780.

10. S. R. Butler et al., "Maternal Behavior as a Regulator of Polyamine Biosynthesis in Brain and Heart Rate of Two-Week-Old Rat Pups," *Science* 179 (1978): 445–47; R. Ader and S. B. Friedman, "Social Factors Affect Emotionality and Resistance to Disease in Animals," *Psychosom. Med.* 27, no. 2 (1965): 119–21;

S. E. Keller et al., "Effect of Premature Weaning on Lymphocyte Stimulation in the Rat," *Psychosom. Med.* 45 (1983): 75.

11. H. B. Slade and S. A. Schwartz, "Mucosal Immunity: The Immunology of Breast Milk," *J. Allergy Clin. Immunol.* 80 (1987): 348–58; A. Bertotto et al., "Lymphocytes Bearing T Cell Receptor Gamma Delta in Human Breast Milk," *Arch. Dis. Child* 65, no. 11 (1990): 1274–75; I. N. Mbawuike et al., "Vaccination with Inactivated Influenza A During Pregnancy Protects Neonatal Mice Against Lethal Challenge by Influenza A," *J. Virol.* 64, no. 3 (1997): 1370–74.

12. J. Bowlby, *Attachment and Loss,* vol. 1, *Attachment* (New York: Basic Books, 1969).

13. M. A. Hoffer, "Relationship as Regulators: A Psychobiologic Perspective in Bereavement," *Psychosom. Med.* 46, no. 3 (1984): 183–97.

14. C. B. Thomas, K. R. Duszynski, and J. W. Shaffer, "Family Attitudes Reported in Youth as Potential Predictors of Cancer," *Psychosom. Med.* 41 (1979): 287–302; C. B. Thomas and K. R. Duszynski, "Closeness to Parents and Family Constellation," *J. Hopkins Med. J.* 134 (1974): 251–70; C. B. Thomas and R. L. Greenstreet, "Psychobiological Characteristics in Youth as Predictors of Five Disease States," *J. Hopkins Med. J.* 132 (1973): 16–43.

15. J. S. House et al., "Social Relationship and Health," *Science* 241 (1988): 540–45; J. S. House et al., "Social Ties and Susceptibility to the Common Cold," *JAMA* 277, no. 24 (1997): 1940–44.

16. L. D. Egbert et al., "Reduction of Post-operative Pain by Encouragement and Instruction of Patients," *NEJM* 270 (1964): 825–27.

17. S. Cohen et al., "Social Ties and Susceptibility to the Common Cold," *JAMA* 277, no. 24 (1997): 1940–44.

18. S. B. Friedman et al., "Differential Susceptibility to a Viral Agent in Mice Housed Alone or in Groups," *Psychosom. Med.* 32, no. 3 (1970): 285–99; L. F. Berkman and S. L. Syme, "Social Networks, Host Resistance, and Mortality," *Am. J. Epidem.* 109 (1979): 185–204; T. M. Vogt et al., "Social Networks as Predictors of Ischemic Heart Disease, Cancer, Stroke, and Hypertension," *J. Clin. Epidemiol.* 45 (1992): 659–66.

19. L. LeShan and R. E. Worthington, "Some Psychologic Correlates of Neoplastic Disease," *J. Clin. & Exper. Psychopath.* 16 (1955): 281; M. Irwin et al., "Impaired Natural Killer Cell Activity During Bereavement," *Brain Behav. Immunity* 1 (1987): 98–104; M. Irwin et al., "Plasma Corded and Natural Killer Cell Activity during Bereavement," *Biol. Psychiatry* 24 (1988): 173–78; R. W. Bartrop et al., "Depressed Lymphocyte Function after Bereavement," *Lancet* 1 (1977): 834–36; P. J. Clayton, "Mortality and Morbidity of the First Year of Widowhood," *Arch. Gen. Psychiatry* 30 (1974): 747–50; M. L. Laudenslager et al., "Suppressed Immune Response in Infant Monkeys Associated with Paternal Separation," *Behav. Neurobiol.* 36 (1982): 40–48; T. J. Jacobs and E. Charles, "Life Events and the Occurrence of Cancer in Children," *Psychosom. Med.* 42, no. 1 (1980): 10–23; A. H. Schmale, "The Relationship of Separation and Depression to Disease," *Psychosom. Med.* 20 (1958): 259; K. J. Helsing et al., "Causes of Death in

a Widowed Population," *Am. J. Epidem.* 116 (1982): 524–32; R. B. Shekelle et al., "Psychological Depression and 17-Year Rise of Death from Cancer," *Psychosom. Med.* 43 (1981): 117–25; S. J. Schleifer et al., "Suppression of Lymphocyte Stimulation Following Bereavement," *JAMA* 250 (1983): 374–77.

20. R. P. Greenberg and P. T. Dattore, "The Relationship between Dependency and the Development of Cancer," *Psychosom. Med.* 43, no. 1 (1981): 35–43.

21. G. H. Frank, "A Review of Research with Measures of Ego Strength Derived from MMPI and the Rorschach," *J. Gen. Psychol.* 77 (1967): 183–206; S. C. Kobasa et al., "Hardiness and Health. A Prospective Study," *J. Personal. & Social Psychology* 42 (1982): 168–77; S. C. Kobasa, "Stressful Life Events, Personality, and Health. An Inquiry into Hardiness," *J. Personal. & Social Psychology* 27, no. 1 (1979): 1–11.

SEVEN. THE SEX ORGANS AND LOWER BACK

1. B. Eisner, "Some Psychological Differences between Fertile and Infertile Women," *J. Clin. Psychol.* 19 (1963): 391; J. Greenhill, "Emotional Factors in Women with Infertility," *Obstet. Gynecol.* 7 (1956): 602–6; B. Sandler, "Emotional Stress and Infertility," *J. Psychosom. Res.* 12 (1968): 51; B. E. Meaning, "The Emotional Needs of Infertile Couples," *Fertil. Steril.* 34 (1980): 313–19.

2. S. Segal et al., "Serotonin and 5-hydroxyindole Acid in Fertile and Subfertile Men," *Fertility & Sterility* 26, no. 4 (1975): 314–16.

3. E. Havelock, *Studies in the Psychology of Sex* (Philadelphia: Davis, 1928); T. H. Van der Veld, *Fertility and Sterility in Marriage* (New York: Covies Fried, 1931); E. Hufez, "Sperm Transport," in S. Behrman and R. Kistner, eds., *Progress in Infertility,* 2d ed. (Boston: Little, Brown, 1975); R. L. Vanden Burgh et al., "Emotional Illness in Habitual Aborters Following Suturing of Incompetent Os," *Psychosom. Med.* 26, no. 3 (1966): 257–63; R. J. Weil and C. Tupper, "Personality, Life Situation and Communication: A Study of Habitual Abortion," *Psychosom. Med.* 22, no. 6 (1960): 448–51; A. Domar et al., "The Prevalence and Predictability of Depression in Infertile Women," *Fertility & Sterility* 58 (1992): 1158–63; P. A. Van Keep and H. Schmidt-Elmendorff, "Partnesschaft in der Sterilen Ehe," *Med. Monnatsschr.* 28 (1974): 523–27; B. Sandler, "Conception after Adoption," *Fertility & Sterility* 16 (1965): 313–21; P. Slade, "Sexual Attitudes and Social Role in Infertile Women," *J. Psychosom. Res.* 25, no. 3 (1981): 183–86.

4. D. Levy, "Maternal Overprotection," *J. Psychiatry* 2 (1939): 563; R. P. Knight, "Some Problems in Selecting and Rearing Adopted Children," *Bull. Menninger Clinic* 5 (1941): 65; N. Payne, *The Language of Fertility* (New York: Harmony Books, 1997); P. Kemeter, "Studies on Psychosomatic Implications of Infertility on Effects of Emotional Stress on Fertilization and Implantation in In Vitro Fertilization," *Human Reprod.* 3, no. 3 (1988): 341–52; L. Jeker et al., "Wish for a Child and Infertility: Study on 116 Couples," *Int. J. Fertil.* 33, no. 6 (1988): 411–20.

5. T. Benedek, "Some Emotional Factors in Infertility," *Psychosom. Med.* 15, no. 5 (1953): 485–98.

6. C. L. Northrup, *Women's Bodies, Women's Wisdom* (New York: Bantam, 1994), 353.

7. K. Menninger, "Somatic Correlations with the Unconscious Repudiation of Femininity in Women," *J. Nerv. Ment. Dis.* 89 (1939): 514; T. Benedek and B. Rubenstein, "Correlations between Ovarian Activity and Psychodynamic Processes: The Ovulatory Phase," *Psychosom. Med.* 1, no. 2 (1939): 245–70; A. Mayer, "Sterility in Women as a Result of Functional Disturbance," *JAMA* 105 (1935): 1474; A. D. Domar and M. M. Seibel, *The Emotional Aspects of Infertility,* in M. Seibel, ed. (Norwalk, Conn.: Appleton, Lange, 1989); P. R. Koninckyx and I. A. Brosens, "Clinical Significance of the Luteinized Unruptured Follicle Syndrome as a Cause of Infertility," *Eur. J. Obstet. Gynecol. Reprod. Biol.* 13 (1982): 355; R. F. Harrison et al., "Intermittent Hyperprolactemia and the Unexplained Infertile Couple," *Infertility* 9 (1986): 1; B. Hochstaedt and G. Langer, "Psychoendocrine Factors in Sterility," *Int. J. Fertil.* 4 (1959): 255; K. S. Moghissi and E. E. Wallach, "Unexplained Infertility," *Fertility & Sterility* 39 (1983): 5; P. Mosley, "Psychophysiologic Infertility: An Overview," *Clin. Obstetr. Gynecol.* 19 (1976): 407; A. D. Domar, M. M. Seibel, and H. Bensen, "The Mind/Body Program for Infertility: A New Behavioral Treatment Approach for Women with Infertility," *Fertility & Sterility* 53, no. 2 (1990): 246–49.

8. K. J. Helzlsoner et al., "Serum Gonadotropins and Steroid Hormones and the Development of Ovarian Cancer," *JAMA* 274, no. 24 (1995): 1926–30; R. E. Bristow and B. Karlan, "Ovulation and Induction: Infertility and Ovarian Cancer Risk," *Fertility & Sterility* 66, no. 4 (1996): 449–507; R. Harris et al., "The Collaborative Ovarian Cancer Group Characteristics Relating to Ovarian Cancer Risk," *Am. J. Epidemiol.* 136 (1972): 1204–11; M. Booth, U. Beral, and P. Smith, "Risk Factors for Ovarian Cancer: A Case Control Study," *Brit. J. Cancer* 60 (1989): 592–98.

9. J. J. Casagrande, "Incessant Ovulation and Ovarian Cancer," *Lancet* 2 (1979): 170–72.

10. D. H. Hellhammer et al., "Male Infertility: Relationship Among Gonadotropins, Sex Steroids, Seminal Parameters and Personality Attitudes," *Psychosom. Med.* 47, no. 1 (1985): 58–66; R. L. Ursy, "Stress and Infertility," in A. T. K. Cockett and R. L. Ursy, eds., *Male Infertility* (New York: Grune & Stratton, 1977), 145–62.

11. M. Stauber, *Psychosomatik der Sterilin Ehe* (Berlin: Grosse Verlag, 1979).

12. H. F. Dunbar, *Emotions and Bodily Changes* (New York: Columbia University Press, 1935), 595; R. L. Dickerson, "Medical Analysis of 1,000 Marriages," *JAMA* 97 (1931): 529; C. C. Norris, "Sterility in the Woman without Gross Pathology," *Surgery, Gynecology, and Obstetrics* 15 (1912): 706.

13. J. Axerod, "Neurotransmitters," *Sci. Am.* 230 (1974): 59–71; J. Greenhill, "Emotional Factors in Women with Infertility," *Obstet. Gynecol.* 7 (1956): 602–6; M. Helman, "Reproduction, Emotions, and Hypothalamus," *Fertility & Sterility* 10 (1959): 162; F. Fachinetti, M. L. Matteo et al., "An Increased

Vulnerability to Stress Associated with a Poor Outcome in In Vitro Fertilization–Embryo Transfer Treatment," *Fertility & Sterility* 67, no. 2 (1997): 309–14.

14. K. D. Kinley et al., "Dissatisfaction, a Gene Involved in Sex-Specific Behavior and Neural Development of Drosophilia Melanogaster," *Proc. Natl. Acad. Sci. USA* 94, no. 3 (1997): 913–18.

15. B. B. Bark and C. T. Javert, "Stress and Habitual Abortion," *Obstet. & Gynecol.* 3 (1954): 298; C. L. Northrup, *Women's Bodies, Women's Wisdom* (New York: Bantam, 1994), 362–64; V. Laukaran and C. Van den Berg, "The Relationship of Attitude to Pregnancy Outcomes and Obstetric Complications," *Am. J. Obstet. Gynecol.* 139 (1981): 956; R. MacDonald, "The Role of Emotional Factors in Obstetrics Complications," *Psychosom. Med.* 30 (1968): 222; M. D. De Muyloer, "Psychological Factors and Preterm Labor," *J. Reprod. Psychol.* 7 (1989): 55; R. Meyers, "Maternal Anxiety and Fetal Death," in L. Zichella and P. Pancheri, eds., *Psychoneuroendocrinology and Reproduction* (New York: Elsevier, 1979); E. Muller-Tyl and B. Wimmer-Puchinger, "Psychosomatic Aspects of Toxemia," *J. Psychosom. Ob. Gyn.* 1, nos. 3–4 (1982): 111–17; C. Ringrose, "Psychosomatic Influence in the Genesis of Toxemia in Pregnancy," *Canad. Med. Assn. J.* 84 (1961): 647; A. J. Copper, "Psychosomatic Aspects of Pre-eclamptic Toxemia," *J. Psychosom. Res.* 2 (1958): 24.

16. E. R. Grimm, "Psychological Investigation of Habitual Abortion," *Psychosom. Med.* 24, no. 4 (1962): 369–78; E. C. Mann, "The Role of Emotional Determinants in Habitual Abortion," *Surg. Clinics in N. A.* 37 (1957): 447.

17. N. Shainess, "Pregnancy, Psychiatric Aspects," in B. B. Wolman, ed., *International Encyclopædia of Psychiatry, Psychology, Psychoanalysis, Neurology* (New York: Aesculapius, 1977); J. Tolchin and B. B. Wolman, "Fears in Childhood and Pregnancy," in B. B. Wolman, ed., *Psychological Aspects of Gynecology and Obstetrics* (Orndell, N.J.: Medical Economics, 1978), 169–76.

18. A. Blau et al, "The Psychogenic Etiology of Premature Births," *Psychosom. Med.* 25, no. 3 (1963): 201–11.

19. B. B. Wolman, "Psychosomatic Issues in Diabetes, Arthritis, Thyroid Diseases, Muscular Tensions, and Infectious Diseases," in *Psychosomatic Disorders* (New York: Plenum Med., 1988); T. C. Dorpat and T. H. Holmes, *Psychosomatic Obstetrics, Gynecology, and Endocrinology* (Springfield, Ill.: Thomas, 1963); T. H. Holmes and H. G. Wolff, "Life Situations, Emotions, and Backache," *Psychosom. Med.* 14 (1952): 18; S. Kasl, S. Gore, and S. Cobb, "The Experience of Losing a Job: Reported Changes in Health, Symptoms, and Illness Behavior," *Psychosom. Med.* 37, no. 2 (1975): 106–22; S. Cobb, "Physiological Changes in Men Whose Jobs Were Abolished," *J. Psychosom. Res.* 18 (1974): 245–48.

20. A. Amkraut and G. F. Soloman, "Stress and Murine Sarcoma Virus (Maloney)–Induced Tumors," *Cancer Research* 32 (1972): 1428–33; P. Ebbson and R. Rask-Nielsen, "Influence of Sex-Aggregate Grouping and of Inoculation and Subcellular Leukemic Material on Development of Non-leukemic Lesions in DAB/2 and BALB/c Mice," *J. Nat. Cancer Instit.* 39 (1967): 917–32.

21. B. L. Bloom, S. J. Asher, and S. W. White, "Marital Disruption as a Stressor: A Review and Analysis," *Psychol. Bull.* 85 (1978): 867–94; J. K. Kiecolt-Glaser et al., "Marital Quality, Marital Disruption, and Immune Function," *Psychosom. Med.* 49, no. 1 (1987): 13–34.

22. S. Saarijarni et al., "Couple Therapy Improves Mental Wellbeing in Chronic Lower Back Pain Patients: A Controlled Five-Year Follow-up Study," *J. Psychosom. Res.* 36, no. 7 (1992): 651–56.

23. J. W. Mason, "Psychological Stress and Endocrine Function," in E. J. Sachar, ed., *Topics in Psychoendocrinology* (New York: Grune, 1975), 1–18.

24. A. J. Pereyra, "The Relationship of Sexual Activity to Cervical Cancer," *J. Obstetr. Gynecol.* 17 (1961): 154–59; M. Tarlan and I. Smalheiser, "Personality Patterns in Patients with Malignant Tumors of the Breast and Cervix," *Psychosom. Med.* 13 (1951): 117; C. R. Wira and C. Kauschic, "Mucosal Immunity in the Female Reproductive Tract: Effect of Sex Hormones on Immune Recognition and Responses," in *Mucosal Vaccines* (New York: Academic Press, 1996).

25. A. H. Schmale and H. Iker, "Hopelessness as a Predictor of Cervical Cancer," *Soc. Sci. Med.* 5 (1971): 95; J. I. Wheeler and B. Caldwell, "Psychological Evaluation of Women with Cancer of the Breast and Cervix," *Psychosom. Med.* 17 (1955): 256; A. H. Schmale and H. Iker, "The Psychological Setting of Uterine and Cervical Cancer," *Ann. N.Y. Acad. Sci.* 125 (1966): 807; K. Goodkin, M. H. Antoni, and P. Blaney, "Stress and Hopelessness in the Promotion of Cervical Intraepithelial Neoplasms in Invasive Squamous Cell Carcinoma of the Cervix," *J. Psychosom. Res.* 30 (1986): 67–76.

26. J. H. Stephenson and W. Grace, "Life Stress and Cancer of the Cervix," *Psychosom. Med.* 16, no. 4 (1954): 287–94.

27. A. H. Schmale and H. Iker, "The Psychological Setting of Uterine and Cervical Cancer," *Ann. N.Y. Acad. Sci.* 125 (1966): 807–13.

28. M. H. Antoni and K. Goodkin, "Host Moderator Variables in the Promotion of Cervical Neoplasia—I: Personality Facets," *J. Psychosom. Res.* 32, no. 3 (1988): 327–38.

29. F. H. Lindberg and L. J. Distad, "Post Traumatic Stress Disorders in Women Who Experienced Childhood Incest," *Child Abuse & Negl.* 9 (1985): 329; M. A. Sedney and B. Brooks, "Factors Associated with History of Childhood Sexual Experience in a Non-clinical Female Population," *J. Am. Acad. Child Psychiatry* 23 (1984): 215; G. L. Engel, "Psychogenic Pain and the Pain Prone Patient," *Am. J. Med.* 26 (1959): 899.

30. G. L. Bachman et al., "Childhood Sexual Abuse and Consequences in Adult Women," *Obstet. & Gynecol.* 71, no. 4 (1988): 631–40; R. C. Reiter et al., "Correlation between Sex Abuse and Somatization in Women with Somatic and Non-somatic Pain," *Am. J. Obstet. & Gynecol.* 165, no. 1 (1991): 104; R. C. Reiter and J. C. Gambora, "Demographic and Historical Variables in Women with Idiopathic Chronic Pelvic Pain," *Obstet. & Gynecol.* 75, no. 3 (1990): 428–32; A. J. Rapkin, "Adhesions and Pelvic Pain: A Retrospective Study," *Obstet. & Gynecol.*

68 (1986): 13; R. D. Reiter, "Occult Somatic Pathology in Women with Chronic Pain," *Clin. Ob. Gynecol.* 33, no. 1 (1990): 154–60; R. Cross et al., "Borderline Syndrome and Incest in Chronic Pelvic Pain Patients," *Int. J. Psychiatry Med.* 10 (1990): 74; J. Herman, *Father-Daughter Incest* (Cambridge, Mass.: Harvard Univ. Press, 1981); R. Fry, "Adult Physical Illness and Childhood Sex Abuse," *J. Psychosom. Med.* 37, no. 2 (1993): 89–103.

31. R. M. Rose et al., "Plasma Testosterone in the Male Rhesus: Influence of Sexual and Social Stimuli," *Science* 178 (1972): 643–45; R. M. Rose, S. Bernstein, and T. P. Gordon, "Consequences of Social Conflict on Plasma Testosterone Levels in Rhesus Monkeys," *Psychosom. Med.* 37, no. 1 (1975): 50–61; K. Matsymoto et al., "Plasma Testosterone Levels Following Surgical Stress in Male Patients," *Acta Endocrinol.* 65 (1970): 11; L. E. Kreuz et al., "Suppression of Plasma Testosterone Levels and Psychological Stress: A Longitudinal Study of Young Men in Officer Candidate School," *Arch. Gen. Psychiatry* 26 (1972): 479–82; R. M. Rose et al., "Androgen Responses to Stress," *Psychosom. Med.* 31 (1969): 408–36.

32. N. Angier, "In Fish, Social Status Goes Right to the Brain," *New York Times,* Nov. 12, 1991; S. Winberg et al., "Effect of Social Rank on Brain Mono-Aminergic Activity in a Ciclid Fish," *Brain Behav. Evol.* 49, no. 4 (1997): 230–36; J. W. Mason, "Organization of Psychoendocrine Mechanisms," *Psychosom. Med.* 30 (1968): 565–80; D. S. Sade, "Seasonal Cycle in Size of Testes of Free Ranging *Macaca malatta,*" *Folia Primat.* 2 (1964): 171–80; J. P. Gordon et al., "Seasonal Changes in Sexual Behavior and Plasma Testosterone Levels of Group Living Monkeys," *Am. Zool.* 13 (1973): 1267.

33. W. R. Paré, "Premature Aging as a Function of Long-term Environmental Stress," *J. Geriatr. Psychol.* 104 (1964): 185; S. G. Johnson, "Abnormal Urinary Androsterone Etiocholanalone Ratio in Hypothalamic Disturbances in Men," *Acta Endocrinol.* 57 (1968): 576–614.

EIGHT. THE GASTROINTESTINAL TRACT

1. I. K. Barker et al., "Observations on Spontaneous Stress-Related Mortality among Males of the Dasyurid *Antechinus stuartii* (MACKAY)," *Australian J. Zoology* 26 (1978): 435–44; J. L. Barnett, "A Stress Response in *Antechinus stuartii* (MACKAY)," *Australian J. Zoology* 21 (1973): 501–13; A. J. Bradley et al., "Stress and Mortality in the Small Marsupial (*Antechinus stuartii* [MACKAY])," *Gen. & Comp. Endocrinol.* 40 (1980): 188–200.

2. W. C. Alvarez, *Nervous Indigestion and Pain* (New York: Hoeber, 1943); F. Draper and G. A. Touraine, "The Man, Environment, and Peptic Ulcers," *Arch. Intern. Med.* 49 (1932): 615; Dunbar, *Emotions and Body Changes,* 3d ed. (Columbia, N.Y., 1947).

3. F. Alexander, "The Influence of Psychological Factors upon Gastrointestinal Disturbances," *Psychoanal. Quart.* 3 (1934): 501–39; F. Alexander, "A Case of Peptic Ulcer and Personality Disorder," *Psychosom. Med.* 9 (1947): 320–30.

4. P. G. Hencke, "Stomach Pathology and the Amygdala," in *The Amyg-*

dala: Neurobiological Aspects of Emotion, Memory, and Mental Dysfunction (New York: Williams & Wilkins, 1992), 323–38; R. N. Sen and B. K. Anand, "Effect of Electrical Stimulation of the Limbic System of the Brain ('Visceral Brain') on Gastric Secretory Activity and Ulceration," *Ind. J. Med. Res.* 45 (1967): 515–21; C. N. Shealy and T. L. Peele, "Studies on Amygdaloid Nucleus in the Cat," *J. Neurophysiol.* 20 (1957): 125–39; E. J. Zawalski, "Gastric Secretory Response of the Unrestrained Cat Following Electrical Stimulation of the Hypothalamus, Amygdala, and Basal Ganglia," *Exp. Neurol.* 17 (1967): 128–39; P. G. Hencke, "The Amygdala and Restraint Ulcers in Rats," *J. Comp. Physiol. Psychol.* 94 (1980): 313–23.

5. E. M. Goldberg, *Family Influences and Psychosomatic Illness* (London: Invistock, 1958); L. K. Trejdosiewicz et al., "Gamma-Delta T-Cell Receptor (t) Cells of the Human Gastrointestinal Mucosa: *Heliobacter pylori* Associated Gastritis, Celiac Disease, and Inflammatory Bowel Disease," *Clin. Exp. Immunol.* 84, no. 3 (1991): 440–44.

6. R. Ader, "Effects of Early Experience and Differential Housing on Susceptibility to Gastric Erosions in Lesion-Susceptible Rats," *Psychosom. Med.* 32, no. 6 (1970): 569–79; G. B. Glavin, "Restraint Ulcer: History of Current Research and Future Implications," *Brain Res. Bull.* (suppl. 1) 5 (1980): 51–55.

7. D. N. Steward and D. M. Winser, "Incidence of Prefrontal Peptic Ulcers: Effect of Heavy Air-Raids," *Lancet* 1 (1942): 259; P. G. Hencke, "Hippocampal Pathway to the Amygdala and Stress Ulcer Development," *Brain Res. Bull.* 25 (1990): 691–95.

8. E. J. Pinter et al., "The Influence of Emotional Stress on Fat Mobilization: The Role of Endogenous Catecholamines and β-Adrenergic Receptors," *Am. J. Med. Sci.* 254 (1967): 634.

9. H. Weiner et al., "Etiology of Duodenal Ulcer. I. Relation of Specific Psychological Characteristics to Rate of Gastric Secretion (Serum Pepsinogen)," *Psychosom. Med.* 19 (1957): 1–10; G. F. Mahl, "Anxiety, HCl, Serotonin and Peptic Ulcer Etiology," *Psychosom. Med.* 12 (1950): 158–69; R. K. Gundry et al., "Pattern of Gastric Acid Secretion in Patients with Clinical and Personality Features," *Gastroenterology* 52 (1967): 176–84; A. Stenbach, "Gastric Neurosis, Pre-ulcers, Conflict and Personality Duodenal Ulcers," *J. Psychosom. Res.* 4 (1960): 282–96; W. B. Cannon, "The Influence of Emotional States on the Function of the Alimentary Canal," *Am. J. Med. Sci.* 137 (1909): 480–87.

10. B. Mittlemann and H. G. Wolfe, "Emotions and Gastroduodenal Function," *Psychosom. Med.* 4 (1942): 5.

11. Pietro Castelnuovo-Tedesco, "Emotional Antecedents of Perforation of Ulcers of the Stomach and Duodenum," *Psychosom. Med.* 24 (1962): 398–416.

12. G. L. Engel, "Studies of Ulcerative Colitis. IV: The Nature of Psychologic Process," *Am. J. Med.* 19 (1955): 231; J. J. Green and J. M. Van der Valk, "Psychosomatic Aspects of Ulcerative Colitis," *Gastroenterology* 86 (1966): 591.

13. S. Minuchin et al., *Psychosomatic Families, Anorexia Nervosa in Context* (Cambridge, Mass.: Harvard Univ. Press, 1978), 23–29; G. L. Engel, "Studies of

Ulcerative Colitis. V: Psychological Aspects and Their Implications for Treatment," *Am. J. Digestive Dis.* 3 (1968): 315–37.

14. P. V. Cardon and P. S. Mueller, "A Possible Mechanism: Psychogenic Fat Mobilization," *Ann. N.Y. Acad. Sci.* 125 (1966): 924–27; P. V. Cardon and R. A. Gordon, "Rapid Increase in Plasma Unesterified Fatty Acids in Men During Fear," *J. Psychosom. Res.* 4 (1959): 5; M. D. Bogdonoff, E. H. Estes, and D. Trout, "Acute Effect of Psychologic Stimuli upon Plasma Non-esterified Fatty Acid Level," *Proc. Soc. Exp. Biol. Med.* 100 (1959): 503.

15. R. N. Melmed et al., "The Influence of Emotional Stress on Mobilization of Marginal Pool Leukocytes after Insulin-induced Hypoglycemia," *Ann. N.Y. Acad. Sci.* 496 (1987): 467–76; A. Meyer et al., "Correlation between Emotions and Carbohydrate Metabolism in Two Cases of Diabetes Mellitus," *Psychosom. Med.* 7 (1945): 335–41.

16. A. M. Jacobson and J. B. Leibovitch, "Psychological Issues in Diabetes Mellitus," in W. Dorfman and L. Cristofar, eds., *Psychosom. Illness Review* (New York: Macmillan, 1985).

17. H. Rosen and T. Lidz, "Emotional Factors in Precipitation of Recurrent Diabetic Acidosis," *Psychosom. Med.* 11 (1949): 211–15.

18. K. Uvnäs-Moberg et al., "Personality Traits of Groups of Individuals in Functional Disorders of the GI Tract and Their Correlation with Gastrin, Somatostatin, and Oxytocin Levels," *J. Psychosom. Res.* 35 (1991): 515–23.

19. D. E. Johnson, "Etiology and Mechanisms in Development of Gastrointestinal Reactions," in J. H. Nodine and J. H. Moyer, eds., *Psychosomatic Medicine,* 117; S. L. Werkman and S. S. Greenberg, "Personality and Interest Patterns in Obese Adolescent Girls," *Psychosom. Med.* 29, no. 1 (1967): 72–78.

20. S. LeVay, *The Sexual Brain* (Cambridge, Mass.: MIT Press, 1993), 47–61.

NINE. THE HEART, LUNGS, AND BREASTS

1. R. M. Nerem, M. J. Levesque, and J. T. Cornell, "Social Environment as a Factor in Diet-Induced Atherosclerosis," *Science* 208, no. 4451 (1980): 1475–76.

2. W. B. Cannon, *Bodily Changes in Pain, Hunger, Fear and Rage* (Boston: Charles T. Bradford, 1953), 226.

3. L. L. Hay, *Heal Your Body* (Carson, Calif.: Hay House, 1984), 39; L. L. Hay, *You Can Heal Your Life* (Carlsbad, Calif.: Hay House, 1987), 168.

4. W. T. Tallman, "Cardiovascular Regulation and Lesions of the CNS," *Annals of Neurol.* 18 (1985): 1–12; P. D. Wall and G. D. Davis, "The Cerebral Cortical Systems Affecting Autonomic Function," *J. Neurophysiol.* 14 (1951): 507–17.

5. M. M. Linehan, *Skills Training Manual for Treatment of Borderline Personality Disorder* (New York: Guilford, 1993), 135–64.

6. I. Pilowski et al., "Hypertension and Personality," *Psychosom. Med.* 35, no. 1 (1973): 50–56; J. P. Henry and J. C. Cassel, "Psychosocial Factors and Essen-

tial Hypertension: Recent Epidemiologic and Experimental Evidence," *Am. J. Epidemiol.* 90 (1969): 171.

7. T. Theorell and R. H. Rabe, "Psychosocial Factors and Myocardial Infarction," *J. Psychosom. Res.* 15 (1971): 25; R. H. Rabe and E. Lind, "Psychosocial Factors and Sudden Death: A Pilot Study," *J. Psychosom. Res.* 15 (1971): 19; U. Lundberg, T. Theorell, and E. Lind, "Life Changes and Myocardial Infarction: Individual Differences in Life Change Scale," *J. Psychosom. Res.* 19 (1975): 27; E. Weiss et al., "Emotional Factors in Coronary Occlusion," *Arch. Intern. Med.* 99 (1957): 628.

8. W. D. Rees and S. G. Lutkins, "Mortality and Bereavement," *Brit. Med. J.* 4 (1967): 13, 43; M. Young et al., "Mortality among Widowers," *Lancet* 2 (1963): 424; C. M. Parkes and R. J. Brown, "Health after Bereavement: A Controlled Study of Young Boston Widows and Widowers," *Psychosom. Med.* 34, no. 5 (1972): 460–90; C. M. Parkes, B. Benjamin, and R. G. Fitzgerald, "'Broken Heart,' A Statistical Study of Increased Mortality among Widowers," *Brit. Med. J.* 1 (1969): 740; P. J. Clayton, "Mortality and Morbidity after the First Year of Widowhood," *Arch. Gen. Psychiatry* 30 (1974): 747–50; M. Seiler et al., "Cardiac Arrhythmias in Infant Pigtail Monkeys Following Maternal Separation," *Psychophysiology* 16 (1979): 130–35.

9. C. L. Northrup, "Your Emotions and Your Heart: Learning to Heed Their Messages Could Save Your Life," *Health Wisdom for Women* 4, no. 8 (1997): 1–4.

10. G. R. Elliot and C. Eisdorfer, *Stress and Human Health: Analysis and Implications of Research* (New York: Springer, 1982).

11. L. Musante et al., "Potential for Hostility and Dimensions of Anger," *Health Psychol.* 8 (1989): 343; M. A. Mittleman et al., "Triggering of Acute MI Onset of Episodes of Anger," *Circulation* 92 (1995): 1720–25; G. Ironson et al., "Effects of Anger on Left Ventricle Ejection Fraction in Coronary Artery Disease," *Am. J. Cardiol.* 70 (1992): 281–85; M. D. Boltwood, "Anger Reports Predict Coronary Artery Vasomotor Response to Mental Stress in Atherosclerotic Segments," *Am. J. Cardiol.* 72 (1993): 1361–65; R. B. Shekelle et al., "Hostility, Risk of Heart Disease and Mortality," *Psychosom. Med.* 45, no. 2 (1983): 109–14; K. F. Helmers, "Hostility and MI in Coronary Artery Disease Patients: Evaluation by Gender and Ischemic Index," *Psychosom. Med.* 55 (1993): 29–36; P. P. Vitaliano et al., "Plasma Lipids and Their Relationship with Psychosocial Factors in Older Patients," *J. Gerontol. B. Psychol. Sci. Soc. Science* 50, no. 1 (1995): 18–24; M. A. Chesney, "Behavioral Barriers to Cardiovascular Health in Women," *CVR&R,* March 1994: 19–33; D. S. Krantz and D. C. Glass, "Personality Behavioral Patterns and Physical Illness Conceptual and Methodological Issues," in W. D. Gentry, ed., *Handbook of Behavioral Medicine* (New York: Guilford, 1984), 63–88; K. A. Lawler, "Gender and Cardiovascular Responses: What Is the Role of Hostility," *J. Psychosom. Res.* 37, no. 6 (1993): 603–13; S. B. Manuck et al., "An Animal Model of Coronary-Prone Behavior," in M. A. Chesney and R. H. Rosenman, eds., *Anger & Hostility in Cardiovascular and Behavioral Disorders*

(Washington, D.C.: Hemisphere, 1985), 187–202; I. Kawachi et al., "A Prospective Study of Anger and Coronary Heart Disease," *Circulation* 94 (1996): 2090–95; M. Koskenuuo et al., "Hostility as a Risk Factor for Mortality and Ischemic Heart Disease in Men," *Psychosom. Med.* 50 (1988): 153–64; T. M. Dembroski, ed., *Proceedings for the Forum on Coronary Prone Behavior* (Washington, D.C.: U.S. Government Printing Office, 1977); N. Lundberg et al., "Type A Behavior in Healthy Men and Women as Related to Physiological Reactivity and Blood Lipids," *Psychosom. Med.* 51 (1989): 113–22; G. Weidner et al., "The Role of Type A Behavior and Hostility in an Elevation of Plasma Lipids in Adult Men and Women," *Psychosom. Med.* 49 (1987): 136–45; L. H. Powell et al., "Can the Type A Behavior Patterns Be Altered after Myocardial Infarction? A Second-Year Report for the Recurrent Coronary Prevention Project," *Psychosom. Med.* 46, no. 9 (1984): 293–313; M. Friedman and R. H. Rosenman, "Association of Specific Overt Behavior with Cardiovascular Findings," *JAMA* 162 (1959): 1286–96; B. L. Kalis et al., "Personality and Life History Factors in Persons Who Are Potentially Hypertensive," *J. Nerv. Ment. Dis.* 132 (1961): 457; F. Alexander, *Psychosomatic Medicine* (London: George Allen, 1952).

12. S. Greer, T. Morris, and K. W. Pettingale, "Psychological Response to Breast Cancer: Effect of Outcome," *Lancet* 2 (1979): 785–87; D. Razavi, C. Farvacques, N. Delvaux, and T. Beffort, "Psychosocial Correlates of Estrogen and Progesterone Receptors in Breast Cancer," *Lancet* 335 (1990): 931–33; A. Brémond, G. Kane, and C. B. Bahnson, "Psychosomatic Factors in Breast Cancer Patients: Results of a Case Control Study," *J. Psychosom. Ob/Gyn* 5 (1986): 127–36; K. W. Pettingale, S. Greer, and D. E. H. Tee, "Serum IgA and Emotional Expression in Breast Cancer Patients," *J. Psychosom. Res.* 21 (1977): 395; K. W. Pettingale, S. Greer et al., "Mental Attitudes to Cancer: An Additional Prognostic Factor," *Lancet* 1 (1985): 750; M. Wirshung et al., "Psychological Identification of Breast Cancer Patients before Biopsy," *J. Psychosom. Res.* 26, no. 1 (1982): 1–10; L. LeShan, "Psychological States as Factors in the Development of Malignant Disease: A Critical Review," *JNCI* 22 (1959): 1–18; M. Jansen and L. R. Muenz, "A Retrospective Study of Personality Variables Associated with Fibrocystic Breast Disease and Breast Cancer," *J. Psychosom. Med.* 28, no. 1 (1984): 35–42.

13. S. M. Levy, R. Herberman, M. Lippman, and T. D'Angelo, "Correlation of Stress Factors with Sustained Depression of Natural Killer Cell Activity and Predicted Prognosis in Patients with Breast Cancer," *J. Clin. Oncol.* 5, no. 3 (1987): 348–53; S. M. Levy, R. B. Herberman, T. Whiteside, K. Sanzo, J. Lee, and J. Kirkwood, "Perceived Social Support and Tumor Estrogen/Progesterone Receptor Status as Predictors of Natural Killer Cell Activity in Breast Cancer Patients," *Psychosom. Med.* 52 (1990): 73–85.

14. T. M. Dembroski et al., "Components of Hostility as Predictors of Sudden Death and MI," *Psychosom. Med.* 51 (1989): 514–22; M. Friedman and R. H. Rosenman, "Association of Specific Overt Behavior with Cardiovascular Findings," *JAMA* 162 (1959): 1286–96.

15. S. G. Haynes et al., "The Relationship of Psychological Factors for

Coronary Heart Disease in the Framingham Study. Part III: Eight-Year Incidence of Coronary Heart Disease," *Am. J. Epidemiol.* 3 (1980): 37–58; K. Matthews et al., "Competitive Drive, Pattern A, and Coronary Heart Disease," *J. Chron. Dis.* 30 (1977): 489–98.

16. I. Pilowsky et al., "Hypertension and Personality," *Psychosom. Med.* 35, no. 1 (1973): 50–56; L. F. Van Egeron, "Social Interactions, Communications, and Coronary-Prone Behavior Pattern: A Psychophysiology Study," *Psychosom. Med.* 41, no. 1 (1979): 2–18.

17. K. Lorenz, *On Aggression* (London: Methuen, 1966); L. Tiger and R. Fox, *The Imperial Animal* (New York: Holt, Rinehart & Winston, 1971).

18. R. D. Lane and G. E. Schwartz, "Induction of Lateralized Sympathetic Input to the Heart by the Central Nervous System during Emotional Arousal: A Possible Neurophysiological Trigger of Sudden Cardiac Death," *Psychosom. Med.* 49 (1987): 274–84; W. K. Smith, "The Functional Significance of the Rostral Cingulate as Revealed by Its Responses to Electrical Stimulations," *J. Neurophysiol.* 8 (1945): 241–55.

19. B. A. Shaywitz and S. E. Shaywitz, "Sex Differences in the Functional Organization of the Brain for Language," *Nature* 373 (1995): 607–9.

20. C. L. Bacon, R. Renneker, and M. Cutler, "A Psychosomatic Survey of Cancer of the Breast," *Psychosom. Med.* 14, no. 6 (1952): 453–60.

21. O. Muhlbock, "A Hormonal Genesis of Mammary Cancer," in J. P. Greenstein and A. Hanlon, eds., *Advances in Cancer Research,* vol. 4 (New York: Academic Press, 1956), 371; T. Marchant, "The Effects of Different Social Conditions in Breast Cancer Induction in Three Genetic Types of Mice," *Brit. J. Cancer* 21 (1967): 576–85; J. P. Henry, V. P. Stephens, and F. M. Watson, "Forced Breeding, Social Disorder, and Mammary Tumor Formation in CBA/USC Mouse Colonies: A Pilot Study," *Psychosom. Med.* 37, no. 3 (1975): 277–83.

22. C. L. Bacon, R. Renneker, and M. Cutler, "A Psychosomatic Survey of Cancer of the Breast," *Psychosom. Med.* 14, no. 6 (1952): 453; M. Tarlau and M. A. Smalheiser, "Personality Patterns in Patients with Malignant Tumors of the Breast and Cervix," *Psychosom. Med.* 13 (1981): 117; M. Wirshung et al., "Psychological Identification of Breast Cancer Patients before Biopsy," *J. Psychosom. Res.* 26, no. 1 (1982): 1–10.

23. C. Nadelson et al., "Psychosomatic Aspects of Obstetrics and Gynecology," in W. Dorfman and L. Cristofar, eds., *Psychosomatic Illness Rev.* (New York, Macmillan, 1985), 162–79.

24. J. P. Wheeler and B. Caldwell, "Psychological Evaluation of Women with Cancer of the Breast and the Cervix," *Psychosom. Med.* 17 (1955): 256.

25. C. M. Reznikoff, "Psychological Factors in Breast Cancer: A Preliminary Study of Personality Trends in Patients with Cancer of the Breast," *Psychosom. Med.* 17 (1955): 96.

26. S. M. Levy, "Survival Hazards Analysis in Recurrent Breast Cancer Patients: Seventh-Year Follow-up," *Psychosom. Med.* 50 (1988): 520–28; L. Derogatis et al., "Psychological Coping Mechanisms and Survival Time in Metastatic

Breast Cancer," *JAMA* 242 (1979): 1504–9; S. M. Levy, R. Heberman, A. Maluish et al., "Prognostic Risk Assessment in Primary Breast Cancer by Behavioral and Immunological Parameters," *Health Psychol.* 4 (1985): 99–113.

27. K. W. Pettingale, S. Greer et al., "Mental Attitudes to Cancer: An Additional Prognostic Factor," *Lancet* 1 (1985): 750; C. C. Chen et al., "Adverse Life Events and Breast Cancer: A Case Control Study," *Br. Med. J.* 311 (1995): 1527–30.

28. S. M. Levy, R. B. Herberman, T. Whiteside, K. Sanzo, J. Lee, and J. Kirkwood, "Perceived Social Support and Tumor Estrogen/Progesterone Receptor Status as Predictors of Natural Killer Cell Activity in Breast Cancer Patients," *Psychosom. Med.* 52 (1990): 59–72, 73–85; S. M. Levy, R. Herberman, M. Lippman, and T. D'Angelo, "Correlation of Stress Factors with Sustained Depression of Natural Killer Cell Activity and Predicted Prognosis in Patients with Breast Cancer," *J. Clin. Oncol.* 5, no. 3 (1987): 348–57; S. M. Levy, R. Herberman, A. Maluish et al., "Prognostic Risk Assessment in Primary Breast Cancer by Behavioral and Immunological Parameters," *Health Psychol.* 4 (1985): 99–113; K. W. Pettingale, S. Greer et al., "Mental Attitudes to Cancer: An Additional Prognostic Factor," *Lancet* 1 (1985): 750.

29. D. Spiegel et al., "Effect of Psychosocial Treatment on Survival of Patients with Metastatic Breast Cancer," *Lancet,* October 14, 1989: 888–90.

30. L. LeShan, "Psychological States as Factors in the Development of Malignant Disease: A Critical Review," *JNCI* 22 (1959): 1–18; H. Becker, "Psychodynamic Aspects of Breast Cancer: Differences in Younger and Older Patients," *Psychotherapy Psychosom.* 32 (1978): 287–96; Guy Richard, *An Essay on Scirrhous Tumors and Cancers* (London: 1759); M. Tarlau and M. A. Smalheiser, "Personality Patterns in Patients with Malignant Tumors of the Breast and Cervix," *Psychosom. Med.* 13 (1981): 137; H. Snow, *Clinical Notes on Cancer* (London: 1883); H. Snow, *The Proclivity of Women to Cancerous Disease* (London: 1891); C. Jasmin et al., "Evidence of a Link between Certain Psychological Factors and the Risk of Breast Cancer in a Case Control Study," *Ann. Oncol.* 1, no. 1 (1990): 22–29.

TEN. THE THYROID, THROAT, AND NECK

1. N. Sonino et al., "Life Events in the Pathogenesis of Graves' Disease: A Controlled Study," *Acta Endocrinologica* 128 (1993): 293–96; E. Morillo and L. I. Gardner, "Actuation of Latent Graves' Disease in Children: A Review of Psychosomatic Mechanisms," *Clin. Pediatri. Philol.* 19, no. 3 (1980): 160–63; E. Morillo and L. I. Gardner, "Bereavement as an Antecedent Factor in Thyrotoxicosis of Childhood: Four Case Studies," *Psychosom. Med.* 41, no. 7 (1979): 545–55; H. M. Voth et al., "Thyroid Hot Spots in Relationship to Life Stress," *Psychosom. Med.* 32, no. 6 (1970): 561–68; R. S. Wallerstein et al., "Thyroid Hot Spots: A Psychophysiological Study," *Psychosom. Med.* 27, no. 6 (1965): 508–23; B. Winsa et al., "Stressful Life Events and Graves' Disease," *Lancet* 338 (1991): 1475–79; S. A. Weisman, "Incidence of Thyrotoxicosis among Refugees from Nazi Prison

Camps," *Ann. Intern. Med.* 48 (1958): 747–52; W. Cannon, *Bodily Changes in Pain, Hunger, Fear, and Rage* (Boston: Charles T. Bradford, 1953).

2. A. W. Bennett and C. G. Cambor, "Clinical Study of Hyperthyroidism," *Arch. Gen. Psychiatry* 4 (1961): 160; W. T. Brown and E. A. Gildea, "Hyperthyroidism and Personality," *Am. J. Psychiatry* 94 (1937): 59.

3. S. K. Gupta et al., "Thyroid Gland Responses to Intermale Aggression in an Inherently Aggressive Wild Male," *Endokrinologie* 80, no. 3 (1982): 350–52.

4. I. L. D. Houtman and F. C. Bakker, "Individual Differences in Reactivity to and Coping with the Stress of Lecturing," *J. Psychosom. Res.* 35, no. 1 (1991): 11–24; R. J. Martin et al., "Paroxysmal Vocal Cord Motion in Presumed Asthmatics," *Seminars Respir. Med.* 8 (1987): 332–37.

5. F. Adams, *The Genuine Works of Hippocrates* (London: Sydenham Society, 1849); I. J. Cock et al., "Upper Esophageal Sphincter Time and Reactivity to Stress in Patients with a History of Globus Sensation," *Dig. Dis. Sci.* 34 (1989): 672–76; J. P. Glaser and S. L. Engel, "Psychodynamics, Psychophysiology and Gastrointestinal Symptoms," *Clinics in Gastroenterology* 6 (1977): 507–37.

6. J. Purcell, *The Treatise of Vapours on Hysteric Fits,* 2d ed. (London, 1707).

7. G. Johansson et al., "Examination Stress Affects Plasma Levels of TSH and Thyroid Hormones Differently in Women and Men," *Psychosom. Med.* 49 (1987): 390–96.

8. J. Sherman, *Sex Related Cognitive Differences: An Essay on Theory* (Springfield, Ill.: Charles C. Thomas, 1978).

9. AAUW, *Shortchanging Girls, Shortchanging America* (Washington, D.C.: AAUW, 1991).

10. D. Kimura, "Sex Differences in Cerebral Organization for Speech and Praxic Function," *Canad. J. Psychol.* 37 (1983): 19–35; J. L. Griffith and M. G. Griffith, *The Body Speaks: Therapeutic Dialogues for Mind-Body Problems* (New York: Basic Books, 1994), 204–5.

11. C. Armengol, personal communication.

ELEVEN. THE BRAIN AND SENSORY ORGANS

1. H. O. Barber, "Psychosomatic Disorders of the Ear, Nose, and Throat," *Postgraduate Medicine,* May 1970, 156–59; I. Pilowsky et al., "Hypertension and Personality," *Psychosom. Med.* 35, no. 1 (1973): 50–56.

2. L. F. Van Egeron, "Social Interactions, Communications, and Coronary- Prone Behavior Pattern: A Psychophysiology Study," *Psychosom. Med.* 41, no. 1 (1979): 2–18.

3. S. D. Stephens, "Personality Tests in Ménière's Disease," *J. Laryngol. & Otol.* 89, no. 5 (1975): 479–90; F. E. Lucente, "Psychiatric Problems in Otolaryngology," *Ann. Otol., Rhino., & Laryngol.* 82, no. 3 (1973): 340–46; M. J. Martin, "Functional Disorders in Otorhinolaryngology," *Arch. Otolaryngol.* 91, no. 5 (1970): 1457–59.

4. C. Martin et al., "Ménière's Disease: A Psychosomatic Disease," *Rev.*

Laryngol., Otol., & Rhinol. 112, no. 2 (1991): 109–11; C. Martin et al., "Psychologic Factor in Ménière's Disease," *Ann. Otolaryngol. Chir. Cervicofac.* 107, no. 8 (1990): 526–31.

5. N. J. Coker et al., "Psychological Profile on Patients with Ménière's Disease," *Arch. Otolaryngol. Head & Neck Surg.* 115 (1989): 1355–57; J. Weiner, "Looking Out and Looking In: Some Reflections on 'Body Talk' in the Consulting Room," *J. Anal. Psychol.* 39, no. 3 (1994): 331–50; R. Hinchcliffe, "Emotion as Precipitating Factor in Ménière's Disease," *J. Laryngol. Otol.* 81 (1967): 471–75; U. Sitrala and K. Gelhar, "Further Studies on the Relationship between Ménière's Psychosomatic Constitution and Stress," *Acta Otolaryngol.* 70 (1970): 142–47.

6. B. Minnigerode and M. Harbrecht, "Otorhinolaryngologic Manifestations of Masked Mono- and Oligosymptomatic Depressions," *HNO* 36, no. 9 (1988): 383–85; C. Martin et al., "Psychologic Factor in Ménière's Disease," *Ann. Otolaryngol. Chir. Cervicofac.* 107, no. 8 (1990): 526–30.

7. M. Rigatelli et al., "Psychosomatic Study of 60 Patients of Vertigo," *Psychother. Psychosom.* 41, no. 2 (1984): 91–99; C. Martin et al., "Ménière's Disease: A Psychosomatic Disease," *Rev. Laryngol., Otol., & Rhinol.* 112, no. 2 (1991): 109–11; J. J. Groen, "Psychosomatic Aspects of Ménière's Disease," *Acta Otolaryngol. Stockh.* 95, nos. 5–6 (1983): 407–16.

8. W. G. Crary and M. Wexler, "Ménière's Disease: A Psychosomatic Disorder," *Psychol. Rep.* 41 (1977): 603–45; L. Yardley, "Prediction of Handicap and Emotional Distress in Patients with Recurrent Vertigo Symptoms, Coping Strategies, Control Beliefs, and Reciprocal Causation," *Soc. Sci. Med.* 39, no. 4 (1994): 573–81.

9. C. L. Schmidt, "Medical Treatment of Ménière's Disease," *Laryngol. Rhinol. & Otol. Stuttgart* 56, no. 5 (1977): 407–9; S. I. Erlandsson et al., "Psychological and Audiological Correlates of Perceived Tinnitus Severity," *Audiology* 31, no. 3 (1992): 168–79; S. I. Erlandsson et al., "Ménière's Disease: Trauma, Disease, and Adaptation Studied through Focus Interview Analyses," *Scand. Audiol. Suppl.* 43 (1996): 45–56.

10. K. Czubulski et al., "Psychological Stress and Personality in Ménière's Disease," *J. Psychosom. Res.* 20 (1976): 187–91.

11. G. W. Paulson and N. Dadmehr, "Is There a Premorbid Personality Typical for Parkinson's Disease?" *Arch. Neurol.* 41, no. 2 (1991): 73–76; I. Sands, "The Type of Personality Susceptible to Parkinson's Disease," *J. Mt. Sinai Hosp.* 9 (1942): 792–94; P. Mouren et al., "Personality of the Parkinsonian," *Ann. Med. Psychol.* (Paris) 141, no. 2 (1983): 153–67; M. Mitscherlich, "The Psychic State of Patients Suffering from Parkinsonism," *Adv. Psychosom. Med.* 1 (1960): 317–24.

12. R. C. Davoisin et al., "Twin Study of Parkinson's Disease," *Neurology* 31 (1981): 77–80; A. H. Robins, "Depression in Patients with Parkinsonism," *Br. J. Psychiatry* 128 (1976): 141–45.

13. C. D. Camp, "Paralysis Agitans, Multiple Sclerosis and Their Treatment," in M. A. White et al., eds., *Modern Treatment of Nervous and Mental Diseases,* vol. 2 (Philadelphia, 1913), 651–67; G. Booth, "Psychodynamics in

Parkinsonism," *Psychosom. Med.* 10 (1948): 1–14; W. Poewe, "Premorbid Personality of Parkinson Patients," *J. Neurol. Transm.* 19, suppl. (1983): 215–24.

14. S. E. Jellife, "The Parkinsonian Body Posture: Some Considerations of Unconscious Hostility," *Psychoanalyst Rev.* 27 (1940): 467–79.

15. J. J. G. Prick, "Genuine Parkinsonism. A Psychosomatic, Anthropological Psychiatric Approach," *Abs. World Congress of Psychiatry Sandorama,* Special no. 4 (1966); I. Sands, "The Type of Personality Susceptible to Parkinson's Disease," *J. Mt. Sinai Hosp.* 9 (1942): 792–94.

16. R. C. Cloninger, "A Systematic Method for Clinical Description and Classification of Personality Variants," *Arch. Gen. Psychiatry* 44 (1987): 573–88; M. A. Menza and M. H. Mark, "Parkinson's Disease and Repression: Relationship to Disability and Personality," *J. Neuropsychiatry and Clinical Neurosciences* 6 (1994): 165–69; R. C. Cloninger, "Brain Network Underlying Personality Development," in B. J. Carroll and J. E. Barrett, eds., *Psychopathology and the Brain* (New York: Raven, 1991), 183–208; M. A. Menza et al., "Dopamine Related Personality Traits in Parkinson's Disease," *Neurology* 43 (1993): 505–8; W. Poewe et al., "The Premorbid Personality of Patients with Parkinson's Disease: A Comparative Study with Healthy Controls and Patients with Essential Tremor," *Adv. Neurol.* 83 (1990): 339–42; V. M. Eatough et al., *Premorbid Personality and Idiopathic Parkinson's Disease: Anatomy, Pathology, and Therapy* (New York: Raven, 1990), 335–37.

17. G. Booth, "Personality and Chronic Arthritis," *J. Nerv. Ment. Dis.* 85 (1937): 637; G. Booth, "The Psychological Approach in the Therapy of Chronic Arthritis," *Rheumatism* 1 (1939): 48.

TWELVE. THE MUSCLES, CONNECTIVE TISSUES, AND GENES

1. E. R. MacDonald et al., "Survival in Amyotrophic Lateral Sclerosis: The Role of Psychological Factors," *Arch. Neurol.* 51 (1994): 17–23.

2. S. Warren, S. Greenhill, and K. G. Warren, "Emotional Stress and the Development of Multiple Sclerosis: A Case Control Evidence of a Relationship," *J. Chronic Dis.* 35 (1982): 821–31; G. S. Philippoulos, E. R. Wittkower, and A. Cousineau, "The Etiologic Significance of Emotional Factors in Onset and Exacerbation of Multiple Sclerosis," *Psychosom. Med.* 20 (1958): 458–74; V. Mei-Tal, M. D. Meyerwitz, and G. Engel, "The Role of Psychological Process in a Somatic Disorder: Multiple Sclerosis," *Psychosom. Med.* 32 (1970): 67–86; J. M. Charcot, *Lectures on the Diseases of the Nervous System,* delivered at the Salpêtrière, 1868, G. Sigerson Lectures, trans. (London: New Sydenham Society, 1877); S. Warren et al., "Emotional Stress and Coping in Multiple Sclerosis Exacerbations," *J. Psychosom. Res.* 35, no. 1 (1991): 37–47; D. McAlpine and N. D. Compston, "Some Aspects of the Natural History of Multiple Sclerosis," *Quart. J. Med.* 21 (1952): 135–67.

3. D. Firth, *The Case of Augustus d'Este* (Cambridge, England: Cambridge Univ. Press, 1948); J. M. Charcot, *Leçons sur les Maladies du Système Nerveux* (Paris: de la Haye, 1872).

4. J. S. Russell, in C. Allbutt and C. Rolleston, eds., *A System of Medicine,* vol. 7 (London: Macmillan, 1911), 809; B. Beamwell, "The Prognosis of Disseminated Sclerosis," *Edinburgh Med.* 18 (1917): 16–19; D. McAlpine and N. D. Compston, "Some Aspects of the Natural History of Disseminated Sclerosis," *Quart. J. Med.* 21 (1952): 135–67; D. K. Adams et al., "Early Clinical Manifestation of Multiple Sclerosis," *Brit. Med. J.* 2 (1950): 431–37.

5. W. Moxon, "Eight Cases of Insular Sclerosis of the Brain and Spinal Cord," *Guys Hosp. Rep.,* 3d series 20 (1875): 437–70; W. Moxon, "Case of Insular Multiple Sclerosis of Brain and Spinal Cord," *Lancet* 1 (1873): 236.

6. V. Mei-Tal, M. D. Meyerwitz, and G. L. Engel, "The Role of Psychological Process in a Somatic Disorder: Multiple Sclerosis," *Psychosom. Med.* 32, no. 1 (1970): 67–86.

7. G. S. Philippoulos, E. R. Wittkower, and A. Cousineau, "The Etiologic Significance of Emotional Factors in Onset and Exacerbation of Multiple Sclerosis," *Psychosom. Med.* 20 (1958): 458–74; O. R. Langworthy, L. C. Kolb, and B. Androp, "Disturbance of Behavior in Patients with Disseminated Sclerosis," *Am. J. Psychiatry* 98 (1941): 243–49; O. R. Langworthy, "Relationship of Personality Problems to Onset and Progress of Multiple Sclerosis," *Arch. Neurol. Psychiatry* 59 (1948): 13–28.

THIRTEEN. YOUR INTUITIVE IDENTITY

1. C. Darwin, *The Origin of the Species* (New York: D. Appleton, 1889).

2. R. C. Gur et al., "Sex and Handedness Differences in Cerebral Blood Flow during Rest and Cognitive Activity," *Science* 217 (1982): 659–60; J. McGlone, "Sex Differences in Human Brain Asymmetry: A Critical Survey," *Behav. Brain Sci.* 3 (1980): 215–63.

3. C. De La Coste-Utamsing and R. L. Holloway, "Sexual Dimorphism in the Corpus Callosum," *Science* 216 (1982): 1431–32; S. F. Witelson, "The Brain Connection: The Corpus Callosum Is Larger in Left-handers," *Science* 229 (1985): 665–68.

4. D. Kimura, "Sex Differences in Cerebral Organization for Speech and Praxic Functions," *Canad. J. Psychol.* 37 (1983): 19–35; N. Geschwind, "The Anatomical Basis of Hemispheric Differentiation," in S. J. Dimond and J. G. Beaumont, eds., *Hemispheric Function in the Human Brain* (New York: John Wiley, 1974).

5. D. McGuiness, *When Children Don't Learn* (New York: Basic Books, 1985); M. Corballis and I. Beale, *The Psychology of Left and Right* (New York: Erlbaum/John Wiley, 1976).

6. I. Gerendai, "Chapter 11: Lateralization of Neuroendocrine Control," in N. Geschwind and A. M. Galaburden, eds., *Cerebral Dominance: Biological Foundation* (Cambridge, Mass.: Harvard Univ. Press, 1984), 167–78.

7. S. E. Shaywitz and B. A. Shaywitz, "Sex Differences in the Functional Organization of the Brain for Language," *Nature* 373 (1995): 607–9.

8. S. Witelson, "Sex and the Single Hemisphere," *Science* 193 (1976): 425–27.

9. Thatcher, R. W., et al., "Human Cerebral Hemispheres Develop at Different Rates and Ages," *Science* 236 (1987): 1110–13.

10. C. N. Northrup, *Women's Bodies, Women's Wisdom,* rev. ed. (New York: Bantam, 1998), 95–103. Dr. Christiane Northrup and I first elucidated the relationship of FSH, LH, the menstrual cycle, and intuition while doing research for her first book.

11. M. Altemus, B. Wexler, and N. Bonlis, "Neuropsychological Correlates of Menstrual Mood Changes," *Psychosom. Med.* 51 (1989): 329–36; H. A. Sackeim et al., "Hemispheric Asymmetry in the Expression of Positive and Negative Emotions: Neurologic Evidence," *Arch. Neurol.* 39 (1982): 210.

12. J. Borysenko, personal communication. For more information, refer to *A Woman's Book of Life* (New York: Riverhead Books, 1996) for a complete discussion of the biology and physiology of women throughout their life.

13. M. B. Denckla, "The Child with Developmental Disabilities Grown Up: Adult Residua of Childhood Disorders," *Neurologic Clinics of North America* 11, no. 1 (1993): 105–26.

14. S. Minuchin et al., *Psychosomatic Families* (Cambridge, Mass.: Harvard Univ. Press, 1978), 23–29.

15. L. R. Baxter et al., "Local Cerebral Glucose Metabolic Rates in Obsessive-Compulsive Disorder," *Arch. Gen. Psychiatry* 44 (1987): 211–18; L. R. Baxter et al., "Cerebral Glucose Metabolic Rates in Non-depressed Patients with Obsessive-Compulsive Disorder," *Am. J. Psychiatry* 145 (1988): 1560–63.

16. P. E. Sifneos et al., "The Phenomenon of Alexithymia: Observations in Neurotic and Psychosomatic Patients," *Psychotherapy and Psychomatics* 28 (1977): 47–57; P. D. MacLean, "Psychosomatic Disease and the Visceral Brain," *Psychosom. Med.* 11 (1949): 338; J. C. Nemiah, "Alexithymia: Present, Past—And Future?" *Psychosom. Med.* 58 (1996): 217–18; R. D. Lane et al., "Impaired Verbal and Non-verbal Emotion Recognition in Alexithymia," *Psychosom. Med.* 58 (1996): 203–10; W. D. Ten Houten et al., "Alexithymia and the Split Brain: VI. Electroencephalographic Correlates of Alexithymia," *Psychiatric Clinics of North America* 11, no. 3 (1988): 317–29; P. E. Sifneos, "Alexithymia and Its Relationship to Hemispheric Specialization, Affect, and Creativity," *Psychiatric Clinics of North America* 11, no. 3 (1988): 287–92; R. Dewaraja and Y. Sasaki, "A Left and Right Hemisphere Callosal Transfer Deficit of Non-Linguistic Information in Alexithymia," *Psychother. Psychosom.* 54, no. 4 (1990): 201–7.

FOURTEEN. YOUR INTUITIVE PROFILE

1. B. Fallik and J. Eliot, "Intuition, Cognitive Style, and Hemispheric Processing," *Perceptual Motor Skills* 60 (1985): 683–97.

INDEX

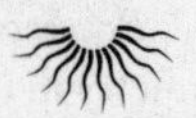

About the Author

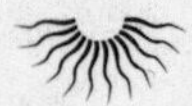

Mona Lisa Schulz, M.D., Ph.D., is a neuropsychiatrist, scientist, and medical intuitive. Dr. Schulz received her doctorate in behavioral neuroscience from Boston University School of Medicine in 1993, along with her M.D., and completed a residency program in psychiatry at Maine Medical Center in Portland.

In addition to her extensive background in clinical medicine and brain research, Dr. Schulz has been a practicing medical intuitive for over a decade.

One of the many joys in her life is teaching health care professionals and others how to acknowledge, trust, and develop their intuitive skills. She is also the research editor for Dr. Christiane Northrup's *Health Wisdom for Women,* a monthly women's health newsletter. She lives in Yarmouth, Maine, with her two cats, Dina and Emily.